# Williams Syndrome across Languages

## Language Acquisition & Language Disorders

Volumes in this series provide a forum for research contributing to theories of language acquistion (first and second, child and adult), language learnability, language attrition and language disorders.



**Volume 36**

Williams Syndrome across Languages
Edited by Susanne Bartke and Julia Siegmüller

# Williams Syndrome across Languages

*Edited by*

Susanne Bartke
University of Giessen

Julia Siegmüller
University of Potsdam

John Benjamins Publishing Company
Amsterdam / Philadelphia

The paper used in this publication meets the minimum requirements of American National Standard for Information Sciences – Permanence of Paper for Printed Library Materials, ANSI Z39.48-1984.

**Library of Congress Cataloging-in-Publication Data**

Williams Syndrome across Languages / edited by Susanne Bartke and Julia Siegmüller.
p. cm. (Language Acquisition & Language Disorders, ISSN 0925–0123 ; v. 36)
Includes bibliographical references and indexes.
1. Williams syndrome--Patients--Language--Case studies. 2. Language disorders in children--Case studies. I. Bartke, Susanne. II. Siegmüller, Julia. III. Series.

RJ506.W44W557 2004
618.92'855-dc22 2003063747
ISBN 90 272 5295 5 (Eur.) / 1 58811 494 5 (US) (Hb; alk. paper)



John Benjamins Publishing Co. · P.O. Box 36224 · 1020 ME Amsterdam · The Netherlands
John Benjamins North America · P.O. Box 27519 · Philadelphia PA 19118-0519 · USA

# Table of contents

# Tables and figures

## Tables

## Figures

# List of contributors

Susanne Bartke
Special Education of Language and Speech Pathology
University of Giessen
35 394 Giessen, Germany
Susanne.Bartke@erziehung.uni-giessen.de

Angela M. Becerra
Department of Psychological & Brain Sciences
University of Louisville
Louisville, KY 40292, USA
ambece01@gwise.louisville.edu

Marita Böhning
Department of Linguistics
University of Potsdam
PO 601553
14415 Potsdam, Germany
boehning@kronos.ling.uni-potsdam.de

Olga Capirci
Institute of Cognitive Sciences and Technology
Italian National Research Council CNR
00137 Rome, Italy
capirci@ip.rm.cnr.it

Maria Cristina Caselli
Institute of Cognitive Sciences and Technology
Italian National Research Council CNR
00137 Rome, Italy
caselli@ip.rm.cnr.it

Harald Clahsen
Department of Linguistics
University of Essex
Colchester CO4 3SQ, UK
harald@essex.ac.uk

Karl-Heinz Grzeschik
Department of Human Genetics
University of Marburg
35037 Marburg, Germany
grzeschi@Mailer.Uni-Marburg.de

Bonita P. Klein-Tasman
Department of Psychology
University of Wisconsin-Milwaukee
PO Box 413
Milwaukee, WI 53201, USA
bklein@uwm.edu

Marion Krause
Department of Linguistics
University of Duesseldorf
40255 Duesseldorf, Germany
Krause@phil-fak.uni-duesseldorf.de

Yonata Levy
Department of Psychology
The Hebrew University
Jerusalem, 91905, Israel
msyonata@mscc.huji.ac.il

Ágnes Lukács
Center for Cognitive Science
Budapest University of Technology and Economics
Stoczek u. 3, ST Building III./311
H-1111 Budapest, Hungary
lukacs@itm.bme.hu

Steve Majerus
Department of Cognitive Sciences
University of Liège
4000 Liège 1, Belgium
smajerus@ulg.ac.be

Carolyn B. Mervis
Department of Psychological & Brain Sciences
University of Louisville
Louisville, KY 40292, USA
cbmervis@louisville.edu

Martina Penke
Department of Linguistics
University of Duesseldorf
40255 Duesseldorf, Germany
penke@phil-fak.uni-duesseldorf.de

Csaba Pléh
Center for Cognitive Science
Budapest University of Technology and Economics
Stoczek u. 3, ST Building III./311
H-1111 Budapest, Hungary
pleh@itm.bme.hu

Mihály Racsmány
Center for Cognitive Science
Budapest University of Technology and Economics
Stoczek u. 3, ST Building III./311
H-1111 Budapest, Hungary
racsmany@itm.bme.hu

Melanie Ring
Department of Linguistics
University of Essex
Colchester CO4 3SQ, UK
mjring@essex.ac.uk

Byron F. Robinson
Department of Psychology
Georgia State University
Atlanta, GA 30303-3082, USA
bfrobinson@gsu.edu

Melissa L. Rowe
Department of Psychological & Brain Sciences
University of Louisville
Louisville, KY 40292, USA
mlthom06@gwise.louisville.edu

Chris Schaner-Wolles
Department of Linguistics
University of Wien
1090 Wien, Austria
christiane.schaner-wolles@univie.ac.at

Julia Siegmüller
Department of Linguistics
University of Potsdam
PO 601553
14415 Potsdam, Germany
siegmuel@kronos.ling.uni-potsdam.de

Franziska Starke
School of Logopedics
Ottilientraße 5
03050 Cottbus, Germany
franziska.starke@web.de

Stavroula Stavrakaki
Center for Developmental Language Disorders and Cognitive Neuroscience
University College London
London WC 1 N 1PF, UK
s.stavrakaki@ucl.ac.uk
svoula@enl.auth.gr

Christine Temple
Department of Psychology
University of Essex
Colchester, CO4 3 SQ, UK
tempc@essex.ac.uk

Stefano Vicari
Children's Hospital Bambino Gesù
00165 Rome, Italy

Virginia Volterra
Institute of Cognitive Sciences
and Technology
Italian National Research Council
00137 Rome, Italy
volterra@www.ip.rm.cnr.it

Jürgen Weissenborn
Department of Linguistics
University of Potsdam
PO 601553
14415 Potsdam, Germany
weissenb@rz.uni-potsdam.de

# Williams syndrome

## An introduction

Susanne Bartke and Julia Siegmüller
Justus-Liebig University Giessen / University of Potsdam

Williams syndrome (WS) resp. Williams-Beuren syndrome is known about for some 40 years. A couple of years ago the cause of this developmental disorder has been detected: a microdeletion on chromosome 7, more specifically at the region of chromosome 7q11.23 (Brøndum-Nielsen et al. 1997; Korenberg et al. 2000; Doll & Grzeschik 2001). The cognitive and behavioral profile in WS is characterized by a marked discrepancy between verbal and non-verbal skills combined with relatively spared linguistic skills. Research made considerable progress in defining the areas of intactness in linguistic abilities. Consequently this volume presents not only an overview of the psycholinguistic research undertaken in this field, but it also opens up new perspectives and insights through the presentation of new data and analyses.

Williams syndrome (WS), sometimes also called Williams-Beuren syndrome, has been known about for some 40 years. In the first descriptions by Williams and his colleagues, respectively by Beuren and his team, that appeared in the sixties of the twentieth century, the emphasis was foremost on clinical characteristics such as heart defects, idiopathic hypercalcemia and special facial features, a so-called elfin-like facial appearance (Williams et al. 1961; Beuren et l. 1962). Additionally, mental retardation was noticed. For a while the belief reigned that an excessive vitamin D intake either during infancy or taken by mothers during pregnancy caused WS (cf. discussion in Beuren et al. 1966; Grimm & Wesselhoeft 1980; Wesselhoeft et al. 1980; Jones 1990). Then the focus of attention shifted to a connection with a calcitonin-gene-related peptide, with the result that a genetic basis at chromosome 11 or chromosome 15 was suspected. Nowadays, the etiology is identified as a microdeletion on chromosome 7, more specifically at the region of chromosome 7q11.23 (Brøndum-Nielsen et al. 1997; Korenberg et al. 2000; Doll & Grzeschik 2001). Soon peaks and valleys of the cognitive and behavioral profile in WS were noticed: a marked discrepancy between verbal and non-verbal skills combined with relatively spared linguistic skills. In the meantime, some less limited areas within the domain of non-verbal skills are detected as for example face recognition abilities (cf. Tager-Flusberg 1999; Bellugi et al. 2000). However, recent research challenges the view of spared linguistic abilities and the literature shows how intact the abilities with respect to syntactic, morphological or semantic knowledge really are. For nearly each topic there is more or less controversial evidence. To date, new discoveries in the field of WS continue to be made and the discussions generated by these new finding are very much part of the contributions to this volume. Consequently this volume presents not only an overview of the psycholinguistic research undertaken in this field, but it also opens up new perspectives and insights through the presentation of new data and analyses. The motivation for further research is twofold. First of all, a lot can be learned about the language processing and language development in people with WS. Knowledge that will be of help to all parties involved, medical, therapeutical, and educational staff, parents, and of course, the individual with WS. Secondly, learning about WS means learning about the language faculty itself: what are the building blocks of the language faculty and how are they linked to each other. Therefore, this book will be of interest to researchers of applied cognitive science and to those occupied with theoretical research.

Williams syndrome is a field of strong interdisciplinary research and practical work. Thus, this book intends to cross borders, i.e. readers from other disciplines concerned with WS in applied or theoretical ways will also benefit from the research concentrated in this book. Each chapter will be of special interest to medical doctors, psychologists, speech therapists, and educational staff. The group of researchers investigating language in Williams syndrome, i.e. psycholinguists and psychologists is rather small. Therefore, collecting and concentrating the current knowledge of the cross-linguistic research on WS offers a special opportunity of information for everybody working in this interdisciplinary area.

Next to providing an overview of clinical and cognitive characteristics, this volume aims to give a survey of the general language development in WS as well as to shed light on the linguistic competence of certain grammatical phenomena. Thus, the contributions will range from early linguistic abilities, vocabulary acquisition, morphology, and morphosyntax up to various aspects of syntax. Most research so far has been done on English speaking individuals with WS, but this volume will provide data from studies concerning other languages, too. This book presents a unique collection of cross-linguistic research, offering analyses from no less than seven languages. Next to English, data from WS individuals with French, German, Greek, Hebrew, Hungarian, and Italian as their first language will be reported. This cross-linguistic perspective allows insight into language competence under special circumstances and into human language capacity in general. Further, the cross-linguistic research presented here adds to special theoretical discussions such as for example the nature of the mental lexicon.

Before turning to the linguistic topics, the reader will be provided with an introduction on the clinical aspects of Williams syndrome that is forming the first part of the book. **Siegmüller and Bartke** will begin with introducing the phenotype of WS individuals, i.e. a description of physiological, social, cognitive, and neurophysiological characteristics of WS. Here, first peaks and valleys of the cognitive profile of WS individuals become clear.

In the subsequent chapter, **Grzeschik** provides insights into the molecular genetics underlying WS. A detailed and all-embracing review of current research provides the reader with up-to-date information on what is currently known about the molecular genetic basis of this syndrome.

The following second part of the book concentrates on cognitive abilities, more specifically on language development and language competence in WS. This part is opened by two studies linking language and cognition. **Mervis, Robinson, Rowe, Becerra and Klein-Tasman** report from their large-sample studies (ranging from 50 up to 250 English speaking participants) on the general performance on a variety of standardized assessments measuring language and cognition: DAS, K-BIT, Mullen measures, PPVT-III, EVT, TRC, TROG, and the Vineland measures. In light of these results, the authors address the relation of general control processes (e.g. auditory working memory) to the intellectual abilities of WS individuals, specifically to language abilities of school age children and adolescents. Guiding question is if language and cognition are independent of each other or not. The authors argue that cognitive and language abilities cannot get regarded as decoupled. **Schaner-Wolles** discusses language acquisition in light of the question whether it is guided by domain specific or domain general cognitive capacities. Her analyses are based on a detailed case study of a child with WS and on data from a group of 82 children with Down syndrome (DS), all acquiring German as their first language. Her conclusion is that the uneven profile within the linguistic domain has to be interpreted as a consequent effect of the general cognitive profile.

The following two chapters will concentrate on early language acquisition, namely babbling, phonological processing, and lexical development. **Majerus** puts forward the hypothesis that over-detailed phonological representations slow down the developmental process of children with WS. His conclusions are based on data from a group of French-speaking children with WS. He further relates phonological processing to short-term memory. **Böhning, Starke and Weissenborn** present data on the process of learning new words from a German child with WS. Data of vocabulary acquisition are examined on the background of the current fast mapping research. While the fast mapping process is reported being normal, results suggest limited memory capacities. Instead long term memory is assumed of being the source for a delay in vocabulary acquisition as well as a probable different organization of the mental lexicon.

**Volterra, Capirci, Caselli and Vicari** present data from preschoolers: language capacities of Italian speaking children with WS are compared to a group of Italian speaking children with DS as well as to typically developing children. Vocabulary acquisition, morphological and syntactical aspects are finally discussed in light of the relation of general cognition and language competence.

The following chapters will be concerned with the organization of the mental lexicon. **Lukács, Pléh and Racsmány** present results from a study on Hungarian children with WS. The study includes vocabulary (naming), morphology (regularly/irregularly inflected nouns) and spatial postpositions. Contrary to findings reported elsewhere, irregular morphology is found to be intact. Instead, the Hungarian WS children show a selective deficit in naming and in spatial language. **Clahsen, Ring and Temple** put further the discussion on the distinction between regular and irregular morphology, i.e. whether regular morphological operations are intact in contrast to deficits in lexical access. English WS children and a control group of typically developing children are tested on past tense formation and comparative adjective formation. The results of a selective lexical impairment are discussed on the background of whether the linguistic system of children with WS reflects an atypical developmental path. The study by **Penke and Krause** addresses the same question by analyzing data from German-speaking individuals with WS. When examining regularly and irregularly inflected German plurals a selective impairment for irregular forms is observed. Further, because of the peculiarities of the German plural formation the influence of the morphophonological component is discussed.

In analyzing data from Hebrew-speaking children with WS **Levy** provides in-depth insights into the development of language beginning with first word combinations, followed by the acquisition of morphology and syntax. Results are taken as evidence that Williams syndrome as an example for congenital brain pathology does not lead to atypical developmental trajectories.

The following three papers are investigating aspects in the domain of syntax. **Stavrakaki** investigates the production of *wh*-questions in Greek-speaking children with WS, DS, and specific language impairment (SLI). While the WS children are reported as having full knowledge of *wh*-questions, the SLI children display severe problems with *wh*-question formation. Therefore, the author argues for residual competence as far as the computational component of language is concerned. **Siegmüller and Weissenborn** present data from German children with WS of higher chronological and mental age as it was the case in the sample presented by Stavrakaki. Here, comprehension of different kinds of *wh*-questions is under investigation. Finally, **Bartke** presents data on passives as an example for another computational process of language competence. Data from German WS children are discussed in light of the hypothesis that computational processes present a spared ability in WS while actions correlated to lexical access are impaired.

In sum, the volume will present a profile of language development and language competence in Williams syndrome across languages while discussing the modularity of mind in general, the relation of cognition and language, and whether children with WS follow a different developmental trajectory than typically developing children or whether language development in WS could be best captured in terms of a delay.

Next to the children and parents who participated in all the studies presented here, thanks go to the contributors themselves who not only contributed a chapter but who also participated in the review process of another chapter. Special thanks go to all the people who were willing to work as an independent reviewer: Sonja Eisenbeiss, Detlef Hansen, Barbara Höhle, David Ingram, Christina Kauschke, Rainer Pankau, Monika Rothweiler, Matthias Schlesewsky, Ingrid Sonnenstuhl-Henning, Andrew Spencer, Helen Tager-Flusberg, Gerd Utermann, Spyridoula Varlokosta, and Andrea Zukowski. Further we want to thank the series editors Harald Clahsen and Lydia White for accepting this book project as part of their series. We thank them both for their patience and helpful advices.

## References

Bellugi, U., L. Lichtenberger, W. Jones, Z. Lai, & M. St. George (2000). "The Neurocognitive Profile of Williams Syndrome: A Complex Pattern of Strenghts and Weaknesses". *Journal of Cognitive Neuroscience 12*, Supplement 1, 7–29.

Beuren, A. J., J. Apitz, & D. Harmjanz (1962). "Supravalvular Aortic Stenosis in Association with Mental Retardation and a Certain Facial Appearance." *Circulation, 26*, 1235–1240.

Beuren, A. J., J. Apitz, J. Stoermer, B. Kaiser, H. Schlange, W. v. Berg, G. Jörgensen (1966). "Vitamin D-hypercalcämische Herz- und Gefäßerkrankung". *Monatsschrift für Kinderheilkunde, 114*, 457–470.

Brøndum-Nielsen, K., B. Beck, J. Gyftodimou, H. Hørlyk, U. Liljenberg, M. Bloch Petersen, W. Pedersen, M. B. Petersen, A. Sand, F. Skovby, G. Stafanger, P. Zetterqvist, & N. Tommerup (1997). "Investigation of deletions at 7q11.23 in 44 patients referred for Williams-Beuren syndrome, using FISH and four DNA polymorphisms". *Human Genetics, 99*, 56–61.

Doll, A. & K.-H. Grzeschik (2001). "Characterization of two novel genes, WBSCR20 and WBSCR22, deleted in Williams-Beuren syndrome." *Cytogenetic Cell Genetics, 95*, 20–27.

Grimm, T. & H. Wesselhoeft (1980). "Zur Genetik des Williams-Beuren-Syndroms und der isolierten Form der supravalvulären Aortenstenose. Untersuchungen von 128 Familien." *Zeitschrift für Kardiologie, 69*, 168–172.

Jones, K. L. (1990). "Williams Syndrome: An Historical Perspective of Its Evolution, Natural History, and Etiology." *American Journal of Medical Genetics*, Supplement 6, 89–96.

Korenberg, J. R., X.-N. Chen, H. Hirota, Z. Lai, U. Bellugi, D. Burian, B. Roe, & R. Matsuoka (1997). "Genome Structure and Cognitive Map of Williams Syndrome." *Journal of Cognitive Neuroscience, 12*, Supplement 1, 89–107.

Tager-Flusberg, H. (1999). "Language in atypical children." In M. Barrett (Ed.), *The Development of Language* (pp. 311–348). Hove: Psychology Press.

Wesselhoeft, H., F. Salomon, & T. Grimm (1980). "Spektrum der supravalvulären Aortenstenose: Untersuchungsergebnisse bei 150 Patienten mit Williams-Beuren-Syndrom und der isolierten Form der supravalvulären Aortenstenose. *Zeitschrift für Kardiologie, 69*, 131–140.

Williams, J. C. P., B. G. Barratt-Boyes, & J. B. Lowe (1961). "Supravalvular Aortic Stenosis." *Circulation, 24*, 1311–1318.

Part I

# Phenotype and genotype in Williams syndrome

# Williams syndrome from a clinical perspective

Julia Siegmüller and Susanne Bartke
University of Potsdam / Justus-Liebig University Giessen

The aim of the opening chapter of the volume is to provide an overview on the non-language phenotypical features of Williams syndrome (WS). The review of clinical aspects in WS begins with a display of the first cases described in the 60ies of the 20th century and lead to modern ways of diagnosis (FISH, fluorescent in situ hybrid). This genetically based exceptional development urges for a discussion of the link between phenotype and genotype, which will be given subsequently. For this purpose, the chapter also provides a review of the current state of research on brain characteristics, the neurological, and neuropsychological profile in WS. More specifically, findings concerning general cognitive and social abilities, auditory and visual perception, face processing, and numeracy are discussed. In sum, at the same time this chapter implies the introduction to and the complement of the aim of the book representing on what is known about WS to date.

## 1. Identifying Williams syndrome (WS): The first cases

The syndrome was initially described as a cardiological disease by Williams et al. (1961) and Fanconi (1952). Williams and colleagues identified a group of four mentally retarded children on the basis of their heart condition, specifically supravalvular aortic stenosis, and specific facial features. At the same time, Beuren et al. (1962, 1966) reported similar observations made in four other children. They added further physical characteristics to the list of symptoms, e.g. small widely spaced teeth and pulmonic valvular stenosis. Some time later, Black and Bonham-Carter (1963) drew a link between the physical symptoms and an alteration of metabolism, i.e. (transient) hypercalcemia. Martin et al. (1984) also concluded that infantile hypercalcemia and Williams syndrome might be the same condition due to the characteristic features of children receiving either one or the other diagnosis. Since then the clinical picture, also formerly known as idiopathic infantile hypercalcemia (IIH), is called Williams syndrome (WS), alternatively Williams-Beuren syndrome. However, Crisco et al. (1988) proposed that infantile hypercalcemia, in contrary to Williams syndrome, might be a metabolically caused disorder, leading to a similar phenotype as Williams syndrome. They suggested that the metabolic disorder had a different etiology than Williams syndrome which was said to be based on mental retardation. Therefore they assumed two different underlying causes.

Since Crisco et al. (1988) questioned whether Williams syndrome and infantile hypercalcemia are two names for the same condition, the term infantile hypercalcemia has become more and more uncommon as a synonym for Williams syndrome. The discussion finally died as the gene locus for Williams syndrome was found. As the research concerning the genotype will get reviewed in a special chapter, we will directly go to the findings concerning the phenotype.

## 2. Physical features

The phenotype of Williams syndrome is complex and multi-dimensional in its profile. In the following section findings from the current literature will be reviewed. Firstly, the connection between genetic impairment and phenotypical symptoms will be discussed. Subsequently, physical characteristics will be documented. Finally, we will discuss the cognitive manifestations of the mental retardation including first insights into the linguistic skills of individuals with Williams syndrome. In a final step, we will provide a survey of the work and research results related to linguistic development and linguistic competence in Williams syndrome to date. This survey will be short and in form of a summary as the contributors themselves will provide insights into these areas of cognitive ability in Williams syndrome within this volume.

From the first case studies on, children with WS are reported to show particular facial features, described as "elf-like or elfish faces" (Jones & Smith 1975; Pagon et al. 1987; Bellugi et al. 1988; Morris et al. 1988; Lopez-Rangel et al. 1992; Gosch & Pankau 1995; Bellugi et al. 2000). These features are quite distinctive, many parents of WS children report a first diagnostic consideration due to the facial expression (St. George & Bellugi 2000:4). The facial features include asynchronous growth of the upper and lower jowl, a flat nasal bridge and prominent ear lobes. They show characteristic dental malformations, sometimes known as "mice-teeth". The eyes are almost always blue or green and show a stellate iris pattern, coupled with farsightedness (Pagon et al. 1987). Winter et al. (1996) find strabismus in about 50% of their sample whereas Morris and Mervis (1999:559) report 30–70% from their sample. Strabismus is often seen more frequently in children with impaired neurodevelopment, thus Morris and Mervis (1999) propose that the strabismus in Williams syndrome may be related to abnormalities of the central visual pathways (Morris & Mervis 1999:559).

These commonly found features can be observed from quite early on in life. Morris et al. (1988) report characteristic facial dysmorphies in four-months old children. Berthold and Seidel (2002) report of a 10-week-old girl with these facial features who was suspected of having Williams syndrome; this suspicion was then confirmed by FISH (fluorescent in situ hybrid).

A low birth weight is often seen in Williams syndrome (see Pagon et al. 1987; but Lopez-Rangel et al. 1992 find heterogeneous evidence). Subsequently in the first four years of life WS children show statural deficiency (Jones & Smith 1975). They catch up later in life with some of them showing a spurt in growth between the tenth and 13th year, usually reaching low-normal adult height (Jones & Smith 1975; Pagon et al. 1987; Pankau et al. 1992). Older children often develop hypertonia. The WS infant has hyperextensible joints which partly contribute to delayed walking. Persistent toe walking in early childhood is reported coupled with orientation problems as well as difficulties in sensory integration (Morris et al. 1999). Physiotherapy is often required to strengthen knee muscles. Children often complain of leg pains or cramps following days in which high physical activity has occurred (Morris et al. 1988).

About 50% of the adults show contractures of the joints leading to gross and fine motor disability (Kaplan et al. 1989). Scoliosis is also often reported (Lopez-Rangel et al. 1992; Gosch & Pankau 1995). Somatic symptoms include kidney diseases and major difficulties with calcitonin metabolism; bowel and bladder diseases are also common. Adults often report of chronic abdominal pain (Morris & Mervis 1999:561). Two typical heart conditions – pulmonary or supravalvular aortic stenosis – have also been reported (Lopez-Rangel et al. 1992). In a study by Gosch and Pankau (1995) only one child of a group of 20 WS children did not show one of these typical heart conditions. In later childhood and adulthood hypertension is common. In some cases hypertension is due to a narrowing of the renal artery which increases with age (Morris et al. 1999). This suggests that the risk of narrowed arteries is not restricted to the aorta, although it seems not to occur in neurovascular regions (Morris & Mervis 1999:560). Broder et al. (1995) suggest that high blood pressure, in Williams syndrome is due to increased rigidity of the artery walls, i.e. hypertension might be a secondary symptom. Another alternative is suggested by Calamandrei et al. (2000) as they find correlations between high-circulating neurotrophin nerve growth factors (NGF) levels and hypertension caused by an elevated NGF level in later childhood and adolescence in WS subjects.

Transient Infantile hypercalcemia is reported by Grimm and Wesselhoeft (1980). It is documented in about 15% of the WS population and is characterized by abdominal pain, polyuria, constipation which may lead to feeding problems and failure to thrive (Morris et al. 1988; Morris & Mervis 1999). Feeding difficulties are documented in 70% of the children (Morris et al. 1988).[1] The majority of the children show failure to thrive due to poor feeding, increased vomiting, constipation and increased number of cases of colics (Sarimski 1997). Udwin (1990) even reports that 95.5% of her survey sample had been suffering from feeding problems during infancy. The parents reported that problems had "begun at a mean age of two month (range birth to 11 month) and [...] continued for a mean age of 21 months (range one to 230 months)" (Udwin 1990: 131). A first study, considering a possible intervention strategy was recently published by O'Reilly and Lancioni (2001).

Sleeping difficulties are also often reported (Udwin 1990; Gosch & Pankau 1994; Morris et al. 1999). The reports suggest that this difficulty decreases with age. For a summary of the major medical features see the Table 1.

**Table 1.** Summary of major medical features in Williams syndrome (based on Bellugi et al. 2000 and Morris et al. 1999)

| | |
|---|---|
| *Neurological features* | *Cardiovascular features* |
| – average IQ 55 (range 40–90)<br>– diagnosis of mental retardation: ca. 75% (Morris et al. 1999)<br>– poor coordination<br>– hypersensitivity to sounds (hyperacusis)<br>– hoarse voice (Gosch et al. 1994)<br>– microcephaly<br>– reduced motor cortex<br>– enlargement of neo-cerebellar areas | – supravalvular aortic stenosis<br>– pulmonary artery stenosis<br>– ventricular / atrial-septal defects<br>– risk of narrowing of any artery<br>– hypertension in later childhood and in adults |
| *Other physical features* | *Facial features* |
| – hypotonia<br>– developmental delay in height and weight (infants)<br>– recurrent otitis media | – full prominent lips<br>– stellate iris pattern (Winter et al. 1996)<br>– strabismus<br>– prominent ear lobes<br>– wide mouth<br>– small, widely spaced teeth<br>– medial eyebrow flare<br>– flat nasal bridge<br>– short nose<br>– anteverted nares |
| *Somatic features* | |
| – kidney diseases (asymmetric kidney growth, Pober et al. 1993)<br>– transient infantile hypercalcemia | |

**Table 2.** Symptoms related to hemizygosity of elastin (based on Morris & Mervis 1999:557)

- generalized arteriopathy (including supravalvular aortic stenosis)
- hernias
- bowel and bladder diverticulae
- premature aging of the skin
- hyperextentibility of joints in young children
- contractures of joints in adults
- hoarse voice
- some facial dysmorphies (periorbital fullness, full cheeks in infants and toddlers)

## 3. A link between genetics and phenotype

The genetic bases and the cognitive profile of Williams syndrome offers the basis for investigating the relationship between phenotype and genetic encoding. However, size and pattern of the deletion in this region of chromosome 7 may differ. Moreover, a deletion in region 7q11.23 not necessarily leads to the classical profile of Williams syndrome. Differing observations revive the discussion about the genetic basis of Williams syndrome, although Meng et al. (1998) published a complete map of the common deletion in Williams syndrome. However, genetic research is still making progress as documented by the ongoing publication of new (deleted) genes being involved in Williams syndrome (cf. e.g. Cairo et al. 2001; Doll & Grzeschik 2001; Grzeschik this volume).

The loss of the elastin gene, which usually determines the production of the protein Elastin, is made responsible for many of the phenotypical symptoms of Williams syndrome. Most importantly, deprivation of elastin leads to the typical metabolic disorders seen in Williams syndrome. Also the characteristic cardiological disease of supravalvular aortic stenosis is at least partly caused by deprived elastin levels (Gosch & Pankau 1996; Morris & Mervis 1999, for a more detailed listing of symptoms caused by deprivation of elastin see Table 2).

Another gene (LIM kinase 1) has been found to be responsible for neurologically deviant development, in particular abnormalities of myelinic development (Tassabehji et al. 1996).

Furthermore, Mervis et al. (2000) also assume the elastin gene LIM kinase 1 to be critical for specific deficits of the cognitive profile in Williams syndrome. LIM kinase 1 hemizygosity is assumed to contribute to deficits in visuo-spatial construction (Frangiskakis et al. 1996). The gene is part of a cascade of genes involved in normal development of visual constructive abilities. Mervis et al. (2000) therefore suggest that a disruption of a gene of this cascade, most likely the deletion of LIM kinase 1, may lead to specific deficits in visuo-spatial construction as observed in Williams syndrome. Additionally, Mervis et al. (1997) argue that individuals with an especially large deletion in the region of 7q11.23 share some features with the phenotype of Williams syndrome, but they do not fit the classical profile of Williams syndrome. Therefore, additional deletions as mentioned above have to be taken into account when discussing the underlying genetics of Williams syndrome. Furthermore, Mervis et al. (1999) report on two families with small deletions of chromosome 7q11.23, but who are not diagnosed as having Williams syndrome. Similar findings are reported by Frangiskakis et al. (1996) who observed deletions of the same genetic material without a developed profile of Williams syndrome in some of their subjects.

Korenberg et al. (1997) tested whether the size of the deletion might explain the observed cognitive variability in the phenotype. In their study of 40 WS subjects they found no correlation between deletion size and cognitive outcome. However, a promising correlation between cognitive behavior and parental origin was found when the mutated gene was of maternal origin. Flint (1996) claims in contrast to Korenberg et al. (1997) that different IQ outcomes and degree of deletion size are related. He explains that sequence differences at equivalent places of the same chromosome are to be interpreted as allelic variation. In this sense, genetic variation may be responsible for behavioral differences in complex cognitive behavior, such as intelligence. The severity of the mental retardation of a child is therefore at least in part "…the consequence of differences in the combination of alleles at these loci" (Flint 1996: 362).

A different perspective on cognitive development is taken by Karmiloff-Smith (1999). By implementing the *model of representational redescription* (RR model) she proposes a learning model of developmental phases that are not age-related. "Representational redescription […] is hypothesized to occur recurrently within microdomains throughout development, as well as in adulthood for some kinds of new learning" (Karmiloff-Smith 1999: 18). The motor of development is seen by redescriptive processes that change implicit knowledge already in the mind into explicit knowledge to the mind (cf. p. 17f.). However, when discussing domain specificity, different examples of abnormal development as e.g. Williams syndrome, Down syndrome and autism, different developmental courses of mastery (resp. of non-mastery) of domains become apparent (cf. pp. 168ff). One might conclude from these results that different genetic causes could lead to different levels of mastery of domains.

The conclusion so far has to be that the locus of the exact genes still has to be identified and that the relation between genetics and cognition is open to discussion – probably to a greater extent than ever before.

## 4. Neurological profile and brain characteristics

In 1990, Bellugi and colleagues started a longitudinal examination of the neurological and neuropsychological characteristics of people with Williams syndrome (Bellugi et al. 1990). In an initial study, six adolescent WS subjects, with a chronological age of 10 to 17 years were matched with adolescents with Down syndrome (DS) for chronological age and IQ-score. They underwent a complete standard neurological examination form, including gross motor, oromotor, fine motor, cerebellar, language, and mental status. Bellugi et al. (1990) found dolichocephaly in the WS population, whereas DS subjects showed microcephaly. Morris et al. (1988) report microcephaly in the first four years of life, but children catch up in later childhood, with little or no microcephaly in adulthood.

Recent findings regarding neuronal anatomy in Williams syndrome report a complex pattern of abnormalities as well as normally developed parts of the brain within these subjects. Some of these results come from post-mortal investigations of the brains of WS subjects (e.g. Galaburda & Bellugi 2000). However, nowadays they are mostly reports from studies which have used the nuclear magnetic resonance tomography (NMR) method or high-resolution magnetic resonance imaging (MRI) scans.

Bellugi et al. (1990) were among the first to use MRI scans with WS subjects. Their study revealed that the WS subjects appear to have decreased posterior width of the cortex and elongated posterior to anterior length of the cortex compared to the norm. The overall brain volume of the WS subjects reaches up to 80% of normal cerebrum volume. They also show decreased myelination, a finding which was further confirmed in the study by Galaburda et al. (1994). The cerebellum and the brain stem of the WS subject group reached 99% of the normal size, while results in the DS group revealed a dramatic reduction (Bellugi et al. 1990: 122). Reiss et al. (2000) find evidence for a disproportionate reduction of the brain stem tissue. Considering all different findings, the reduction of the total brain size in Williams syndrome appears to display an asynchronous pattern. The reduced parts of the left hemisphere seem to cluster in the parietal and occipital regions. In contrary, the frontal and temporal lobes, the hippocampus, parahyppocampal gyrus, the amygdala, and the cerebellum are relatively spared or even larger than observed in normal development (Reiss et al. 2000). When investigating four brains from autopsies, Galaburda et al. (1994) report normal size and configuration for three of the subjects. However, the forth brain was characterized by a marked reduction of the parietal, posterior temporal, and occipital regions. Bellugi et al. (1999) suggest that this reduction might be seen as the cytoarchitectonic correlate of severe visuo-spatial deficits observed in Williams syndrome.

Lenhoff et al. (1998) and Jernigan and Bellugi (1990) find normal anterior and temporal limbic cortices. The overall size of the cerebellum has been found to be normal, due to better preservation of the neocerebellum (Mervis et al. 2000).

A recent study by Schmitt et al. (2001) examines size reduction and disproportional reduction in different sub-parts of the corpus callosum. The study is based on the claim by Reiss et al. (2000) that the white matter is more affected in Williams syndrome than the gray matter. The corpus callosum is critical to the higher cognitive processes of bilateral sensory integration, such as language and visuo-spatial processing (Thompson 1994:32). Abnormal growth rate of the corpus callosum might therefore be a critical neuroanatomical factor in the unusual development in WS individuals. The subject sample consisted of 20 WS adults and 20 normal adults as controls. The controls were individually matched for age and sex. Their results suggest a reduction of the total corpus callosum in the Williams syndrome group. Closer fractionation of the corpus callosum into different sub-parts revealed disproportional reduction sizes in the posterior regions of the corpus callosum: the isthmus and the splenium. Anterior and middle part regions were not significantly reduced (Schmitt et al. 2001). These findings agree with earlier results of the same research group (Bellugi et al. 1990). Jernigan and Bellugi (1990) also report normal anterior portions of the corpus callosum. They find evidence for a correlation between apparent visuo-spatial deficits and abnormal parts of the corpus callosum in WS subjects.

Lenhoff et al. (1998) compare the brain size of DS subjects with WS subjects. They report decreased volume of the neocerebellum in Down syndrome whereas in Williams syndrome the volume of the neocerebellum seems to be normal. Bellugi et al. (1999a, b) emphasize the fact that neocerebellum and frontal cortex are mostly preserved in Williams syndrome and link it to a model of language representation that relates a fronto-cortico-cerebellar system with language functions. Nevertheless, Lenhoff et al. (1998) report that both populations display a decreased size of the neocortex in comparison to normal controls of the same age. Jernigan and Bellugi (1994), as well as Lenhoff et al. (1998) find individuals in their WS population that show an even more strongly developed neocerebellum than a normal development would predict. In another study, Galaburda and Bellugi (2000) present data from four brains of WS individuals in comparison to control brains of DS individuals. The data suggest subtly different brain shapes in these two populations, although a similar weight reduction is observed. The brains of WS individuals appear curtailed from top to bottom, with a particularly strong curtailment in the posterior portions of the hemispheres. The central sulcus in the WS brains ends before the midline of the brain, where it usually (in normal brains) proceeds in a posteriorly curved direction. This abnormality is responsible for an unusual configuration of the dorsal-central region, including the dorsal portions of the superior-parietal lobule and the dorsal-frontal gyrus (Galaburda & Bellugi 2000:86).

Reiss et al. (2000) relate the disproportionate reduction of the gray and white matter in Williams syndrome to the deletion region on chromosome 7. One of the genes, which is usually included in the deletion, is LIM kinase 1. It is claimed that the missing protein which is usually controlled by the gene, plays an important role in synapse formation and intracellular signaling. In other words, a direct relation is stated between the neurodevelopmental disorder and a genetic basis. This view corresponds to the approach of cognitive neuroscience, wherein a clinical condition affects genes that in turn modify the building of cognitively relevant brain structures and their lifelong configuration.

Evidence for morphological/chemical abnormalities in the brain development in Williams syndrome is reported by Calamandrei et al. (2000). They find high NGF levels in three age groups with Williams syndrome, ranging from 6 years to adolescence.[2] In the normal control group, a much earlier decrease of the NGF level was observed. The authors suggest several consequences from this finding, such as sympathetic hypertrophy, hyperinnervation of target organs, and general nerve dysfunction. Furthermore, hormonal and immunological consequences might occur. In general, the authors state that the increased NGF level is indicative of a general alteration of various developmental processes, which occur outside the brain (Calamandrei et al. 2000: 749).

Morphological investigation of the amygdalar nuclei in one WS brain revealed a substantially diminished volume of the amygdala, to about 50% of the normal size (Galaburda & Bellugi 2000). In the same specimen, the temporal horn is more dorsally placed than in normal brains. No evidence for morphological changes in the right hemisphere in Williams syndrome has been found in studies from the Salk institute (Bellugi et al. 1994; Jernigan & Bellugi 1994).

The cytoarchitecture of the frontal cortical areas in Williams syndrome brains appears normal (Galaburda & Bellugi 2000). Evidence was found for enlarged neuron size in WS brains (measured in area 17). Furthermore, the histometric observations reveal abnormal neuron sizes in some layers, normal size in others. The question of cell packing density was not sufficiently answered. The authors recall findings from MRI studies, suggesting increased cell-packing density (Tassabehji et al. 1999). They carry out a histomorphometric analysis that has suggested decreased cell packing density in some layers, as a general observation they state that the variability in Williams syndrome is much broader than in normal subjects, regarding this question. Galaburda and Bellugi (2000) suggest that the combination of decreased cell density and increased neuron size might result in higher subcortical connectivity in WS brains.

In summary, several observations in WS brains suggest abnormal development and maintenance in this population. Proponents of two different approaches have investigated the brains of WS subjects and found evidence for modified brains as a consequence from deletion of genes. The overall findings are that the WS brain is smaller and of lower weight than normal brains. However, the brain reductions show certain asynchronical patterns affecting the parietal and occipital regions of the neocortex more strongly than the frontal and temporal regions. In addition, subcortical structures appear affected in differing strengths. Morphological, chemical and histometric analyses suggest abnormal building of cytoarchitectonics. Altogether, the findings strongly suggest that genetic syndromes affect the development of the brain on various levels of development and configuration. However, the exact relationship between the underlying genetic disorder, cognitive behavior and development still remains highly unclear. Other approaches, such as Elman et al. (1996), do not assume a direct relation between a genetic disorder and a neural manifestation.

When evaluating the discussion regarding genetic disorders and brain size with respect to neural correlates, one has to keep in mind that the data are based on very few cases. These few cases display high variability (cf. for a summery Bellugi et al. 1999a). In spite of this fact, sometimes reports are based on single-case examinations (Bellugi et al. 1999a, b). As insightful and valuable as these research results may be, it remains for future research to show if the knowledge obtained so far can be generalized across subjects.

## 5. The neuropsychological profile of Williams syndrome

### General cognitive abilities

Studies examining the cognitive abilities of WS children have used a great range of different full scale IQ-tests: Udwin et al. (1987) and Pagon et al. (1987) for instance, administered the WISC-R, Greer et al. (1997) the Stanford-Binet Intelligence Scale, Gosch and Pankau (1995) the German Münchener Funktionale Entwicklungsdiagnostik (MFED), Volterra et al. (1996) the Leiter International Performance Scale (LIPS). The mean IQ of the different subject groups reported in these studies is typically around 55, with a range from 40 to 90, the latter corresponds to low, normal intelligence (Jones & Smith 1975; Karmiloff-Smith et al. 1997; Jarrold et al. 1998; Mervis et al. 1999; Bellugi et al. 2000). According to the WHO, this score puts the subjects with Williams syndrome in the range of severe or moderate to mild mental retardation. The IQ is confirmed in studies using developmental scales, for example those in German, the Münchener Funktionale Entwicklungsdiagnostik (MFED, Süss-Burghart 1993; see Gosch & Pankau 1995 for German data).[3] Individual cases in some studies show normal cognitive abilities (Morris & Mervis 1999; Bellugi et al. 2000).[4] Morris and Mervis (1999) report that a syndrome-specific pattern of cognitive strengths and weaknesses can already be observed at the chronological age of 4 and younger and they presume the profile to be similar to that of older children. In accordance with these findings and citing Mervis et al. (1999), verbal subtests are slightly better than non-verbal subtests but significantly better than visuo-spatial construction tasks (Morris & Mervis 1999: 575). Although the importance of the administration of a full scale IQ test for children with neurodevelopmental impairments is stressed, Morris and Mervis (1999) suggest that for clinical work the focus should be on the different sub-scales of the test rather than on the overall IQ (see e.g. the argumentation in Mervis et al. 2000).

Crisco (1990) briefly reports from a longitudinal study on the stability of the global intelligence in 14 WS children. The children were investigated twice, once at pre-school age, mean age 4;3, and a second time five years later. The results suggest a steady and consistent rate of cognitive development, i.e. the WS children's delays appear equally severe at both times. This is interesting to note because it provides evidence that the rate of development in this subject group is no slower than in normal children, if it were the case, then the scores of the WS children would be lower at the second time of investigation, compared to the norm group for the assessment tool used. Crisco (1990) argues that the WS children show lower ability levels but appear as stable in their developmental rate as normal children.[5] Bellugi et al. (2000) report from their various lab studies that the level of the general cognition of WS adolescents is similar to DS subjects (Bellugi et al. 2000: 9). In their findings, subscales for verbal and non-verbal abilities did not differ significantly. This is one of the main reasons why Bellugi and collaborators usually include a DS subject group in studies concerning Williams syndrome. Bellugi et al. (1992, 1994) administered some Piagetian tasks of conservation (including numbers, weight and substance) additionally to the tasks investigating the general cognitive development of WS and DS adolescents. No difference between the two groups could be documented.

## Social abilities

People with Williams syndrome are described as being very sociable and friendly (e.g. Gosch & Pankau 1994). All of them seem to have the same kind of friendly nature – "they love everyone, are loved by everyone, and are very charming" (Beuren et al. 1962: 1235). There is broad consensus in the literature about this feature (e.g. Bellugi et al. 1988; Morris et al. 1988; van Lieshout et al. 1998; Morris & Mervis 1999), although some reports describe negative temperament characteristics in Williams syndrome, i.e. displaying a difficult temperament leading to problems in making and also keeping friends (cf. Dilts et al. 1990). The behavioral phenotype as implemented as a diagnostic instrument by Dilts et al. (1990) also includes this observation and usually goes together with strong talkativeness (Gosch & Pankau 1994). Some scholars relate this feature to the linguistic domains of pragmatics and syntax (e.g. Stojanovik et al. 2001), and argue that this behavioral pattern may be responsible for the good language performance. Several studies claim that children and adults with Williams syndrome overdo social behavior and therefore appear socially less well adjusted than normal children. They often show a marked friendliness towards strangers (Gosch & Pankau 1994), which may tend to cause problems in everyday life.

## Cognitive profile

From early on, the scientific discussion turned to the uneven profile within non-verbal cognition in this group of subjects. The initial observation of asynchronous performance patterns on the different cognitive domain levels in Williams syndrome came from Bellugi et al. (1988), who described face processing as being the only preserved ability in non-verbal cognition. Crisco et al. (1988), Mac Donald and Roy (1988) and Udwin and Yule (1991) were among the first to investigate this claim. Broad consensus exists regarding the main dissociation lying between visual and verbal/auditory memory and performance skills. Visual perception and construction may be a weak point in the cognitive profile of Williams syndrome, while auditory immediate performance, as well as short-term memory functions, are superior to their non-verbal mental age.

In a follow-up study Udwin et al. (1996) examined whether the IQ of WS adults changes over time. The interval between the two test times was about 8 years, 10 months on average. In other genetic syndromes, such as Fragile-X syndrome, a decline in IQ over time had been reported (Hagerman et al. 1989), although findings were not entirely consistent (cf. Mazzocco & Reiss 1999). Udwin et al. (1996) did not confirm this finding for Williams syndrome. In contrast to Fragile-X syndrome, the WS group showed an increase in IQ scores. Thus, they emphasize that WS adults follow the same trend of IQ development as the normal population.

In the following sections strengths and weaknesses of different perceptual domains in Williams syndrome will be reviewed in more detail.

## Auditory perception

The results of several studies during the last ten years suggest that phonological short-term memory (often synonymously used with verbal memory) is a relative strength in WS individuals (a definite strength, according to Mervis et al. 1999). This has a certain impact on their linguistic development. It is often reported for different domains of language that WS subjects rely more heavily on phonological factors and less on semantic factors than the norm (e.g. Thomas et al. 2001). The same is reported for auditory short term memory (Vicari et al. 1996b; Vicari et al. 2000; Zukowski 2001).

The abilities in auditory short-term memory appear extremely well developed when compared to disordered spatial memory performance. In a basic study, Wang and Bellugi (1994) matched WS adults with DS subjects individually for age and IQ in a forward digit span task, taken from WISC-R. In this task, digits were presented at a rate of one digit per second. The results suggested significant differences between auditory rote memory abilities in Williams and Down syndrome. While this task proved to be very difficult for DS subjects, WS adults showed significantly better performances (Wang & Bellugi 1994: 319). Mervis et al. (1999) tested digit spans more rapidly with two digits per second. This was taken from the Differential Ability Scale (DAS, Elliot 1990). Two digits per second resemble the rate of natural speech more closely. Mervis et al. (1999) interpret that the auditory rote memory abilities provide an excellent base for both vocabulary and grammatical development. This interpretation may serve as an explanation for the superior language abilities of people with Williams syndrome.

Udwin and Yule (1991) tested 20 WS children on the Rivermead Behavioural Memory Test (RBMT, Wilson et al. 1985). When compared to control groups with mixed etiologies (all mentally retarded without a known cause), WS children again scored significantly better than the control children in recalling the verbal material from the RBMT (Udwin & Yule 1991).

Other researchers state that the well-developed verbal memory is a result of the normal developmental pathway and normal developmental rate in phonology (Vicari et al. 1996b). They suggest that phonological disorders might affect the short-term memory, while semantic disorders are more likely to produce a long-term memory deficit (as it has been described by Barisnikov et al. 1996 for a single case with Williams syndrome). Vicari et al. (1996b) confirm that WS subjects show a dissociation between normal short-term memory and deficient long-term memory for verbal material, indicating superior phonological abilities in Williams syndrome.

However, there is some evidence that auditory short-term memory does not operate on normal frequency and phonological effects. Differently from normal processing, the performances in WS children are not affected by the factor frequency in word span tasks, i.e. the performance does not decrease to the normal degree when the words in the span task become less frequent (Vicari et al. 1996b). The length effect in word span tasks is normal, i.e. the span length decreases when the words in the task become longer. But there is no primacy effect in Williams syndrome, according to the results of Vicari et al. (1996b).

Hypersensitivity to sounds (hyperacusis) is a symptom often reported for WS people (Morris et al. 1988; Klein et al. 1990; Klein & Mervis 1999). Klein et al. (1990) count up to 95% of the population suffering from this phenomenon. Young children tend to be afraid of loud noises (even the vacuum cleaner can cause complaints). Older children and adults are more sensitive to background noises from the environment. Klein et al. (1990) find results in an American sample in full agreement with the findings of Martin et al. (1984), collected in Great Britain. Both studies were carried out by questionnaires sent to families with reported cases of Williams syndrome. Klein et al. (1990) conclude that hyperacusis is a very consistent feature of Williams syndrome, which can be observed in the first year of life and therefore seems to be innate. Morris and Mervis (1999) report one study of Marriage and Barnes (1995) who suggest naming these symptoms phonophobia instead of hyperacusis since it may be much more related to psychological perception of noises than to acoustic facts. An alternative explanation is given in Calamandrei et al. (2000). They relate the symptoms of the hyperacusis directly to the increased NGF levels in WS children. They suggest that a hypersensitivity to sounds might depend upon a peripheral "hyperinnervation" of the inner ear, due to an excess of NGF production by the target organ. Too many neurons processing the information could then cause a stronger receptive experience, in this case the louder perception of sounds. A recent study by Böhning et al. (2002) provided evidence that hyperacusis does not have an impact on oral processing of linguistic stimuli.

Neville et al. (1994) used the technique of event-related potentials (ERP) to investigate a possible influence of hypersensitivity to sounds on subsequent stages of cognitive language processing. To sum up the findings regarding auditory presentation of tones, brain responses suggest that similar brain regions are active in Williams and control subjects. But the brain responses by the individuals with Williams syndrome are characterized by an abnormally large P200. In contrast, brain responses to audibly presented words show a highly different morphology, never observed in normal auditory development. The authors conclude that these results suggest that the systems that mediate the preserved language in WS are not the same as those that operate in normal control subjects (Neville et al. 1994:81). Further, they interpret their findings in such a way that hypersensitivity of the auditory system in WS subjects may in part underlie the sparing of and the precocious and hyperfluent nature of the WS subjects' language, and the fact that this development occurs following abnormal delays in the acquisition of auditory language (Neville et al. 1994:82). It remains to note, that although otitis media is a recurring problem in about 61% of the young WS population, there is no correlation between hearing impairments and chronic otitis media (Klein et al. 1990).

Lenhoff et al. (1998) as well as Gosch and Pankau (1994) report that their subjects with Williams syndrome appear to be very sensitive to music. Gosch and Pankau (1994) find a musical sensitivity in 74% of their sample (N = 25). They suggest using the musical abilities in training programs, supporting motor skills as well as language. There has been little systematic research about unique musical talents in Williams syndrome.

## Visual perception

Visual cognition was identified early on as a particularly deficient domain in Williams syndrome. There are many consistent findings in the literature that describe extreme difficulties with any task involving visuo-spatial construction, such as drawing or pattern construction subtests of various developmental scales (Udwin & Yule 1991; Bellugi et al. 1992; Wang et al. 1995; Bertrand et al. 1997; Klein & Mervis 1999; Mervis et al. 2000; Atkinson et al. 2001). Whether this profile can be considered as Williams syndrome-specific or rather typical for mental retardation in general was investigated by Crisco et al. (1988) and Mac Donald and Roy (1988). They used mentally retarded control groups, matched for general cognitive level. Both studies found specific deficits in Williams syndrome, even in comparison to the other groups of mentally retarded subjects with mixed etiologies. The visuo-spatial deficit in construction tasks of WS subjects is apparently the most homogeneous finding within the cognitive profile of the syndrome. A recent documentation of better visual constructive abilities is reported for a subgroup of the Williams syndrome sample in Mervis et al. (2000). This study examined 84 WS subjects from 3;11 to 46;6 years of age. In this sample 7% of the WS subjects performed at least as well as the mean level of individual performance on the visuo-spatial construction tasks (subtest from the DAS battery, Elliot 1990). Mervis et al. (2000) report that although variability exists in visuo-constructive tasks, the range is not as wide as in other subtests of the DAS. Still, this might indicate that the visuo-spatial deficit may turn out to be a relative rather than an absolute difficulty for individuals with Williams syndrome, showing a within-syndrome variability which is at least partly comparable to the within-syndrome performance variability of language tasks and overall non-verbal cognition.

Among the first studies giving evidence for a visual constructive deficit in Williams syndrome was the work by Bihrle et al. (1989). They compared young WS and DS adults in drawing tests. Their results suggested a double dissociation between the two populations: while DS subjects were able to preserve the rough global form of the objects, WS subjects focused on details in their drawings; the global form of the object being lost. Bihrle et al. (1989) concluded that WS subjects showed a global perception deficit. However, simple visual recognition tasks do not reveal greater difficulties than the non-verbal mental age of the subject is presumed to have. A more recent study examines the visuo-spatial short-term memory in adolescents of WS cases (Jarrold et al. 1999). The experiment included a Corsi span as well as a digit span task. Jarrold et al. (1999) compared the WS subjects with a group of DS subjects and adolescents with mild learning disabilities. One goal of this study was to find supportive evidence for a specific, isolated deficit in a specific processing domain, or alternatively to find a broader learning and processing difficulty in both syndromes. In order to distinguish between relative or absolute strengths and weakness in Williams syndrome and Down syndrome, the third control group was necessary. The results suggest further evidence for the findings of Wang and Bellugi (1993). These authors suggested a double dissociation between Down syndrome and Williams syndrome in two different domains of cognition. WS subjects showed relatively good performance in verbal memory, but deficits in visual memory span. DS subjects' performance suggested a severe deficit in verbal memory with relatively good skills in visuo-spatial tasks. These results are supported by a longitudinal case study in a girl (Elisa) with Williams syndrome which was conducted in order to examine her drawing abilities (Stiles et al. 2000). They followed her for a period of about four years starting at the age of 2;5 years, continuing to 6;7 years. To pool their observations, Elisa's drawings (spontaneous drawings as well as drawings elicited by standardized tests) improved over time, but marked difficulties persisted.

Regarding these results, the WS subject group showed a rather severe deficit in visuo-spatial tasks. However, the difference to the matched DS subjects appeared to be smaller than expected. According to Jarrold et al. (1999) it remains unclear what the primary deficit in Williams syndrome might be. Firstly, the visuo-spatial short-term memory deficit could be the consequence of general low non-verbal abilities. Secondly, the visuo-spatial short-term memory deficit could be more fundamental than the general non-verbal deficit and therefore be the cause of the low performance on non-verbal tasks.

A more recent study is concerned with the relationship between visuo-spatial deficits and the underlying general problems in visual perception (Atkinson et al. 2001). In a large sample of 73 children, aged from 0;8 to 13;8 years (mean CA 7;3) orthopedic examination measures are combined with visual perception tasks and tasks of visuo-spatial cognition. Some language tasks (BPVS and TROG) are also administered in order to confirm the distinct profile of each subject. The results for visuo-spatial cognition indicate a growing difference between the age-equivalent mean and the performance of the WS children. The authors suggest that the WS children are not only delayed in their performance but show severe basic visual deficiencies. This deficiency has not been observed for the administered language tasks in the same children. Since this finding is consistent with the characteristic profile of WS subjects, the authors conclude from their data that WS children have a higher incidence of basic visual deficiencies together with a severe delay in visuo-spatial tasks. Apart from this rather general claim, no direct interaction between sensory visual problems and the performance on visuo-spatial tasks was found. The authors propose that if the cause of the visuo-spatial disorder in

WS children is not the result of basic visual problems, the development of neural mechanisms critical for processing and transforming spatial information must be involved. Atkinson et al. (2001) find evidence for deficiencies in dorsal-stream processing of visual information yet better ventral-stream processing. Böhning et al. (2002) investigate the so-called McGurk effect in a sample of 13 WS subjects (CA 10;1–50;9). The operating of the McGurk effect in Williams syndrome means that visual and auditory information interact in the perception of sounds, subjects listen to and see them articulated at the same time. In Williams syndrome it can be suspected that the interaction of the two perceptual modalities might not be the same as in the norm since visual perception (in this case lip reading) seems to be disordered. Normal subjects get confused when the person they see says different sound than the sound they hear. The question addressed in this study has been whether WS subjects react in the same way. The WS subjects performed more poorly in visual identification of sounds than the control subjects. This had as a consequence an effect on the integration of processing sound and vision. The poor lip reading abilities in the Williams syndrome subjects made them not as sensitive to the McGurk effect as the normal controls. This result is particularly noteworthy for another interesting point regarding the cognitive profile of Williams syndrome. As Böhning et al. (2002) mention, the WS population is said to be very interested in faces. However, as the results of this study indicate, the looking at faces itself might not have a positive effect on the quality of face processing.

## Face processing

Face recognition appears to be an area of particular strength in Williams syndrome (Karmiloff-Smith et al. 1995). Bellugi et al. (1992) found that young WS children seemed to be extremely interested in faces of fellow men. Their subjects fixated another person's face longer relative to a group of children with Fragile X syndrome. Tager-Flusberg and Sullivan (1998) report that this extreme social interest seemed quite inappropriate in quantity and quality, since WS children spend more time looking at faces than normal children (Tager-Flusberg & Sullivan 1998:214).

However, a recent study by Deruelle et al. (1999) provides evidence for an abnormal development of face processing in Williams syndrome. Deruelle et al. (1999) as well as Karmiloff-Smith (1997) assume a local processing bias for the face processing tasks which does not exist to the same extent in normal face processing. This claim gets support from the finding that inverted faces show a lower face recognition effect in Williams syndrome, indicating that the WS subjects react more similarly to mental age-matched children than to chronologically age-matched controls. In the Deruelle et al. (1999) study the WS subjects (5–23 years) performed efficiently on the given task, however they still did not reach their chronologically age-matched normal controls; instead, the WS subjects performed on the level of the controls of the same verbal IQ.

## Numeracy

The studying of numerical abilities in Williams syndrome is still a rather rare research topic. But in spite of the lack of a long history of research, arithmetic is typically reported as a field of extreme difficulty in Williams syndrome (e.g. Zukowski 2001). There are some anecdotal reports on the numerical abilities in children and adults with Williams syndrome. For example, Bellugi et al. (2000) report severe problems in their Williams syndrome subjects in the handling of money. Zukowski (2001) also states that similar problems are common in the Williams syndrome subjects in her studies. There are some older, more structured findings reported by Udwin (1990). The survey with WS adults (n = 119) provides evidence for severe problems in numeracy. The majority of her subjects show basic skills in numeracy (81.3%). However, there are also 18.5% (which is a total of 22 persons) of adults who still can only count up to ten or even perform less well than that (Udwin 1990: 133). Only six per cent of Udwin's (1990) subjects were reported to use money without the help of caregivers. This report suggests that in arithmetic abilities there might also be a great variation within the syndrome. This is confirmed by Bellugi et al. (2000), who, alongside the documentation of severe difficulties, state that some of their subjects are able to perform quite well on tasks assessing the four fundamental operations of arithmetic.

Pagon et al. (1987) also find that arithmetic is the weakest subject in school for their whole sample. They observe that it is even more apparent in the more capable children who display quite good reading abilities. This finding might suggest a dissociative acquisition of different academic achievements in Williams syndrome. Relying on subtests of the Wechsler Intelligence Scale (WISC-III UK), Howlin et al. (1998) have to conclude that arithmetic skills together with reading, spelling and social adaptation remain at a low level. They investigated the cognitive profile in 62 adults with Williams syndrome, aged from 19 years to 39 years. The results obtained by several standardized tests concerning arithmetic, reading, and spelling skills revealed an age equivalent of 6–8 years (cf. Howlin et al. 1998: 185, Table 3).

## Language: A brief overview

Only little is known about the preverbal development of WS children. The first words are reported to emerge around the 20th month of life (Morris et al. 1988 document 21.6 months; Lenhoff et al. 1998 report a range between 18th and 24th month of life; Pankau et al. 2000 report the prospective mean age for the emergence of the first words is 20 months). Before the emergence of words, normally developing children run through the different stages of babbling with canonical babbling as the end state of preverbal prosodic development. In a recent study, Masataka (2001) reports the emergence of canonical babbling in a Japanese sample of eight WS children. The study provides longitudinal data from the 6th to the 30th month of life. The results suggest that, although delayed, canonical babbling and the emergence of the first words relate in the same way in Williams syndrome as in normal language acquisition.

Following the first steps in language acquisition Mervis and Bertrand (1997) observe a growing of the lexicon in a strong relation to non-verbal abilities, such as joint attention. Other interfaces cannot be confirmed in Williams syndrome. Mervis and Bertrand (1997) find evidence that the WS children show the vocabulary spurt without the ability to map word-forms and the corresponding referents quickly, or to sort objects spontaneously. But the different relations between language and cognition in the WS group show the greater delays in non-verbal aspects. Language seems to be ahead of non-verbal cognition in the WS children of this study. Pankau et al. (2000) report from a follow-up examination of one of the original patients of Beuren (1962). His anamnestic data revealed a delay in producing two-word sentences until five years of age. Prospective results of a study in Kiel (Germany), including data of 218 WS subjects, suggest a mean age for two-word utterances of 36 months, with a range between 18–84 months of life (Pankau et al. 2000: 322).

Linguistic competence can be expected to increase in early school age. Their well-developed language functions are then especially prominent in adolescence in comparison to other mentally retarded subject groups of the same age, e.g. Down syndrome (Sarimski 1996). One of the questions arising from such studies is how reliably results from early developmental stages can predict the developmental progress and the final level of language in the particular individual.

As a result of a survey of WS adults interesting evidence for within-syndrome variation in language acquisition is reported by Udwin (1990). Parents of 119 subjects were asked about the level of language use of their children in adulthood. She found 77% of her subjects using fluent speech and complex sentences. Another three adults were reported to be using primitive phrases and single words only in their speech (Udwin 1990: 134). To the best of our knowledge, this is the only report on severe language difficulties in adult individuals with Williams syndrome.

Fowler (1998) suggests that the linguistic domains of pragmatics and semantics are much more closely related to MA and IQ in mental retardation than the computational domains of syntax and phonology. Dissociative profiles in mentally retarded subjects with spared areas in the language faculty should, according to this view, show strengths particularly in syntax and phonology. This suggestion is in some aspects supported by the findings of WS research. Phonology is a definite strength in children with Williams syndrome (Mervis et al. 1999; Thomas et al. 2001). The statements considering the development of syntax are much more controversial. The initial finding that WS adolescents rely on a totally intact grammar as opposed to gaps in non-verbal cognitive domains as stated by e.g. Bellugi et al. (1990) has been relativised over the last decade and will be documented in greater detail by the contributions to follow. Nevertheless, the more recent studies of Bellugi and colleagues show an unchanging dissociation between grammar and visual cognition (Bellugi et al. 1999a; Bellugi et al. 1999b; Bellugi et al. 2000). More informal evidence of "normal" grammar in a large WS sample is reported in Morris et al. (1988). They state that "speech of the individuals sounded appropriate for their age" (Morris et al. 1988: 321). Controversial evidence is provided by Volterra et al. (1996). They investigate 17 WS children (CA 4;10–15;3) and 17 control children of the same mental age. The results revealed lexical abilities on mental age level, while grammar appeared delayed compared to mental age in receptive as well as productive analyses.

Other researchers do not agree with the position of Bellugi and colleagues and suggest some grammatical difficulties, such as Karmiloff-Smith et al. (1998). They conclude from a comparison of an on-line word monitoring task and an off-line sentence picture-matching task, that older WS subjects show at least integrational and perhaps also representational impairments in this linguistic domain. In their experiment the WS subjects scored much better in the on-line task, indicating better underlying abilities than performed in a more integrative task, such as a sentence-picture matching task.

In some of the initial studies, WS subjects are sometimes attributed with terms such as "verbose" or "pseudo-mature" (Udwin et al. 1987; Udwin 1990). Usually they were classified as showing a "cocktail party syndrome" or "chatterbox syndrome" (Jones & Smith 1975; Meyerson & Frank 1987; Udwin et al. 1987). Formerly, this condition was described in subjects with hydrocephalus and spina bifida (Tew 1979). In a study by Udwin et al. (1987) verbose and pseudo-mature speech is reported for the whole subject sample. In contrast to the earlier result, Udwin and Yule (1990) find symptoms for chatterbox in only 30% of their subject group, Cromer (1994) again reports chatterbox symptoms in his case study. There is consensus in current literature that besides the questions of verbosity, the speech and talkativeness in individuals with Williams syndrome often lacks deeper meaning. The conversation tends to be repetitive and lacks new ideas. A dialogue is typically marked with excessive use of social phrases and stereotypical utterances (Udwin 1990). Sensitivity to situational reserve is only rarely reported in WS subjects. In contrary, they are typically very interested in disasters or tragedies and tell everyone their most intimate problems. This frequency of inappropriate situational speech behavior grows in early adulthood (Udwin et al. 1987). Observations such as these have led to the idea of an unusual semantic organization in Williams syndrome.

Bellugi and colleagues (Bellugi et al. 1988; Reilly et al. 1990) examined the claim of deviant semantic organization in word fluency tasks for semantic categories. Their results supported the view that adolescents and adults with Williams syndrome show unusually structured semantic knowledge. The most striking symptom was the repeated utterance of infrequent or highly untypical items of a category. There have been several attempts to replicate the results of the Bellugi group. In a more recent study Jarrold et al. (2000) systematically examined a group of WS adolescents and young adults matched to persons with mild learning disabilities, yet with the same abilities of receptive lexicon. Their results indicate no unusual or deviant semantic organization. Rather their subjects tend to utter the same items as the control group, albeit in a slightly different order. Therefore, Jarrold et al. (2000) proposed that WS subjects might show a deficit in the reorganization of semantic structure, which would be a normal result of gaining new information during language development. They stress that this result agrees with the statements that WS subjects are able to enrich the semantic knowledge but struggle in terms of reorganization of the semantic system (Johnson & Carey 1998). Volterra et al. (1996) report that their WS children performed better than mental age-matched normal control children in a phonological fluency task; the level of semantic fluency did not show an advantage for the WS group. The explanation of this finding focuses on the higher chronological age of WS subjects, indicating a greater world knowledge than the younger normal controls. The consequence in the fluency task might be that the WS children just know more words than the younger normal children. As the authors state, another important point of this interpretation is the knowledge of the phonemes of a word form which is, of course, much more elaborated in the WS group because a greater part of the group already attends school.

Pragmatics and dialogue are said to be a strength in WS. They are usually described to be friendly or even over-friendly, very sociable and communicative. But there are hints that their communicative ability is "odd", showing verbosity without comprehension of the context and loquacity. This has led to the idea that WS people might produce something that they do not understand (Udwin & Yule 1990). However it is hard to believe that such a profile is part of a developmental disorder. One asks how the language production should be acquired when the comprehension level is too low to process it. A recent study (Stojanovik et al. 2001) examined the conversational abilities of four WS children (CA 7;6–12;1) more closely, applying the analysis framework of Adams and Bishop (Adams & Bishop 1989; Bishop & Adams 1989). The WS children were matched to four children with specific language impairment (SLI) within the same chronological age range. The conversational analysis revealed that the WS children showed a rather wide variation in conversational abilities and disabilities. The most striking result, in the face of the claim that WS subjects are verbose, is the finding that all children show problems in providing enough information in their utterances. The utterances lack the necessary amount of semantic information and are therefore considered as inappropriate; therefore the four children of this study do not seem, in the pragmatic analysis, to be verbally superior. Stojanovik et al. (2001) emphasize the data of one child who scores within the chronological normal range in grammar comprehension tasks. This child also seems to provide too little information in conversational settings. The authors argue that WS children have too little knowledge of the world to keep up with normal conversation. That is to say they can only keep up an appropriate dialogue when they talk about their favorite topic; nevertheless they show a high willingness to communicate. The authors suggest that this behavior masks linguistic difficulties in these children.

Summing up this section, it becomes obvious that despite the growing number of studies, the language profile of Williams syndrome is far from being fully described. It seems rather as if the cognitive profile in general and linguistic competence in particular, is becoming ever more complex, thus careful consideration of competences and performances is needed. WS children are delayed in the onset of language acquisition. However, in the face of their mental retardation they achieve a high level of language ability. The children seem to catch up in the domains of syntax, semantics, and morphology later on. Differently to other genetic syndromes their phonological domain is rather unaffected and might disclose the possibility for further progress in other domains of language. Strengths and weaknesses in the areas of vocabulary growth, syntax and morphology are to be described and discussed from different languages in full detail in the following chapters.

## Notes

1. Gosch and Pankau (1995) report from a German group of small children with Williams syndrome (N = 20; CA 0;11–5;4) of feeding difficulties in 55% of their subjects. 70% of the children were reported not to drink enough.

2. The NGF plays an important role in the brain development during the prenatal and postnatal period. During these periods the normal development of sympathetic ganglias depends heavily on the chemical signal NGF, which controls the growth of this kind of neurons. In this way the organs can trigger the growing of their corresponding neurons. Higher levels of NGF, as indicated in animal experiments, lead to a strong increase of neuron growth in certain brain areas (Thompson 1994: 350).

3. In the Gosch and Pankau (1995) study, the developmental delay of a WS group (N = 20; CA 0;11–5;4) showed a homogeneous picture on several developmental domains. The mean developmental delay of the subjects, assessed with the German developmental scale MFED, revealed mild deficits in cognition.

4. One of the subjects in the contribution by Siegmüller and Weissenborn, PL, also shows a non-verbal IQ in the boarder range of normal cognition.

5. This result is therefore quite extraordinary, because mental retardation is usually defined on the basis of a decreased developmental rate in childhood. For very small children, Mervis and Bertrand (1997) appear to believe in the same assumption, as indicated by the chronologically age-matched, normal control children in a longitudinal study.

## References

Adams, C. & Bishop, D. (1989). "Conversational characteristics of children with semantic-pragmatic disorder I: exchange structure, turntaking, repairs and cohesion". *British Journal of Disorders of Communication, 24*, 211–239.

Atkinson, J., Anker, S., Braddick, O., Nokes, L., Mason, A., & Braddick, F. (2001). "Visual and visuospatial development in young children with Williams syndrome". *Developmental Medicine and Child Neurology, 43*, 330–337.

Barisnikov, K., Van der Linden, M., & Poncelet, M. (1996). "Acquisition of new words and phonological working memory in Williams syndrome: A case study." *Neurocase, 2*, 395–404.

Bellugi, U., Marks, S., Bihrle, A., & Sabo, H. (1988). "Dissociation between language and cognitive functions in Williams syndrome". In D. Bishop & K. Mogford (Eds.), *Language Development in Exceptional Circumstances* (pp. 132–149). Hillsdale, NJ: LEA.

Bellugi, U., Bihrle, A., Jernigan, T., Trauner, D., & Doherty, S. (1990). "Neuropsychological, neurological and neuroanatomical profile of Williams syndrome". *American Journal of Medical Genetics Supplement, 6*, 764–768.

Bellugi, U., Bihrle, A., Neville, H. J., Doherty, S., & Jernigan, T. (1992). "Language, cognition, and brain organization in a neurodevelopmental disorder". In M. Gunnar & C. Nelson (Eds.), *Developmental Behavioural Neuroscience* (pp. 201–232). Hillsdale, NJ: LEA.

Bellugi, U., Wang, P. P., & Jernigan, T. (1994). "Williams syndrome: An unusual neuropsychological profile". In S. H. Broman & J. Grafman (Eds.), *Atypical Cognitive Deficits in Developmental Disorders: Implications for brain functions* (pp. 23–56). Hillsdale, NJ: LEA.

Bellugi, U., Mills, D. L., Jernigan, T., Hickok, G., & Galaburda, A. (1999a). "Linking cognition, brain structure, and brain function in Williams syndrome". In H. Tager-Flusberg (Ed.), *Neurodevelopmental Disorders* (pp. 111–136). London: Bradford.

Bellugi, U., Lichtenberger, L., Mills, D. L., Galaburda, A., & Korenberg, J. R. (1999b). "Bridging cognition, the brain and molecular genetics: Evidence from Williams syndrome." *Trends in Neuroscience, 22*, 197–207.

Bellugi, U., Lichtenberger, L., Jones, W., Lai, Z., & St. George, M. (2000). "The neurocognitive profile of Williams syndrome: A complex pattern of strengths and weaknesses". *Journal of Cognitive Neuroscience, 12* (Suppl.), 7–29.

Berthold, M. & J. Seidel (2002). "Williams-Beuren-Syndrome. Frühdiagnose bei einem 10 Wochen alten Säugling". *Monatsschrift für Kinderheilkunde, 150*, 736–742.

Bertrand, J., Mervis, C., & Eisenberg, J. D. (1997). "Drawing by children with Williams syndrome: A developmental perspective". *Developmental Neuropsychology, 13*, 41–67.

Beuren, A., Apitz, J., & Harmjanz, D. (1962). "Supravalvular aortic stenosis in association with mental retardation and a certain facial appearance". *Circulation, 26*, 1235–1240.

Bihrle, A., Bellugi, U., Delis, D., & Marks, S. (1989). "Seeing the forest or the trees: Dissociation in visuospatial processing". *Brain and Cognition, 19*, 37–49.

Bishop, D. & Adams, C. (1989). "Conversational characteristics of children with semantic-pragmatic disorder II: What features lead to judgements of inappropriacy?" *British Journal of Disorders of Communication, 24*, 241–263.

Böhning, M., Campbell, R., & Karmiloff-Smith, A. (2002). "Audiovisual speech perception in Williams syndrome". *Neuropsychologia, 1349*, 1–11.

Broder, K., Reinhardt, E., Lifton, R., Tamborlane, W., & Pober, B. (1995). "Ambulatory blood pressure monitoring in Williams syndrome". *Genetic Counselling, 6*, 150–151.

Cairo, S., G. Merla, F. Urbinati, A. Ballabio, & A. Reymond (2001). "WBSCR14, a gene mapping to the William-Beuren syndrome deleted region, is a new member of the Mlx transcription factor network". *Human Molecular Genetics, 10*(6), 617–627.

Calamandrei, G., Alleva, E., Cirulli, F., Queyras, A., Volterra, V., Capirci, O., Vicari, S., Giannotti, A., Turrini, P., & Aloe, L. (2000). "Serum NGF levels in children and adolescents with either Williams syndrome of Down syndrome". *Developmental Medicine and Child Neurology, 42*, 746–750.

Crisco, J. J. & Dobbs, J. M. (1988). "Verbal behaviour of children with Williams syndrome". *Clinical Research, 36*, 403A.

Crisco, J. J., Dobbs, J. M., & Mulhern, R. F. (1988). "Cognitive processing of children with Williams syndrome". *Developmental Medicine and Child Neurology, 30*, 650–656.

Crisco, J. J. (1990). "Rate of cognitive development in young children with Williams syndrome". *Clinical Research, 38*, 536A.

Cromer, R. (1994). "A case study of dissociations between language and cognition". In H. Tager-Flusberg (Ed.), *Constraints on Language Acquisition* (pp. 141–154). Hillsdale, NJ: LEA.

Deruelle, C., Mancini, J., Livet, M. O., Cassé-Perrot, C., & de Schonen, S. (1999). "Configural and local processing of faces in children with Williams syndrome". *Brain and Cognition, 41*, 276–298.

Dilts, C. V., C. A. Morris, & C. O. Leonard (1990). "Hypothesis for development of a behavioral phenotype in Williams syndrome". *American Journal of Medical Genetics* (Supplement 6), 126–131.

Doll, A. & K.-H. Grzeschik (2001). "Characterization of two novel genes, WBSCR20 and WBSCR22, deleted in Williams-Beuren syndrome". *Cytogenetics and Cell Genetics, 95*, 20–27.

Elliot, C. D. 1990. *Differential Ability Scales*. San Diego: Harcourt, Brace, Jovanovich.

Elman, J. L., Bates, E., Johnson, M. H., Karmiloff-Smith, A., Parisi, D., & Plunkett, K. (1996). *Rethinking Innateness*. Cambridge, MA: The MIT Press.

Fanconi, G., Girardet, P., Schlesinger, B., Butler, H., & Black, J. (1952). "Chronische Hypercalcaemie kombiniert mit Osteoklerose, Hyperazotomie, Minderwuchs und kongenitalen Mißbildungen". *Helvetica Paediatrica Acta, 7*, 314–334.

Flint, J. (1996). "Annotation: Behavioural phenotypes: A window onto the biology of behaviour". *Journal of Child Psychology and Psychiatry, 37*, 355–367.

Fowler, A. E. (1998). "Language in mental retardation: Associations with and dissociations from general cognition". In J. A. Burack, R. M. Hodapp, & E. Zigler (Eds.), *Handbook of Mental Retardation and Development* (pp. 290–333). Cambridge: CUP.

Frangiskakis, J. M., Ewart, A., Morris, C. A., Mervis, C., Bertrand, J., Robinson, B. F., Klein, B. P., Ensing, G. J., Everett, L. A., & Green, E. D. (1996). "LIM-Kinase1 hemizygosity implicated in impaired visuospatial constructive cognition". *Cell, 86*, 59–69.

Galaburda, A., Wang, P. P., Bellugi, U., & Rossen, M. (1994). "Cytoarchitectonic anomalies in a genetically based disorder: Williams syndrome". *Neuroreport, 5*, 753–757.

Galaburda, A. & Bellugi, U. (2000). "Multi-level analysis of cortical neuroanatomy in Williams syndrome". *Journal of Cognitive Neuroscience, 12* (Suppl.), 74–88.

Gosch, A. & Pankau, R. (1994). "Social-emotional and behavioural adjustment in children with Williams-Beuren-syndrome". *American Journal of Medical Genetics, 53*, 335–339.

Gosch, A. & Pankau, R. (1995). "Entwicklungsdiagnostische Ergebnisse bei Kindern mit Williams-Beuren-Syndrom." *Kindheit und Entwicklung, 4*, 143–148.

Gosch, A. & Pankau, R. (1996). "Longitudinal study of the cognitive development in children with Williams syndrome". *American Journal of Medical Genetics, 61*, 26–29.

Grant, J., Karmiloff-Smith, A., Berthoud, I., & Christophe, A. (1996). "Is the language of people with Williams syndrome mere mimicry? Phonological short-term memory in a foreign language". *CPC, 15*, 615–628.

Grant, J., Karmiloff-Smith, A., Gathercole, S. A., Paterson, S., Howlin, P., Davies, M., & Udwin, O. (1997). "Phonological short-term memory and its relationship to language in Williams syndrome". *Cognitive Neuropsychiatry, 2*, 81–99.

Greer, M. K., Brown, F., Pai, G. S., Choudry, S. H., & Klein, A. (1997). "Cognitive, adaptive, and behavioural characteristics of Williams syndrome". *American Journal of Medical Genetics, 74*, 521–525.

Grimm, T. & Wesselhoeft, H. (1980). "Zur Genetik des Williams-Beuren-Syndroms und der isolierten Form der supravalvulären Aortenstenose". *Zeitschrift für Kardiologie, 69*, 168–172.

Hagerman, R. J., Schreiner, R. A., Kemper, M. B., Wittenberger, M. D., Zahn, B. & Habicht, K. (1989). "Longitudinal IQ changes in fragile X males". *American Journal of Medical Genetics, 33*, 513–518.

Howlin, P., Davies, B., & Udwin, O. (1998). "Cognitive functioning in adults with Williams syndrome". *Journal of Child Psychology and Psychiatry, 39*, 183–189.

Jarrold, C., Baddeley, A. D., & Hewes, A. K. (1998). "Verbal and nonverbal abilities in the Williams syndrome phenotype: Evidence for diverging developmental trajectories". *Journal of Child Psychology and Psychiatry, 39*, 511–523.

Jarrold, C., Baddeley, A. D., & Hewes, A. K. (1999). "Genetically dissociated components of working memory: Evidence from Down's and Williams syndrome". *Neuropsychologia, 37*, 637–651.

Jarrold, C., Hartley, S. J., Philips, C., & Baddeley, A. D. (2000). "Word fluency in Williams syndrome: Evidence for unusual semantic organisation?" *Cognitive Neuropsychiatry, 5*, 293–319.

Jernigan, T. & Bellugi, U. (1990). "Anomalous brain morphology on magnetic resonance images in Williams syndrome and Down syndrome". *Archives of Neurology, 47*, 529–533.

Jernigan, T. & Bellugi, U. (1994). "Neuroanatomical distinctions between Williams and Down syndromes". In S. H. Broman & J. Grafman (Eds.), *Atypical Cognitive Deficits in Developmental Disorders: Implications for brain functions* (pp. 57–66). Hillsdale, NJ: LEA.

Johnson, S. C. & Carey, S. (1998). "Knowledge enrichment and conceptual change in folkbiology: Evidence from Williams syndrome". *Cognitive Psychology, 37*, 156–200.

Jones, K. L. & Smith, D. W. (1975). "The Williams elfin syndrome: A new perspective". *Journal of Paediatrics, 86*, 718–723.

Kaplan, P., Kirschner, M., Watters, G. V., & Costa, T. (1989). "Contractures in patients with Williams syndrome". *Pediatrics, 84*, 895–897.

Karmiloff-Smith, A., Klima, E., Bellugi, U., Grant, J., & Baron-Cohen, S. (1995). "Is there a social module? Language, face processing, and theory of mind in individuals with Williams syndrome". *Journal of Cognitive Neuroscience, 7*, 196–208.

Karmiloff-Smith, A. (1997). "Crucial differences between developmental cognitive neuroscience and adult neuropsychology". *Developmental Neuropsychology, 13*, 513–524.

Karmiloff-Smith, A., Klima, E., Bellugi, U., Grant, J., & Baron-Cohen, S. (1997). "Language and Williams syndrome: how intact is intact?" *Child Development, 68*, 246–262.

Karmiloff-Smith, A., Tyler, L. K. T., Voice, K., Sims, K., Udwin, O., Howlin, P., & Davies, M. (1998). "Linguistic dissociations in Williams syndrome: Evaluating receptive syntax in on-line and off-line tasks". *Neuropsychologia, 36*, 343–351.

Klein, A., Armstrong, B., Greer, M., & Brown, F. (1990). "Hyperacusis and otitis media in individuals with Williams syndrome". *Journal of Speech and Hearing Disorders, 55*, 339–344.

Klein, B. P. & Mervis, C. B. (1999). "Contrasting patterns of cognitive abilities of 9- and 10-year-olds with Williams syndrome or Down syndrome". *Developmental Neuropsychology, 16*, 177–196.

Korenberg, J. R., Chen, X.-N., Hirota, H., Lai, Z., Yimlamai, D., Bisighini, R., & Bellugi, U. (1997). "Williams syndrome: The search for the genetic origins of cognition". *American Journal of Human Genetics, 61*, 103.

Lenhoff, H. M., Wang, P. P., Greenberg, F., & Bellugi, U. (1998). "Williams-Beuren-Syndrom und Hirnfunktionen". *Spektrum der Wissenschaft*, 62–68.

Lopez-Rangel, E., Maurice, B., McGillivray, B., & Friedman, J. (1992). "Williams syndrome in adults". *American Journal of Medical Genetics, 44*, 720–729.

Mac Donald, G. W. & Roy, D. L. (1988). "Williams syndrome: A neuropsychological profile". *Journal of clinical and experimental Neuropsychology, 10*, 125–131.

Mazzocco, M. & Reiss, A. L. (1999). "Normal variation in size of the FMR2 gene is not related with variation in intellectual performance". *Intelligence, 27*, 175–182.

Marriage, J. & Barnes, N. M. (1995). "Is central hyperacusis a symptom of 5-hydroxytryptamine (5-HT) dysfunction?" *Journal of Laryngology and Otology, 109*, 915–921.

Martin, N., Snodgrass, G., & Cohen, R. (1984). "Idiopathic infantile hypercalcaemia – A continuing enigma". *Archives of Diseases in Childhood, 59*, 605–613.

Masataka, N. (2001). "Why early linguistic milestones are delayed in children with Williams syndrome: Late onset of hand banging as a possible rate-limiting constraint on the emergence of canonical babbling." *Developmental Science, 4*, 158–164.

Meng, X., Lu, X., Li, Z., Green, E. D., Massa, H., Trask, B. J., Morris, C. A., & Keating, M. (1998). "Complete physical map of the common deletion region in Williams syndrome and identification and characterization of three novel genes". *Human Genetics, 103*, 590–599.

Mervis, C. & Bertrand, J. (1997). "Developmental relations between cognition and language". In L. B. Adamson & M. A. Romski (Eds.), *Communication and Language Acquisition* (pp. 75–106). Baltimore, MD: Brookes.

Mervis, C., Morris, C. A., Bertrand, J., & Robinson, B. F. (1999). "Williams syndrome: Findings from an integrated program of research". In H. Tager-Flusberg (Ed.), *Neurodevelopmental Disorders: Contributions to a new framework from cognitive neuroscience* (pp. 65–110). Cambridge, MA: The MIT Press.

Mervis, C., Bertrand, J., Morris, C. A., Klein-Tasman, B. P., & Armstrong, S. C. (2000). "The Williams syndrome cognitive profile". *Brain and Cognition, 44*, 604–628.

Meyerson, M. D. & Frank, R. A. (1987). "Language, speech and hearing in Williams syndrome: Intervention approaches and research needs." *Developmental Medicine and Child Neurology, 29*, 258–270.

Morris, C. A., Demsey, S., Leonard, C., Dilts, C., & Blackburn, B. (1988). "Natural history of Williams syndrome: Physical characteristics". *Journal of Paediatrics, 113*, 318–326.

Morris, C. A. & Mervis, C. (1999). "Williams syndrome". In S. Goldstein & C. R. Reynolds (Eds.), *Handbook of Neurodevelopmental andGenetic Disorders* (pp. 555–590). New York, NY: The Guilford Press.

Morris, C. A., Pober, B., Wang, P. P., Levinson, M., Sadler, L., Kaplan, P., Lacro, R., & Greenberg, F. (1999). "Medical guidelines for Williams syndrome". WSA national office.

Neville, H. J., Mills, D. L., & Bellugi, U. (1994). "Effects of altered auditory sensitivity and age of language acquisition on the development of language-relevant neural systems: Preliminary studies of Williams syndrome". In S. H. Broman & J. Grafman (Eds.), *Atypical Cognitive Deficits in Developmental Disorders: Implications for brain functions* (pp. 67–86). Hillsdale, NJ: LEA.

O'Reilly, M. F. & Lancioni, G. E. (2001). "Treating food refusal in a child with Williams syndrome using the parent as therapist in the home setting". *Journal of Intellectual Disability Research, 45*, 41–46.

Pagon, R. A., Bennett, F. C., LaVeck, B., Stewart, K. B., & Johnson, J. (1987). "Williams syndrome: Features in late childhood and adolescence". *Pediatrics, 80*, 85–91.

Pankau, R., Partsch, C., Gosch, A., Oppermann, H., & Wessel, A. (1992). "Statural growth in Williams-Beuren syndrome". *European Journal of Pediatrics, 151*, 751–755.

Pankau, R., Partsch, C., Gosch, A., Siebert, R., Schneider, M., Schneppenheim, R., Winter, M., & Wessel, A. (2000). "Williams-Beuren syndrome 35 years after the diagnosis of the first Beuren patient." *American Journal of Medical Genetics, 91*, 322–324.

Pérez Jurado, L. A., Peoples, R., Kaplan, P., Hamel, B. C. J., & Francke, U. (1996). "Molecular definition of the chromosome 7 deletion in Williams syndrome and parent-of origin effects on growth". *American Journal of Human Genetics, 59*, 781–792.

Reilly, J., Klima, E. S., & Bellugi, U. (1990). "Once more with feeling: Affect and language in atypical populations". *Development and Psychopathology, 2*, 367–391.

Reiss, A. L., Eliez, S., Schmitt, J. E., Straus, E., Lai, Z., Jones, W., & Bellugi, U. (2000). "Neuroanatomy of Williams syndrome: a high resolution study". *Journal of Cognitive Neuroscience, 12* (Supplement), 65–73.

Sarimski, K. (1996). "Williams-Beuren-Syndrom im Schulalter – Fähigkeitsprofil und Verhaltensbesonderheiten". *Sonderpädagogik, 26*, 124–135.

Sarimski, K. (1997). *Entwicklungspsychologie genetischer Syndrome*. Göttingen: Hogrefe.

Schmitt, J. E., Eliez, S., Warsofsky, I. S., Bellugi, U., & Reiss, A. L. (2001). "Corpus callosum morphology of Williams syndrome: Relation to genetics and behaviour". *Developmental Medicine and Child Neurology, 43*, 155–159.

St. George, M. & Bellugi, U. (2000). "Preface". *Journal of Cognitive Neuroscience, 12* (Suppl.), S1–S6.

Stojanovik, V., Perkins, M., & Howard, S. (2001). "Language and conversational abilities in Williams syndrome: How good is good?" *International Journal of Language and Communication Disorders, 36*, 234–239.

Süss-Burghart, H. (1993). "Die Münchener Funktionelle Entwicklungsdiagnostik 2/3 bei mental retardierten Kindern im Vergleich mit Intelligenztests". *Zeitschrift für Differentielle und Diagnostische Psychologie, 14*, 67–73.

Tager-Flusberg, H. & Sullivan, K. (1998). "Early language development in children with mental retardation". In J. A. Burack, R. M., Hodapp, & E. Zigler. (Eds.), *Handbook of Mental Retardation and Development* (pp. 208–239). Cambridge: CUP.

Tassabehji, M., Metcalfe, K., Fergusson, W. D., Carette, M. J., Dore, J. K., Donnai, D., Read, A. P., Pröschel, C., Gutowski, N. J., Mao, X., & Sheer, D. (1996). "LIM-kinase deleted in Williams syndrome". *Nature Genetics, 13*, 272–273.

Tassabehji, M., Metcalfe, K., Karmiloff-Smith, A., Carette, M. J., Grant, J., Dennis, N., Reardon, W., Splitt, M., Read, A. P., & Donnai, D. (1999). "Williams syndrome: Use of chromosomal microdeletions as a tool to dissect cognitive and physical phenotypes". *American Journal of Human Genetics, 64*, 118–125.

Tew, B. (1979). "The 'Cocktail Party Syndrome' in children with Hydrocephalus and Spina Bifida". *British Journal of Disorders of Communication, 14*, 89–101.

Thomas, M. S. C., Grant, J., Barham, Z., Gsödl, M., Laing, E., Lakusta, L., Tyler, L. K. T., Grice, S., Paterson, S., & Karmiloff-Smith, A. (2001). "Past tense formation in Williams syndrome". *Language and Cognitive Processes, 16*, 143–176.

Thompson, R. F. (1994). *Das Gehirn. Von der Nervenzelle zur Verhaltenssteuerung* (2nd edition). Heidelberg: Spektrum Akademischer Verlag.

Udwin, O., Yule, W., & Martin, N. (1987). "Cognitive abilities and behavioural characteristics of children with idiopathic infantile hypercalcaemia". *Journal of Child Psychology and Psychiatry, 28*, 297–309.

Udwin, O. (1990). "A survey of adults with Williams syndrome and idiopathic infantile hypercalcaemia". *Developmental Medicine and Child Neurology, 32*, 129–141.

Udwin, O. & Yule, W. (1990). "Expressive language of children with Williams syndrome". *American Journal of Medical Genetics Supplement, 6*, 108–114.

Udwin, O. & Yule, W. (1991). "A cognitive and behavioural phenotype in Williams syndrome." *Journal of clinical and experimental Neuropsychology, 13*, 232–244.

Udwin, O., Davies, M., & Howlin, P. (1996). "A longitudinal study of cognitive abilities and educational attainment in Williams syndrome". *Developmental Medicine and Child Neurology, 38*, 1020–1029.

van Lieshout, C. F. M., De Meyer, R. E., Curfs, L. M. G., & Fryns, J. P. (1998). "Family contexts, parental behaviour, and personality profile of children and adolescents with Prader-Willi, Fragile-X, or Williams syndrome". *Journal of Child Psychology and Psychiatry, 39*, 699–710.

Vicari, S., Brizzolara, D., Carlesimo, G. A., Pezzini, G., & Volterra, V. (1996a). "Memory abilities in children with Williams syndrome". *Cortex, 32*, 503–514.

Vicari, S., Carlesimo, G. A., Pezzini, G., & Volterra, V. (1996b). "Short-term memory in children with Williams syndrome: A reduced contribution of lexical-semantic knowledge to word span". *Neuropsychologia, 34*, 919–925.

Vicari, S., Bellucci, S., & Carlesimo, G. A. (2000). "Implicit and explicit memory: A functional dissociation in persons with Down syndrome". *Neuropsychologia, 38*, 240–251.

Volterra, V., Capirci, O., Pezzini, G., Sabbadini, L., & Vicari, S. (1996). "Linguistic abilities in Italian children with Williams syndrome". *Cortex, 32*, 663–677.

Wang, P. P. & Bellugi, U. (1993). "Williams syndrome, Down syndrome, and cognitive neuroscience". *American Journal of Disabled Children, 147*, 1246–1251.

Wang, P. P. & Bellugi, U. (1994). "Evidence from two genetic syndromes for a dissociation between verbal and visual-spatial short-term memory". *Journal of clinical and experimental Neuropsychology, 16*, 317–322.

Wang, P. P., Doherty, S., Rourke, S. B., & Bellugi, U. (1995). "Unique profile of visuo-perceptual skills in a genetic syndrome". *Brain and Cognition, 29*, 54–65.

Williams, J. C. P., Barratt-Boyes, B. G., & Lowe, J. B. (1961). "Supravalvular aortic stenosis". *Circulation, 24*, 1311.

Wilson, B., Cockburn, J., & Baddeley, A. D. (1985). *Rivermead Behavioural Memory Test.* Reading: Thames Valley Test Co.

Winter, M., Pankau, R., Amm, M., Gosch, A., & Wessel, A. (1996). "The spectrum of ocular features in the Williams syndrome". *Clinical Genetics, 49*, 28–31.

Zukowski, A. (2001). Uncovering Grammatical Competence in Children with Williams Syndrome. Boston University, Doctoral dissertation.

# Genetics of Williams-Beuren syndrome

Karl-Heinz Grzeschik
University of Marburg, Germany

Williams-Beuren syndrome (WS) is caused in most cases by a "common" hemizygous de novo deletion of 1.5–1.7 megabases from chromosome 7q11.23 encompassing >20 genes. These genes and their map position are described.

Duplicated chromosome segments flanking the deleted region provoke meiotic or mitotic mispairing. Association of the phenotype with the minimal region affected by atypical smaller deletions indicates that defects of the elastin gene cause the phenotype of supravalvular aortic stenosis whereas the genomic sequences contributing to other WS phenotypic features may lie at the telomeric end of the common deletion. Analysis of the WS-homologous genomic region in the mouse helps in human gene mapping, guides in generating of animal models of WS, and reveals the evolution of the region.

## The common WS-deletion

Williams-Beuren syndrome (WS) is a contiguous gene disorder caused in most of the patients (95%) by a hemizygous de novo deletion of 1.5–1.7 Mb (Megabases, Million base pairs) from chromosome 7q11.23 encompassing approximately > 20 genes including in a central position the elastin (*ELN*) gene (Ewart et al. 1993; Nickerson et al. 1995; Wu et al. 1998) and Figure 1. This genetic rearrangement, extending over a genetic distance of about 2 cM (Wu et al. 1998), is named the "common WS deletion". The deletion is visible on high resolution chromosomes, but only if the relative position of the light-gray-staining sub-band 7q11.22 that subdivides band 7q11.2 is considered (Francke 1999; Perez Jurado et al. 1996). The clinical diagnosis of WS, therefore, is routinely confirmed by fluorescence-in-situ-hybridization (FISH) analysis employing cosmid probes which contain parts of *ELN* (Lowery et al. 1995). Alternatively, the search for hemizygosity on polymorphic microsatellite loci using polymerase chain reaction (PCR) followed by various methods of allele detection or quantitative analysis of gene copy number by Southern-blot experiments can be applied to find deletions.

The breakpoints of the common deletion are observed within flanking blocks of DNA of near-identical sequence (Perez Jurado et al. 1996; Robinson et al. 1996; Valero et al. 2000). The majority of WS-region interstitital deletions (~67%) have been shown to be due to unbalanced recombination during meiosis (interchromosomal rearrangement); fewer (~33%) seem to arise due to intrachromosomal recombination (Baumer et al. 1998; Dutly & Schinzel 1996; Peoples, R. et al. 2000; Urban et al. 1996). The deletions arise equally often from both paternal and maternal meiosis, although a potential role for genomic imprinting in clinical features of WS (Perez Jurado et al. 1996; Wu et al. 1998) remains controversial (Francke 1999; Wang, M. S. et al. 1999).

Few familial cases of WS with the common deletion have been reported (Ounap et al. 1998; Pankau et al. 2001; White & Preus 1977; White et al. 1977). Affected family members typically show varying clinical expression of the phenotype. Recurrent WS in a sibship suggestive of maternal germ-line mosaicism has been described by Kara-Mostefa and co-workers (Kara-Mostefa et al. 1999). Two affected sibs failed to inherit a maternal allele at the elastin and D7S1870 loci although heterozygosity at both loci was observed in the leukocytes of their mother. Similarly, FISH indicated, that the deletion which was observed in both affected children, could not be detected in maternal blood. Apart from gonadal mosaicism, an undetected constitutive structural defect of the maternal chromosome 7 could theoretically account for the recurrence of the elastin deletion in sibs. A cryptic 7q11.23 rearrangement in a maternal homologue, such as an inversion or an insertion, could interfere with meiotic pairing, thus leading to recurrence of unequal crossover in distinct meioses and greatly enhancing the possibility of a deletion (Osborne, L. R. et al. 2001). The data available so far are insufficient to assess the potential impact of cryptic rearrangements or of gonadal mosaicism on the overall recurrence risk of WS.

## Haploinsufficiency of genes affected by the deletion as a cause for individual WS symptoms

Since 1993 it is known that there is a connection between isolated supravalvular aortic stenosis (SVAS) and WS which shares SVAS as one of its major symptoms. In both cases *ELN* appears to be critically affected (Morris et al. 1993). While isolated SVAS is attributed to disruption of the *ELN* gene by translocation, partial deletion or mutations leading to premature stop codons (Ewart et al. 1994; Ewart et al. 1993; Li & Toland 1997; Li et al. 1997; Tassabehji et al. 1997), in WS, one copy of the

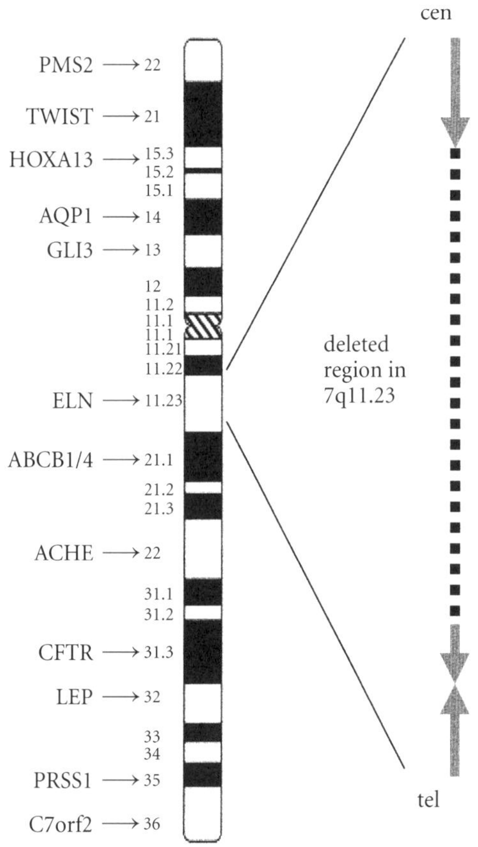


**Figure 1.** Ideogram of human chromosome 7 showing the map position of several selected genes of medical relevance. PMS2 = postmeiotic segregation increased (S. cerevisiae)-2; TWIST = TWIST, homolog of Drosophila TWIST, acrocephalosyndactyly type III; HOXA13 = homeo box A13; AQP1 = aquaporin-1, blood group Colton; GLI3 = GLI-Krüppel family member 3, Pallister-Hall syndrome, Greig cephalopolysyndactyly syndrome, postaxial polydactyly typA1; ELN = elastin, Williams-Beuren syndrome, SVAS; ABCB1/4 = P-glycoprotein-1 and 3; ACHE = acetylcholinesterase; CFTR = cystic fibrosis; LEP = leptin; PRSS1 = serine protease 1, hereditary pancreatitis; C7orf2 = acheiropody.
The position of the genes is indicated according to "Genes, locations and genetic disorders in chromosome 7" in the GDB database (http://www.gdb.org/gdbreports/Chr.7.omim.html). The chromosome region 7q11.23 encompassing the region commonly deleted in WS is extended. The position and orientation of the major LCRs harbouring the deletion breakpoints is indicated.

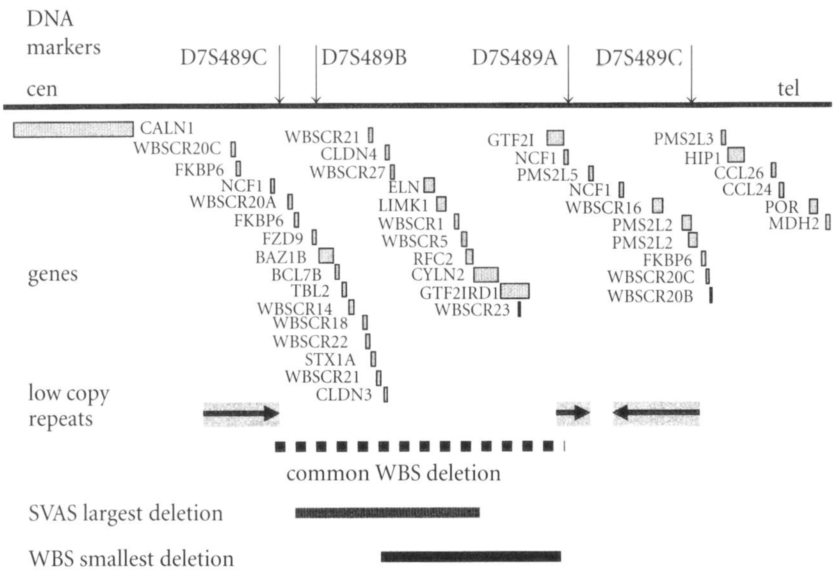


**Figure 2.** Physical map of the Williams-Beuren syndrome region derived from the UCSC Genome Browser database (http://genome.ucsc.edu/index.html) (Karolchik et al. 2003; Kent et al. 2002). Relative to the chromosome 7 interval q11.23 from centromere (cen) to q-telomere (tel) the position of polymorphic microsatellite markers D7S489, of genes including duplicated copies, of the flanking low copy repeats, of the common deleted region, and of particular deletions in SVAS or WS are shown (from top to bottom). Gene symbols are explained in Table 1. The map in the database as well as a detailed annotation of this segment derived from comparative mapping (DeSilva et al. 2002) list more loci the existence of which is predicted by sequence annotation programs and is supported by sequence identity with cDNAs. They are not yet included here, since detailed genomic analysis must prove that they are functional.

elastin gene is eliminated as part of a larger deletion which affects other genes, as well (Figure 2). To allocate individual features of WS to specific genes from the ones commonly deleted appeared to be a daunting task in view of the phenotypic heterogeneity of the syndrome and of contradictory results derived from the study of small deletions or other chromosome rearrangements. A wealth of different models and mechanisms has to be considered (Francke 1999). Almost all authors describing an individual gene from within the deletion can not refrain from speculating on its potential specific impact on one or several WS symptoms, mainly based on the prediction of function by sequence comparison. These predictions have been reviewed repeatedly, e.g. (Francke 1999; Osborne 1999).

**Table 1.** Genes from human 7q11.23 including the common WS deletion

| Symbol | Gene | References |
|---|---|---|
| CALN1 | Calneuron 1 | Wu et al. 2001 |
| WBSCR20C | WS chromosome region 20C | Doll and Grzeschik 2001; Merla et al. 2002 |
| FKBP6 | FK506 binding protein 6 | Meng, X., Lu, Morris et al. 1998; Merla et al. 2002; Peoples, R. et al. 2000 |
| NCF1 | Human neutrophil oxidase factor mRNA | Bayarsaihan et al. 2002; DeSilva et al. 2000; Francke et al. 1990 |
| WBSCR20A | WS chromosome region | Doll and Grzeschik 2001; Merla et al. 2002 |
| FZD9 | Human frizzled homolog (FZD3) | Wang, Y. K. et al. 1997 |
| BAZ1B | Bromodomain adjacent to zinc finger domain, 1B; WSTF; WSCR9 / 10 | Lu et al. 1998; Peoples, R. J. et al. 1998 |
| BCL7B | B-cell lymphoma 7B | Jadayel et al. 1998; Meng, X., Lu, Li et al. 1998 |
| TBL2 | Transducin (beta)-like 2 | Meng, X., Lu, Li et al. 1998; Perez Jurado et al. 1999 |
| WBSCR14 | WS chromosome region 14 | Cairo et al. 2001; de Luis et al. 2000; Meng, X., Lu, Li et al. 1998 |
| WBSCR18 | WS chromosome region 18 | Merla et al. 2002 |
| WBSCR22 | WS chromosome region 22 | Doll and Grzeschik 2001; Merla et al. 2002 |
| STX1A | Syntaxin 1A | Nakayama et al. 1997 |
| WBSCR21 | WS chromosome region 21 | Merla et al. 2002 |
| CLDN3/ CPETR1 | Claudin 3 / Clostridium perfringens enterotoxin receptor 1 | Morita et al. 1999 |
| CLDN4/ CPETR2 | Claudin 4 / Clostridium perfringens enterotoxin receptor 2 | Morita et al. 1999 |
| ELN | Elastin | Curran et al. 1993; Emanuel et al. 1985 |
| LIMK1 | LIM domain kinase 1 | Mao et al. 1996; Tassabehji et al. 1996 |
| WBSCR1 | WS chromosome region 1 | Osborne, L. R. et al. 1996 |
| WBSCR5 | WS chromosome region 5 | Doyle et al. 2000 |
| RFC2 | Replication factor C (activator 1) 2 | Okumura et al. 1995; Peoples, R. et al. 1996 |
| CYLN2 | Cytoplasmatic linker protein 2 (CLIP-115 protein) | Hoogenraad et al. 1998; Osborne, L. R. et al. 1996 |
| GTF2IRD1 | General transcription factor 2-I related | Osborne, L. R. et al. 1999; Tassabehji, Carette et al. 1999 |
| WBSCR23 | WS chromosome region 23 | Merla et al. 2002 |
| GTF2I | General transcription factor 2-I | Perez Jurado et al. 1998; Yang and Desiderio 1997 |

Table 1. (*continued*)

| Symbol | Gene | References |
|---|---|---|
| PMS2L5 | PMS1 protein homolog 7 [fragment] | Horii et al. 1994 |
| WBSC2CR16 | WS chromosome region 16 | Merla et al. 2002 |
| PMS2L2 | PMS1 protein homolog 14 | Kondo et al. 1999 |
| WBS2CR20B/C | WS chromosome region 20B | Doll and Grzeschik 2001; Merla et al. 2002 |
| PMS2L3 | PMS1 protein homolog 14 | Horii et al. 1994 |
| HIP1 | Huntingtin interacting protein 1 | Wedemeyer et al. 1997 |
| CCL26 | CCL26, CC chemokine IMAC | Guo et al. 1999 |
| CCL24 | CCL24, CC chemokine ligand 24 | Nomiyama et al. 1998 |
| POR | NADPH-cytochrome P450 reductase | Shephard et al. 1989 |
| MDH2 | Mitochondrial malate dehydrogenase | Habets et al. 1992 |

Here, single and duplicated genes assigned to the common WS deletion and the flanking regions are shown in their map order according to the results compiled by the Human Genome Sequencing Project and accessible in the UCSC Genome Browser database (http://genome.ucsc.edu/index.html) (Karolchik et al. 2003; Kent et al. 2002) (Figure 2). This database as well as DeSilva and colleagues list more genes which are predicted by annotation of contiguous genomic sequence covering most of the region in man or mouse (DeSilva et al. 2002). When these will be confirmed, the total list of deleted functional genes in WS may well exceed the number of 30.

## The WS deletion might result in the loss of regulatory elements governing flanking genes

The search for genes associated with WS has preferentially been focused on the deleted genes. However, chromosomal sequence elements regulating the expression of a gene can be positioned at a distance (> 1 Mb) on the same chromosome. This possibility suggests that genes flanking the common deletion (DeSilva et al. 2002; Osborne, L. R. et al. 2001) should be scrutinized for their association with WS. This approach will involve searching for regulatory elements within the common deletion and analyzing if the expression of individual non-deleted, flanking genes depends on any of those elements. As a step towards this goal, comparative sequence analysis of human and murine DNA from within the WS region has identified sequence elements of high similarity between the species outside the transcribed exons (DeSilva et al. 2002).

## Molecular mechanisms of genomic rearrangements causing WS

Phenotypes which are due to the concomitant loss of several adjacent genes on a chromosome are classified as "contiguous gene syndromes" or more recently as "genomic syndromes". The common mechanism leading to this type of chromosome loss appears to be meiotic or mitotic mispairing of duplicated chromosome segments in cis, i.e. on the same chromosome (Figure 3).

The common chromosome microdeletion in patients with WS is mediated by a flanking large (~400 kb) complex structure of region-specific low-copy repeats (LCRs), also called segmental duplications or duplicons (Peoples, R. et al. 2000) and Figure 2. Each of them contains clusters of up to three transcripts, including at least three duplicons that have sequences related to the *PMS2* mismatch repair

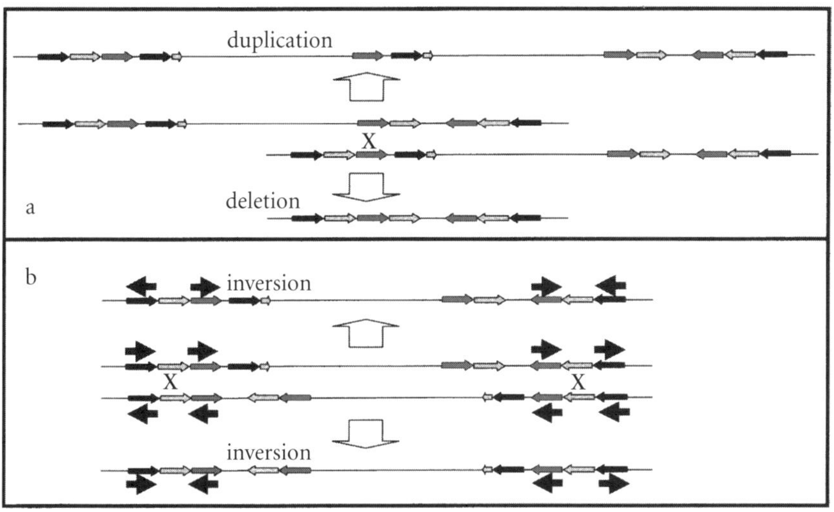


**Figure 3.** Diagram explaining mechanism and outcome of non-homologous recombination between low copy repeats: (a) deletion and duplication; (b) inversion.
Arrows with the same grey shade symbolize duplicons with nearly identical sequence as well as their orientation. X indicates the site of recombination between the homologous chromosomes during meiosis or between sequences on the same chromosome. Black arrows in (b) indicate the orientation of the segment (centromere to telomere) in unrearranged chromosomes.

gene (Osborne, L. R., Herbrick et al. 1997). Two of the duplicons contain copies of the transcription factor *GTF2I*, in which the distal copy is the ancestral *GTF2I* gene with a unique 5′end within the common deletions, whereas the proximal copy represents a truncated, expressed pseudogene (*GTF2IP1*) (Perez Jurado et al. 1998). The neutrophile cytosolic factor 1 (*NCF1*) gene maps telomeric to *GTF2I* in the distal duplicon, whereas an *NCF1* pseudogene is present at both the proximal and the distal duplicons (Hockenhull et al. 1999).

A shared > 3-Mb junction *NotI* fragment in WS deletions indicates clustering of breakpoints (Perez Jurado et al. 1998), suggesting that homologous recombination between the duplicons is responsible for generating the WS deletion, with an interchromosomal event in most cases (Baumer et al. 1998; Dutly & Schinzel 1996).

WS can be taken as a paradigm for genomic syndromes in general. LCRs occur in multiple regions of the human genome. They usually span ~10–400 kb of genomic DNA and share ≥97% sequence identity (Stankiewicz & Lupski 2002a, 2002b). Analysis of the different duplicons involved in human genomic syndromes identifies features that may predispose to recombination, including large size and high sequence identity between the recombining copies, putative recombination promoting features, and the presence of multiple genes/pseudogenes that may include genes expressed in germ cells (Yonggang et al. 2000). Homologous recombination between different duplicon copies leads to chromosome rearrangements, such as deletions, duplications, inversions, and inverted duplications, depending on the orientation of the recombining duplicons (Peoples, R. et al. 2000; Yonggang et al. 2000) and Figure 3. When such rearrangements cause dosage imbalance of a developmentally important gene(s), genetic diseases, now termed genomic disorders, result at a frequency of 0.7–1/1000 births. The rearranged DNA segments usually span several megabases.

Recent estimates suggest that as much as 10% of the human genome might be duplicated (Stankiewicz & Lupski 2002a). LCRs can contain genes, gene fragments, pseudogenes, endogenous retroviral sequences or other fragments. Alternatively, they can contain a series of paralogous genes, in which case they represent repeat gene clusters.

Multiple copies of the duplicons can be present at both breakpoint regions commonly associated with deletions or duplications, elsewhere within the same subchromosomal region or the same chromosome, or on another chromosome. In humans, sequence homologs of yeast mismatch repair genes (*PMS*) map to distinct regions of chromosome 7. In 7q11.23 they are flanking the common WS deletion at three sites, but they are detected in 7p22 and 7q22, as well (Osborne, Herbrick et al. 1997). The *PMS2* gene on 7p22 (Figure 1) may be mutated in hereditary non-polyposis colorectal cancer (Osborne, Herbrick et al. 1997). Such widely distributed duplicons predispose to various types of rearrangements. Larger deletions extending telomerically on 7q, e.g., lead to phenotypes combining WS features and seizure disorders such as infantile spasms with hypsarrhythmia (Francke 1999; Kahler et al. 1995; Mizugishi et al. 1998; Tsao & Westman 1997; Zackowski 1990; Zackowski et al. 1990).

Repeat-rich regions present challenges for hybridization-based physical mapping and computational assemblies, especially LCRs of 100–200 kb in length, which are the same size as the BAC clones that have been preferentially employed in the human genome sequencing effort, and there are limitations in the ability of the human genome draft to provide positional information. Therefore, in particular the characterization of the LCRs in WS consisting of several differently oriented repeat subunits (Figure 2) has proven to be difficult as documented by a successively improving series of physical maps (DeSilva et al. 2002; DeSilva et al. 1999; Doll & Grzeschik 2001; Francke 1999; Hockenhull et al. 1999; Osborne & Pober 2001; Osborne 1999; Osborne, Herbrick et al. 1997; Osborne, L. R. et al. 2001; Osborne et al. 1996; Osborne, Soder et al. 1997; Valero et al. 2000).

In addition to the flanking repeats, LCR within the common WS deletion contain part of the repeated sequences and, therefore, potentially could take part in the unequal exchanges associated with WS. This complex high-order architecture of the LCRs in the WS region can explain why the breakpoints of the deletion can differ between individuals.

Misalignment and unequal cross-over of DNA-sequences positioned in direct orientation within each of the larger duplicons could lead to a deletion as observed in WS or to a duplication which has not yet been observed (Figure 3). Both deletions and duplications are known from other cases of genomic diseases, however, there the gain of genetic material due to a duplication resulted in phenotypes very different from the ones caused by deletion (Stankiewicz & Lupski 2002a, 2002b; Yonggang et al. 2000). It can be predicted that carriers of a duplication of the WS-region, if viable at all, would not show symptoms of WS.

The structural features of the LCRs are not only important for DNA rearrangements associated with WS but also for polymorphic variations of the genome in the human population: Osborne and co-workers could detect hemizygous inversions with breakpoints mapping within the 400-kb repeat interval in 3 of 11 atypical affected individuals which express a subset of the WS phenotypic spectrum but do not carry the typical WS microdeletion, in two of their unaffected parents which transmitted the trait, as well as in approximately 30% of transmitting chromosomes in families with typical WS patients showing the common deletion (Osborne, L. R. et al. 2001). These results suggest the presence of a genomic variant within the population that may primarily result in predisposition to WS-causing microdeletions, but may also cause translocations and inversions. The precise sites of rearrangement could not be determined by these authors because the DNA sequences among the duplicons are nearly identical. The structural changes in the chromosome lead to the generation of novel *NotI* restriction fragments ranging in different individuals in size from 500–600 kb. This variation in size could be due to the breakpoints occurring within different repeated segments of the duplicons. If no chromosome material is lost during the event resulting in an inversion, carriers of this rearrangement might not show phenotypic signs of WS. However, the inversion might predispose to mispairing of the homologous chromosome sequences during meiosis and thus to offspring with chromosome rearrangements causing WS. This notion is corroborated by the finding of Osborne et al. that the longer novel *NotI* fragments of about 600 kb were found in phenotypically normal parents of children with WS. In contrast, an atypical WS individual carried a smaller *NotI* fragment of approximately 500 kb which indicates, in addition to an inversion, the loss of material from the repeating units flanking the WS interval or from elsewhere within this segment. Further studies will confirm if genomic polymorphism may be an important contributor in disease-associated recurrent chromosomal rearrangements that were previously thought to be stochastic in nature (Osborne, L. R. et al. 2001).

### Atypical chromosome rearrangements associated with WS link the distal region of the common deletion with phenotypic peculiarities

Atypical deletions have been described in patients with either supravalvular aortic stenosis (SVAS) or Williams-Beuren syndrome. All of those disrupt or delete one copy of the elastin gene. Some are intragenic, others are larger and encompass other genes. The largest deletion spanning 1 Mb of DNA in a patient with SVAS as the only phenotypic characteristic, removed the DNA between *FZD9* centomeric and *RFC2* telomeric of *ELN*. The smallest atypical deletion in WS, on the other hand, removes the segment from *CLDN3* to the telomeric common breakpoint region (Osborne 1999) (Figure 2). Comparing these two deletions allows the conclusion that hemizygosity for the genes from *FKBP6* to *CLDN3* may not contribute to WS. Instead, the genes contributing to the WS phenotypic features other than SVAS may lie at the telomeric end of the common deletion (Osborne 1999) and Figure 2.

Four chromosome rearrangements, one inversion [inv(7)(q11.23;q21.3)] (Osborne, L. R. et al. 2001), and three translocations t(6;7)(p21.1;q11.23) (Morris et al. 1993), t(6;7)(q27;q11.23) (von Dadelszen et al. 2000) and t(7;16)(q11.23;q13) (Duba et al. 2002), involving 7q11.23, are of particular interest: The individual with the inversion showed in addition to a WS-typical phenotypic profile features known to be associated with 7q21.3 such as ectrodactyly (Osborne, L. R. et al. 2001). Both translocations involving different breakpoints on chromosome 6, in addition to the one in 7q11.23, had SVAS as the only feature from the WS-spectrum of phenotypic peculiarities. Whereas the child with the breakpoint in 6q27 showed in addition a hydrops fetalis and died shortly after birth, the break in 6p21.1 apparently did not cause phenotypic features in addition to the isolated SVAS.

Both the t(6;7)(p21.1;q11.23) and the t(7;16)(q11.23;q13) disrupt chromosome 7 within the *ELN* locus, however, the reciprocal fusion occurred with parts of chromosome 6 or 16, respectively. In both families genes on the second chromosome involved in the translocation obviously do not contribute to the pathological phenotype, since in one case only an isolated SVAS was observed whereas the family carrying the translocation t(7;16) manifested a broad spectrum of clinical phenotypes ranging from a hoarse voice as the only feature to the full WS phenotype, but no peculiarities unrelated to WS (Duba et al. 2002). The mildly affected individuals in this family are puzzling, as in both cases *ELN* was truncated within the translated region. As in the (6;7)-translocation, SVAS should have appeared in all (7;16)-translocation carriers if *ELN* haploinsufficiency would invariably cause SVAS. This observation is compatible with the finding that phenotypic heterogeneity was a frequent observation within and between WS families (Pankau et al. 2001). Of all WS individuals proven to be hemizygous for *ELN*, only 50–60% had documented SVAS (Perez Jurado et al. 1996). Thus, other, undefined factors appear to determine if the single intact copy of *ELN* is sufficient to prevent all or part of the adverse phenotypic consequences attributed to haploinsufficiency.

## Analysis of the WS-homologous region in the mouse helps in human gene mapping and reveals the evolution of the region

There have been numerous attempts at mapping the WS region on the human chromosome interval 7q11.23 in order to identify all genes and pseudogenes, their order, distance, genomic structure, and transcriptional direction (de Luis et al. 2000; Doll & Grzeschik 2001; Hockenhull et al. 1999; Korenberg et al. 2000; Merla et al. 2002; Osborne et al. 1999; Osborne, Herbrick et al. 1997; Osborne, L. R. et al. 2001; Osborne et al. 1996; Osborne, Soder et al. 1997; Peoples, R. et al. 2000; Valero et al. 2000; Wu et al. 2002; Wu et al. 1998). However, significant challenges have been encountered and conflicting results prohibited the establishment of a generally accepted map. A high density of repetitive sequences and the presence of several large closely spaced blocks of DNA with very high sequence similarity hampered the classical approaches of mapping and sequence alignment requiring unique sequence tags. The number of copies of individual polymorphic loci (D7S489 A, B, or C) varies among different individuals in the population (Valero et al. 2000). An inversion polymorphism detected in families with WS employs slightly different breakpoints within the commonly deleted region (Osborne, L. R. et al. 2001). These examples suggest that there may be variability in the population concerning the number and the map order of individual genes or sequence elements. This would prohibit a unique map altogether.

In that situation, comparative mapping proved to be particularly helpful: Clone contig, genetic, and long-range restriction maps of the mouse homologous region on mouse chromosome 5G1-G2 indicated, that the number and order of intradeletion genes appears to be conserved in the mouse. No low-copy number repeats are found in the region. The region is inverted relative to the human map with breakpoints at a position homologous to the common breakpoints in WS (DeSilva et al. 1999; Peoples, R. et al. 2000; Valero et al. 2000). Mapping of individual murine genes within the interval commonly deleted in WS has helped to identify and map human genes (Bayarsaihan et al. 2002; Doll & Grzeschik 2001; Hoogenraad et al. 1998; Martindale et al. 2000; Mizuki 1998). In addition, comparative analysis of ~3.3 Mb completed, annotated mouse DNA from chromosome 5G1-G2 and orthologous human DNA sequences generated by the Human Genome Project has facilitated the identification of nine previously unreported genes (not shown in Figure 2), provided in total detailed sequence-based information regarding 30 genes residing in the region, and revealed a number of potentially interesting conserved noncoding sequences (DeSilva et al. 2002).

These studies have identified an evolutionary inversion with chromosomal breakpoints at the location of the duplicated blocks in the human WS region in 7q11.23 and suggested a model for human chromosome evolution due to serial inversions leading to genomic duplications (Valero et al. 2000).

## Animal models for WS

The high-resolution mouse maps of the region orthologous to the WS region in man provide the framework required for the generation of mouse models for WS mimicking the human molecular defect. The comparison of atypical deletions in WS and deletions observed in several SVAS-individuals suggests that the genes contributing to the majority of the WS phenotypes other than supravalvular aortic stenosis may lie at the telomeric side of *ELN* including *LIMK1*, *CYLN2*, *GTF2IRD1*, and *GTF2I* (Figure 2) (Osborne 1999).

In vitro studies indicated a role for the LIM kinase family in the regulation of cofilin regulation and actin dynamics. The actin cytoskeleton is important for many cellular processes, including cytokinesis, endocytosis, chemotaxis, and neurite outgrowth. Actin remodeling may be particularly important for the establishment and structural modification of dendritic spines on which the great majority of excitatory synapses are formed in the mammalian CNS. In addition, the actin network is directly involved in synaptic regulation at mature synapses including hippocampal long term potentiation (LTP), a form of synaptic plasticity considered critical to learning and memory formation [references in (Meng, Y. et al. 2002)]. *LIMK1* is among the genes deleted in WS which is characterized by mental retardation and profound deficits in visuospatial cognition (Bellugi et al. 1999; Frangiskakis et al. 1996). Therefore it was hypothesized that LIMK1 is critically involved in brain function via regulation of actin dynamics. To test this hypothesis, Meng and colleagues have generated mutant mice deficient in the expression of *LIMK1* (Meng, Y. et al. 2002). Indeed, the knockout mice were altered in ADF/cofilin phosphorylation and the actin cytoskeleton. These mice were also perturbed in synaptic structure and function related to the actin network. Consistent with the physiological deficits, the *Limk1* knockout mice exhibited abnormalities in behavioral responses, including impaired fear conditioning and spatial learning. Visuospatial deficits and hyperactivity are among the hallmarks of the cognitive profile of WS patients, but it remains to be determined whether the behavioral abnormalities in the knockout mice and in human patients are related.

A potential involvement of LIMK1 in the WS phenotype has been questioned based on other SVAS-patients which show a deletion of both *ELN* and *LIMK1* but do not show the impaired visuospatial constructive cognition (Tassabehji, Metcalfe et al. 1999). It is now thought that genes telomeric to *RFC2*, excluding *LIMK1*, are responsible for most of the behavioral abnormalities associated with WS (de Zeeuw 1997; Francke 1999; Osborne 1999).

To analyze the potential role of *CYLN2* (encoding the protein CLIP-115) (Hoogenraad et al. 1998), a further gene located in the WS-region telomeric of *ELN and RFC2* (de Zeeuw 1997), Hoogenraad and colleagues provided evidence that mice with haploinsufficiency for *Cyln2* (heterozygous knockout animals) have features reminiscent of Williams syndrome, including mild growth deficiency, brain abnormalities, hippocampal dysfunction, and particular deficits in motor coordination (Hoogenraad et al. 1998; Hoogenraad et al. 2002). A postnatal growth deficiency has been documented in WPS-individuals (Morris et al. 1988) and has also been observed in *Cyln2*-kockout mice. Data from these mice indicate that a reduction in CLIP-115 levels also affects the morphology of the adult mouse brain. The enlarged ventricle size and smaller corpus callosum in adult *Cyln2*-knockout mice correlates with the increased volume of cerebrospinal fluids in WS-patients (Reiss et al. 2000) as well as with their smaller corpus callosum (Schmitt et al. 2001). Absence of CLIP-115CL did not significantly alter microtubule dynamics, but did enhance accumulation of the related protein CLIP-170 and of dynactin at microtubule tips. CLIP-170 regulates the localization of with LIS1, a protein essential for nuclear migration that modulates dynein function and for several processes mediated by the dynein-dynactin pathway, to microtubule tips. Mutations in the gene LIS1 give rise to lissencephaly, a severe brain disorder (Reiner 1993). Notably, an increase in gyrification of the brain has been reported for WS patients (Schmitt et al. 2002).

Together with the loss of functions specific to CLIP-115, the perturbation of CLIP-like protein distributions at microtubule tips might underlie neurodevelopmental problems in *Cyln2*-knockout mice and individuals with Williams-Beuren syndrome (Hoogenraad et al. 2002).

Integration of a transgene had induced a ~40-kb deletion in mouse chromosome 5G1, starting downstream of the *Cyln2* gene and including the first exon of the *Gtf2ird1* gene. *Gtf2ird1* encodes a polypeptide related to the general transcription factor TFII-I, and it is the mouse orthologue of *GTF2IRD1* (*WSCR11*), one of the genes mapping telomeric of *RFC2* and commonly deleted in WS patients (Durkin et al. 2001). The deletion in this mouse resulted in greatly reduced expression of *Gtf2ird1* mRNA in mice homozygous for the transgene, suggesting that *Gtf2ird1* is not essential for viability. No observations concerning phenotypic peculiarities in line with WS features have been reported for these mice, so far.

Further studies with animal models for WS addressing other candidate genes or groups of genes are required to elucidate in detail the physiological and biochemical changes resulting in the characteristic WS phenotype.

## References

Baumer, A., Dutly, F., Balmer, D., Riegel, M., Tukel, T., Krajewska-Walasek, M., & Schinzel A. A. (1998). "High level of unequal meiotic crossovers at the origin of the 22q11. 2 and 7q11.23 deletions". *Human Molecular Genetics, 7*(5), 887–894.

Bayarsaihan, D., Dunai, J., Greally, J. M., Kawasaki, K., Sumiyama, K., Enkhmandakh, B., Shimizu, N., & Ruddle F. H. (2002). "Genomic organization of the genes Gtf2ird1, Gtf2i, and Ncf1 at the mouse chromosome 5 region syntenic to the human chromosome 7q11.23 Williams syndrome critical region". *Genomics, 79*(1), 137–143.

Bellugi, U., Lichtenberger, L., Mills, D., Galaburda, A., & Korenberg, J. R. (1999). "Bridging cognition, the brain and molecular genetics: evidence from Williams syndrome". *Trends in Neurosciences, 22*(5), 197–207.

Cairo, S., Merla, G., Urbinati, F., Ballabio, A., & Reymond, A. (2001). "WBSCR14, a gene mapping to the Williams-Beuren syndrome deleted region, is a new member of the Mlx transcription factor network". *Human Molecular Genetics, 10*(6), 617–627.

Curran, M. E., Atkinson, D. L., Ewart, A. K., Morris, C. A., Leppert, M. F., & Keating, M. T. (1993). "The elastin gene is disrupted by a translocation associated with supravalvular aortic stenosis". *Cell, 73*(1), 159–168.

de Luis, O., Valero, M. C., & Jurado, L. A. (2000). "WBSCR14, a putative transcription factor gene deleted in Williams-Beuren syndrome: complete characterisation of the human gene and the mouse ortholog". *European Journal of Human Genetics, 8*(3), 215–222.

de Zeeuw, C. I. (1997). "CLIP-115, a novel brain-specific cytoplasmatic linker protein, mediates the localization of dendritic lamellar bodies". *Neuron, 19*, 1187–1199.

DeSilva, U., et al. (2002). "Generation and comparative analysis of approximately 3.3 Mb of mouse genomic sequence orthologous to the region of human chromosome 7q11.23 implicated in Williams syndrome". *Genome Research, 12*(1), 3–15.

DeSilva, U., Massa, H., Trask, B. J., & Green, E. D. (1999). "Comparative mapping of the region of human chromosome 7 deleted in Williams syndrome". *Genome Research, 9*(5), 428–436.

DeSilva, U., Miller, E., Gorlach, A., Foster, C. B., Green, E. D., & Chanock, S. J. (2000). "Molecular characterization of the mouse p47-phox (Ncf1) gene and comparative analysis of the mouse p47-phox (Ncf1) gene to the human NCF1 gene". *Molecular Cell Biology Research Communication, 3*(4), 224–230.

Doll, A. & Grzeschik, K. H. (2001). "Characterization of two novel genes, WBSCR20 and WBSCR22, deleted in Williams-Beuren syndrome". *Cytogenetics and Cell Genetics, 95*(1–2), 20–27.

Doyle, J. L., DeSilva, U., Miller, W., & Green, E. D. (2000). "Divergent human and mouse orthologs of a novel gene (WBSCR15/Wbscr15) reside within the genomic interval commonly deleted in Williams syndrome". *Cytogenetics and Cell Genetics, 90*(3–4), 285–290.

Duba, H. C., Doll, A., Neyer, M., Erdel, M., Mann, C., Hammerer, I., Utermann G., & Grzeschik, K.-H. (2002). "The elastin gene is disrupted in a family with a balanced translocation t(7;16)(q11.23;q13) associated with a variable expression of the Williams-Beuren syndrome". *European Journal of Human Genetics, 10*(6), 351–361.

Durkin, M. E., Keck-Waggoner, C. L., Popescu, N. C., & Thorgeirsson, S. S. (2001). "Integration of a c-myc transgene results in disruption of the mouse Gtf2ird1 gene, the homologue of the human GTF2IRD1 gene hemizygously deleted in Williams-Beuren syndrome". *Genomics, 73*(1), 20–27.

Dutly, F. & Schinzel, A. (1996). "Unequal interchromosomal rearrangements may result in elastin gene deletions causing the Williams-Beuren syndrome". *Human Molecular Genetics, 5*(12), 1893–1898.

Emanuel, B. S., Cannizzaro, L., Ornstein-Goldstein, N., Indik, Z. K., Yoon, K., May, M., Oliver, L., Boyd, C., & Rosenbloom, J. (1985). "Chromosomal localization of the human elastin gene". *American Journal of Human Genetics, 37*(5), 873–882.

Ewart, A. K., Jin, W., Atkinson, D., Morris, C. A., & Keating, M. T. (1994). "Supravalvular aortic stenosis associated with a deletion disrupting the elastin gene". *Journal of Clinical Investigations, 93*(3), 1071–1077.

Ewart, A. K., Morris, C. A., Atkinson, D., Jin, W., Sternes, K., Spallone, P., Stock, A. D., Leppert, M., & Keating, M. T. (1993). "Hemizygosity at the elastin locus in a developmental disorder, Williams syndrome". *Nature Genetics, 5*(1), 11–16.

Francke, U. (1999). "Williams-Beuren syndrome: Genes and mechanisms". *Human Molecular Genetics, 8*(10), 1947–1954.

Francke, U., Hsieh, C. L., Foellmer, B. E., Lomax, K. J., Malech, H. L., & Leto, T. L. (1990). "Genes for two autosomal recessive forms of chronic granulomatous disease assigned to 1q25 (NCF2) and 7q11.23 (NCF1)". *American Journal of Human Genetics, 47*(3), 483–492.

Frangiskakis, J. M. et al. (1996). "LIM-kinase1 hemizygosity implicated in impaired visuospatial constructive cognition". *Cell, 86*(1), 59–69.

Guo, R. F., Ward, P. A., Hu, S. M., McDuffie, J. E., Huber-Lang, M., & Shi, M. M. (1999). "Molecular cloning and characterization of a novel human CC chemokine, SCYA26". *Genomics, 58*(3), 313–317.

Habets, G. G., van der Kammen, R. A., Willemsen, V., Balemans, M., Wiegant, J., & Collard, J. G. (1992). "Sublocalization of an invasion-inducing locus and other genes on human chromosome 7". *Cytogenetics and Cell Genetics, 60*(3–4), 200–205.

Hockenhull, E. L., Carette, M. J., Metcalfe, K., Donnai, D., Read, A. P., & Tassabehji, M. (1999). "A complete physical contig and partial transcript map of the Williams syndrome critical region". *Genomics, 58*(2), 138–145.

Hoogenraad, C. C., Eussen, B. H., Langeveld, A., van Haperen, R., Winterberg, S., Wouters, C. H., Grosveld, F., De Zeeuw, C. I., & Galjart, N. (1998). "The murine CYLN2 gene: Genomic organization, chromosome localization, and comparison to the human gene that is located within the 7q11.23 Williams syndrome critical region". *Genomics, 53*(3), 348–358.

Hoogenraad, C. C., et al. (2002). "Targeted mutation of Cyln2 in the Williams syndrome critical region links CLIP-115 haploinsufficiency to neurodevelopmental abnormalities in mice". *Nature Genetics, 32*(1), 116–127.

Horii, A., Han, H. J., Sasaki, S., Shimada, M., & Nakamura, Y. (1994). "Cloning, characterization and chromosomal assignment of the human genes homologous to yeast PMS1, a member of mismatch repair genes". *Biochemical and Biophysical Reseach Communication, 204*(3), 1257–1264.

Jadayel, D. M., Osborne, L. R., Coignet, L. J., Zani, V. J., Tsui, L. C., Scherer, S. W., & Dyer, M. J. (1998). "The BCL7 gene family: deletion of BCL7B in Williams syndrome". *Gene, 224*(1–2), 35–44.

Kahler, S. G., Adhvaryu, S. G., Helali, N., & Qumsiyeh, M. B. (1995). "Microscopically visible deletion of chromosome 7 in a child with features of Williams syndrome". *American Journal of Human Genetics, 57*, A117.

Kara-Mostefa, A., Raoul, O., Lyonnet, S., Amiel, J., Munnich, A., Vekemans, M., Magnier, S., Ossareh, B., & Bonnefont, J. P. (1999). "Recurrent Williams-Beuren syndrome in a sibship suggestive of maternal germ-line mosaicism". *American Journal of Human Genetics, 64*(5), 1475–1478.

Karolchik, D., Baertsch, R., Diekhans, M., Furey, T. S., Hinrichs, A., Lu, Y. T., Roskin, K. M., Schwartz, M., Sugnet, C. S., Thomas, D. J., Weber, R. J., Haussler, D., & Kent, W. J. (2003). "The UCSC Genome Browser Database". *Nucleic Acids Research, 31*(1), 51–54.

Kent, W. J., Sugnet, C. W., Furey, T. S., Roskin, K. M., Pringle, T. H., Zahler, A. M., & Haussler, D. (2002). "The human genome browser at UCSC". *Genome Research, 12*(6), 996–1006.

Kondo, E., Horii, A., & Fukushige, S. (1999). "The human PMS2L proteins do not interact with hMLH1, a major DNA mismatch repair protein". *Journal of Biochemistry (Tokyo), 125*(4), 818–825.

Korenberg, J. R., Chen, X. N., Hirota, H., Lai, Z., Bellugi, U., Burian, D., Roe B., & Matsuoka, R. (2000). "VI. Genome structure and cognitive map of Williams syndrome". *Journal of Cognitive Neuroscience, 12*, Suppl. 1, 89–107.

Li, D. Y., Toland, A. E., Boak, B. B., Atkinson, D. L., Ensing, G. J., Morris, C. A., & Keating M. T. (1997). "Elastin point mutations cause an obstructive vascular disease, supravalvular aortic stenosis". *Human Molecular Genetics, 6*(7), 1021–1028.

Lowery, M. C., Morris, C. A., Ewart, A., Brothman, L. J., Zhu, X. L., Leonard, C. O., Carey, J. C., Keating, M., & Brothman, A. R. (1995). "Strong correlation of elastin deletions, detected by FISH, with Williams syndrome: evaluation of 235 patients". *American Journal of Human Genetics, 57*(1), 49–53.

Lu, X., Meng, X., Morris, C. A., & Keating, M. T. (1998). "A novel human gene, WSTF, is deleted in Williams syndrome". *Genomics, 54*(2), 241–249.

Mao, X., Jones, T. A., Williamson, J., Gutowski, N. J., Proschel, C., Noble, M., & Sheer D. (1996). "Assignment of the human and mouse LIM-kinase genes (LIMK1; Limk1) to chromosome bands 7q11.23 and 5G1, respectively, by in situ hybridization". *Cytogenetics and Cell Genetics, 74*(3), 190–191.

Martindale, D. W., Wilson, M. D., Wang, D., Burke, R. D., Chen, X., Duronio, V., & Koop, B. F. (2000). "Comparative genomic sequence analysis of the Williams syndrome region (LIMK1-RFC2) of human chromosome 7q11.23". *Mammalian Genome, 11*(10), 890–898.

Meng, X., Lu, X., Li, Z., Green, E. D., Massa, H., Trask, B. J., Morris, C. A., & Keating, M. T. (1998). "Complete physical map of the common deletion region in Williams syndrome and identification and characterization of three novel genes". *Human Genetics, 103*(5), 590–599.

Meng, X., Lu, X., Morris, C. A., & Keating, M. T. (1998). "A novel human gene FKBP6 is deleted in Williams syndrome". *Genomics, 52*(2), 130–137.

Meng, Y., Zhang, Y., Tregoubov, V., Janus, C., Cruz, L., Jackson, M., Lu, W. Y., MacDonald, J. F., Wang, J. Y., Falls, D. L., & Jia, Z. (2002). "Abnormal spine morphology and enhanced LTP in LIMK-1 knockout mice". *Neuron, 35*(1), 121–133.

Merla, G., Ucla, C., Guipponi, M., & Reymond, A. (2002). "Identification of additional transcripts in the Williams-Beuren syndrome critical region". *Human Genetics, 110*(5), 429–438.

Mizugishi, K., Yamanaka, K., Kuwajima, K., & Kondo, I. (1998). "Interstitial deletion of chromosome 7q in a patient with Williams syndrome and infantile spasms". *Journal of Human Genetics, 43*(3), 178–181.

Mizuki, K. (1998). "Funktional modules and expression of mouse p40phox and p67phox, SH3domain-containing proteins involved in the phagocyte NADPH oxidase complex". *Euopean Journal of Biochemistry, 251*, 573–582.

Morita, K., Furuse, M., Fujimoto, K., & Tsukita, S. (1999). "Claudin multigene family encoding four-transmembrane domain protein components of tight junction strands". *Proceedings of National Academic Science USA, 96*(2), 511–516.

Morris, C. A., Demsey, S. A., Leonard, C. O., Dilts, C., & Blackburn, B. L. (1988). "Natural history of Williams syndrome: Physical characteristics". *Journal of Pediatrics, 113*, 318–326.

Morris, C. A., Loker, J., Ensing, G., & Stock, A. D. (1993). "Supravalvular aortic stenosis cosegregates with a familial 6; 7 translocation which disrupts the elastin gene". *American Journal of Medical Genetics, 46*(6), 737–744.

Nakayama, T., Fujiwara, T., Miyazawa, A., Asakawa, S., Shimizu, N., Shimizu, Y., Mikoshiba, K., & Akagawa, K. (1997). "Mapping of the human HPC-1/syntaxin 1A gene (STX1A) to chromosome 7 band q11.2". *Genomics, 42*(1), 173–176.

Nickerson, E., Greenberg, F., Keating, M. T., McCaskill, C., & Shaffer, L. G. (1995). "Deletions of the elastin gene at 7q11.23 occur in approximately 90% of patients with Williams syndrome". *American Journal of Human Genetics, 56*(5), 1156–1161.

Nomiyama, H., Osborne, L. R., Imai, T., Kusuda, J., Miura, R., Tsui, L. C., & Yoshie, O. (1998). "Assignment of the human CC chemokine MPIF-2/eotaxin-2 (SCYA24) to chromosome 7q11.23". *Genomics, 49*(2), 339–340.

Okumura, K., Nogami, M., Taguchi, H., Dean, F. B., Chen, M., Pan, Z. Q., Hurwitz, J., Shiratori, A., Murakami, Y., Ozawa, K., & Eki, T. (1995). "Assignment of the 36.5-kDa (RFC5), 37-kDa (RFC4), 38-kDa (RFC3), and 40-kDa (RFC2) subunit genes of human replication factor C to chromosome bands 12q24.2-q24.3, 3q27, 13q12.3-q13, and 7q11.23". *Genomics, 25*(1), 274–278.

Osborne, L. & Pober, B. (2001). "Genetics of childhood disorders: XXVII. Genes and cognition in Williams syndrome". *Journal of the Amercian Academy of Child and Aolescent Psychiatry, 40*(6), 732–735.

Osborne, L. R. (1999). "Williams-Beuren syndrome: Unraveling the mysteries of a microdeletion disorder". *Molecular Genetics and Metabolism, 67*(1), 1–10.

Osborne, L. R., Campbell, T., Daradich, A., Scherer, S. W., & Tsui, L. C. (1999). "Identification of a putative transcription factor gene (WBSCR11) that is commonly deleted in Williams-Beuren syndrome". *Genomics, 57*(2), 279–284.

Osborne, L. R., Herbrick, J. A., Greavette, T., Heng, H. H., Tsui, L. C., & Scherer, S. W. (1997). "PMS2-related genes flank the rearrangement breakpoints associated with Williams syndrome and other diseases on human chromosome 7". *Genomics, 45*(2), 402–406.

Osborne, L. R., Li, M., Pober, B., Chitayat, D., Bodurtha, J., Mandel, A., Costa, T., Grebe, T., Cox, S., Tsui, L. C., & Scherer, S. W. (2001). "A 1.5 million-base pair inversion polymorphism in families with Williams-Beuren syndrome". *Nature Genetics, 29*(3), 321–325.

Osborne, L. R., Martindale, D., Scherer, S. W., Shi, X. M., Huizenga, J., Heng, H. H., Costa T., Pober, B., Lew, L., Brinkman, J., Rommens, J. R., Koop, B., & Tsui, L. C. (1996). "Identification of genes from a 500-kb region at 7q11.23 that is commonly deleted in Williams syndrome patients". *Genomics, 36*(2), 328–336.

Osborne, L. R., Soder, S., Shi, X. M., Pober, B., Costa, T., Scherer, S. W., & Tsui, L. C. (1997). "Hemizygous deletion of the syntaxin 1A gene in individuals with Williams syndrome". *American Journal of Human Genetics, 61*(2), 449–452.

Ounap, K., Laidre, P., Bartsch, O., Rein, R., & Lipping-Sitska, M. (1998). "Familial Williams-Beuren syndrome". *American Journal of Medical Genetics, 80*(5), 491–493.

Pankau, R., Siebert, R., Kautza, M., Schneppenheim, R., Gosch, A., Wessel, A., & Partsch, C. J. (2001). "Familial Williams-Beuren syndrome showing varying clinical expression". *American Journal of Medical Genetics, 98*(4), 324–329.

Peoples, R., Franke, Y., Wang, Y. K., Perez-Jurado, L., Paperna, T., Cisco, M., & Francke, U. (2000). "A physical map, including a BAC/PAC clone contig, of the Williams-Beuren syndrome-deletion region at 7q11.23". *American Journal of Human Genetics, 66*(1), 47–68.

Peoples, R., Perez-Jurado, L., Wang, Y. K., Kaplan, P., & Francke, U. (1996). "The gene for replication factor C subunit 2 (RFC2) is within the 7q11.23 Williams syndrome deletion". *American Journal of Human Genetics, 58*(6), 1370–1373.

Peoples, R. J., Cisco, M. J., Kaplan, P., & Francke, U. (1998). "Identification of the WBSCR9 gene, encoding a novel transcriptional regulator, in the Williams-Beuren syndrome deletion at 7q11.23". *Cytogenetics and Cell Genetics, 82*(3–4), 238–246.

Perez Jurado, L. A., Peoples, R., Kaplan, P., Hamel, B. C., & Francke, U. (1996). "Molecular definition of the chromosome 7 deletion in Williams syndrome and parent-of-origin effects on growth". *American Journal of Human Genetics, 59*(4), 781–792.

Perez Jurado, L. A., Wang, Y. K., Francke, U., & Cruces, J. (1999). "TBL2, a novel transducin family member in the WBS deletion: characterization of the complete sequence, genomic structure, transcriptional variants and the mouse ortholog". *Cytogenetics and Cell Genetics, 86*(3–4), 277–284.

Perez Jurado, L. A., Wang, Y. K., Peoples, R., Coloma, A., Cruces, J., & Francke, U. (1998). "A duplicated gene in the breakpoint regions of the 7q11.23 Williams-Beuren syndrome deletion encodes the initiator binding protein TFII-I and BAP-135, a phosphorylation target of BTK". *Human Molecular Genetics, 7*(3), 325–334.

Reiner, O. (1993). "Isolation of a Miller-Dieker lissencephaly gene containing G protein ß-subunit-like repeats". *Nature, 364*, 717–721.

Reiss, A. L., Eliez, S., Schmitt, J. E., Straus, E., Lai, Z., Jones, W., & Bellugi, U. (2000). "IV. Neuroanatomy of Williams syndrome: a high-resolution MRI study". *Journal of Cognitive Neuroscience, 12*, Suppl. 1, 65–73.

Robinson, W. P., Waslynka, J., Bernasconi, F., Wang, M., Clark, S., Kotzot, D., & Schinzel, A. (1996). "Delineation of 7q11.2 deletions associated with Williams-Beuren syndrome and mapping of a repetitive sequence to within and to either side of the common deletion". *Genomics, 34*(1), 17–23.

Schmitt, J. E., Eliez, S., Warsofsky, I. S., Bellugi, U., & Reiss, A. L. (2001). "Corpus callosum morphology of Williams syndrome: relation to genetics and behavior". *Developmental Medicine and Child Neurology, 43*(3), 155–159.

Schmitt, J. E., Watts, K., Eliez, S., Bellugi, U., Galaburda, A. M., & Reiss, A. L. (2002). "Increased gyrification in Williams syndrome: evidence using 3D MRI methods". *Developmental Medicine and Child Neurology, 44*(5), 292–295.

Shephard, E. A., Phillips, I. R., Santisteban, I., West, L. F., Palmer, C. N., Ashworth, A., et al. (1989). "Isolation of a human cytochrome P-450 reductase cDNA clone and localization of the corresponding gene to chromosome 7q11.2". *Annual Human Genetics, 53*(Pt 4), 291–301.

Stankiewicz, P. & Lupski, J. R. (2002a). "Genome architecture, rearrangements and genomic disorders". *Trends in Genetics, 18*(2), 74–82.

Stankiewicz, P. & Lupski, J. R. (2002b). "Molecular-evolutionary mechanisms for genomic disorders". *Current Opinion in Genetics and Development, 12*(3), 312–319.

Tassabehji, M., Carette, M., Wilmot, C., Donnai, D., Read, A. P., & Metcalfe, K. (1999). "A transcription factor involved in skeletal muscle gene expression is deleted in patients with Williams syndrome". *European Journal of Human Genetics, 7*(7), 737–747.

Tassabehji, M., Metcalfe, K., Donnai, D., Hurst, J., Reardon, W., Burch, M., & Read, A. P. (1997). "Elastin: Genomic structure and point mutations in patients with supravalvular aortic stenosis". *Human Molecular Genetics, 6*(7), 1029–1036.

Tassabehji, M., Metcalfe, K., Fergusson, W. D., Carette, M. J., Dore, J. K., Donnai, D., Read, A. P., Proschel, C., Gutowski, N. J., Mao, X., & Sheer, D. (1996). "LIM-kinase deleted in Williams syndrome". *Nature Genetics, 13*(3), 272–273.

Tassabehji, M., Metcalfe, K., Karmiloff-Smith, A., Carette, M. J., Grant, J., Dennis, N., Reardon, W., Splitt, M., Read, A. P., & Donnai, D. (1999). "Williams syndrome: Use of chromosomal microdeletions as a tool to dissect cognitive and physical phenotypes". *American Journal of Human Genetics, 64*(1), 118–125.

Tsao, C. Y. & Westman, J. A. (1997). "Infantile spasms in two children with Williams syndrome". *American Journal of Medical Genetics, 71*(1), 54–56.

Urban, Z., Helms, C., Fekete, G., Csiszar, K., Bonnet, D., Munnich, A., Donis-Keller, H., & Boyd, C. D. (1996). "7q11.23 deletions in Williams syndrome arise as a consequence of unequal meiotic crossover". *American Journal of Human Genetics, 59*(4), 958–962.

Valero, M. C., de Luis, O., Cruces, J., & Perez Jurado, L. A. (2000). "Fine-scale comparative mapping of the human 7q11.23 region and the orthologous region on mouse chromosome 5G: the low-copy repeats that flank the Williams-Beuren syndrome deletion arose at breakpoint sites of an evolutionary inversion(s)". *Genomics, 69*(1), 1–13.

von Dadelszen, P., Chitayat, D., Winsor, E. J., Cohen, H., MacDonald, C., Taylor, G., Rose, T., & Hornberger, L. K. (2000). "De novo 46,XX,t(6;7)(q27;q11;23) associated with severe cardiovascular manifestations characteristic of supravalvular aortic stenosis and Williams syndrome". *American Journal of Medical Genetics, 90*(4), 270–275.

Wang, M. S., Schinzel, A., Kotzot, D., Balmer, D., Casey, R., Chodirker, B. N., Gyftodimou, J., Petersen, M. B., Lopez-Rangel, E., & Robinson, W. P. (1999). "Molecular and clinical correlation study of Williams-Beuren syndrome: No evidence of molecular factors in the deletion region or imprinting affecting clinical outcome". *American Journal of Medical Genetics, 86*(1), 34–43.

Wang, Y. K., Samos, C. H., Peoples, R., Perez-Jurado, L. A., Nusse, R., & Francke, U. (1997). "A novel human homologue of the Drosophila frizzled wnt receptor gene binds wingless protein and is in the Williams syndrome deletion at 7q11.23". *Human Molecular Genetics, 6*(3), 465–472.

Wedemeyer, N., Peoples, R., Himmelbauer, H., Lehrach, H., Francke, U., & Wanker, E. E. (1997). "Localization of the human HIP1 gene close to the elastin (ELN) locus on 7q11.23". *Genomics, 46*(2), 313–315.

White, R. A., Preus, M., Watters, G. V., & Fraser, F. C. (1977). "Familial occurrence of the Williams syndrome". *Journal of Pediatrics, 91*, 614–616.

Wu, Y. Q., Bejjani, B. A., Tsui, L. C., Mandel, A., Osborne, L. R., & Shaffer, L. G. (2002). "Refinement of the genomic structure of STX1A and mutation analysis in nondeletion Williams syndrome patients". *American Journal of Medical Genetics, 109*(2), 121–124.

Wu, Y. Q., Lin, X., Liu, C. M., Jamrich, M., & Shaffer, L. G. (2001). "Identification of a human brain-specific gene, calneuron 1, a new member of the calmodulin superfamily". *Molecular Genetics and Metabolism, 72*(4), 343–350.

Wu, Y. Q., Sutton, V. R., Nickerson, E., Lupski, J. R., Potocki, L., Korenberg, J. R., Greenberg, F., Tassabehji, M., & Shaffer, L. G. (1998). "Delineation of the common critical region in Williams syndrome and clinical correlation of growth, heart defects, ethnicity, and parental origin". *American Journal of Medical Genetics, 78*(1), 82–89.

Yang, W. & Desiderio, S. (1997). "BAP-135, a target for Bruton's tyrosine kinase in response to B cell receptor engagement". *Proceedings of the National Academy of Sciences of the USA, 94*(2), 604–609.

Yonggang, J., Eichler, E. E., Schwartz, S., & Nicholls, R. D. (2000). "Structure of chromosomal duplicons and their role in mediating human disorders". *Genome Research, 10*, 597–610.

Zackowski, J. L., Raffel, L. J., Blank, C. A., & Schwartz, S. (1990). "Proximal interstitial deletion of 7q: a case report and review of the literature". *American Journal of Medical Genetics, 36*(3), 328–332.

# Part II

# Language development and language competence in WS

# Relations between language and cognition in Williams syndrome

Carolyn B. Mervis, Byron F. Robinson, Melissa L. Rowe, Angela M. Becerra, and Bonita P. Klein-Tasman
University of Louisville / Georgia State University / University of Louisville / University of Louisville / University of Wisconsin-Milwaukee

We present an overview of our research on the relations between the language and cognitive abilities of individuals with Williams syndrome. First, we describe findings from our large-sample studies of performance on standardized assessments. We then use correlational analyses to consider the relations between language and cognition for school age children and adults. Third, we consider relations between language and cognition during early language acquisition. Fourth, we address the acquisition of grammar and its relation to cognitive abilities. Based on our findings, we discuss the possibility that relative to language acquisition by children who are developing typically, language acquisition by individuals with Williams syndrome may be more dependent on verbal memory and less dependent on more conceptual aspects of cognition.

This research was supported by Grant No. HD29957 from the National Institute of Child Health and Human Development and by Grant No. NS35102 from the National Institute of Neurological Disorders and Stroke. We thank all of the participants and their families. We are grateful to the geneticists, cardiologists, and early intervention agencies who referred individuals with Williams syndrome to our research, as well as to Terry Monkaba, executive director of the National Williams Syndrome Association, who has encouraged and facilitated the conduct of research at regional and national meetings of the Williams Syndrome Association. This chapter is based on Mervis, Robinson, Thomas, Becerra, and Klein-Tasman (2003) and Mervis (1999).

## Relations between language and cognition in Williams syndrome

Williams syndrome (WS) is a neurodevelopmental disorder characterized by a distinctive pattern of dysmorphic facial features, cardiovascular disease, connective tissue abnormalities, delayed development leading to mental retardation (MR) or learning disabilities, a specific cognitive profile, and an unusual personality profile. The syndrome usually occurs sporadically, with an incidence of 1 in 20,000 live births in all ethnic groups. WS is caused by a hemizygous 1.5 megabase microdeletion of chromosome 7q11.23 (Ewart et al. 1993). So far, 17 genes have been mapped to the deleted region (Osborne et al. 2001). More than 98% of individuals with WS have the same deletion breakpoints; the resulting deletion is referred to as the "classic" or "common" WS deletion (Morris & Mervis 2000).

The importance, from a theoretical perspective, of research on language and cognitive aspects of WS was first made clear by Ursula Bellugi, who argued that WS was a paradigmatic example of the independence of language and cognition. In her invited address at the International Conference on Infant Studies in 1990, Elizabeth Bates presented Bellugi's position as follows: Individuals with WS have excellent language abilities, including correct use of complex syntax such as passives, conditionals, relative and embedded clauses, and tag questions. They also have an unusual command of vocabulary. These language abilities occur in the context of profound MR, providing clear evidence of the independence of language from cognition. Upon hearing these claims, which contrasted with her own research on the relation between language and cognition for children with Down syndrome (DS), the first author of this chapter immediately decided to expand her research program to include children with WS. The major findings from this program regarding the relation between language and cognition for individuals with WS are presented in this chapter. We begin by describing findings from our large-sample studies of performance on standardized assessments measuring language and cognition. In the second section, we use correlational analyses to consider the relations between language and cognition for school age children and adults, as measured by several of these standardized assessments. In the third section, we turn to the relations between language and cognition during the early period of language acquisition. In the fourth section, we address the acquisition of grammar by children and adolescents with WS and its relation to cognitive abilities. In the final section, we conclude by summarizing our findings concerning similarities and differences between the language acquisition patterns of children with WS and children with typical development. Based on these findings, we consider the possibility that relative to language acquisition by children who are developing typically, language acquisition by individuals with WS may be more dependent on verbal memory and less dependent on more conceptual aspects of cognition.

## Performance on standardized assessments

We begin our examination of the language and cognitive abilities of individuals with WS by considering their performance on a variety of standardized assessments. Standardized assessments provide important information about these individuals' abilities relative to peers of the same chronological age (CA). Scores on these measures are summarized in Table 1.

When studying a rare syndrome, it is tempting to conduct one's research on small, relatively easily obtained samples of individuals varying widely in CA. We have taken a different approach, seeking large samples across a broad age range for our studies of performance on standardized assessments and smaller but still substantial samples focused on a narrower age range for studies using observational or experimental approaches. To obtain these samples, we have sought referrals from geneticists, cardiologists, early intervention agencies, and parents of individuals with WS in a number of states in the southeast, midwest, and southwest regions of the United States as well as from the National Williams Syndrome Association (WSA). We also have tested as many participants as possible at regional and na-

**Table 1.** Descriptive statistics for standardized assessments[a]

| Measure | N | CA Range | Mean Standard Score | SD | Range |
|---|---|---|---|---|---|
| DAS (School Age): GCA | 50 | 7;0–16;11 | 58.14 | 11.44 | 32–88 |
| Verbal Cluster | 50 | 7;0–16;11 | 70.02 | 13.21 | 51–100 |
| Nonverbal Cluster | 50 | 7;0–16;11 | 67.56 | 12.09 | 52–98 |
| Spatial Cluster | 50 | 7;0–16;11 | 54.74 | 6.07 | 50–79 |
| Pattern Construction T | 210 | 5;0–51;6 | 23.25 | 5.52 | 20–53 |
| Recall of Digits T | 234 | 5;0–51;6 | 32.97 | 9.72 | 20–60 |
| K-BIT: Composite IQ | 250 | 4;0–51;6 | 67.38 | 15.39 | 40–108 |
| Verbal IQ | 250 | 4;0–51;6 | 71.77 | 15.45 | 40–108 |
| Nonverbal IQ | 250 | 4;0–51;6 | 68.52 | 17.12 | 40–108 |
| Mullen: Composite | 34 | 2;9–5;5 | 62.32 | 11.64 | 49–88 |
| Visual Reception T | 34 | 2;9–5;5 | 30.12 | 10.12 | 20–46 |
| Fine Motor T | 34 | 2;9–5;5 | 21.65 | 3.45 | 20–31 |
| Receptive Language T | 34 | 2;9–5;5 | 30.47 | 9.82 | 20–55 |
| Expressive Language T | 34 | 2;9–5;5 | 33.21 | 9.59 | 20–48 |
| PPVT-III | 146 | 4;0–51;6 | 77.91 | 15.38 | 40–120 |
| EVT | 119 | 4;0–49;5 | 64.14 | 19.18 | 40–106 |
| TRC | 40 | 5;0–7;11 | 58.45 | 18.14 | 40–105 |
| TROG | 209 | 5;0–51;8 | 73.67 | 12.54 | 55–112 |

[a] For the general population, mean = 100 and SD = 15 for all measures not labeled "T." For all measures labeled "T," mean = 50 and SD = 10.

tional family meetings of the WSA. Overall, our sample includes individuals from 42 of the 50 states in the United States.

## Differential Ability Scales

The DAS (Elliott 1990) is a full-scale measure of intellectual functioning. The six core subtests included in the School Age form of the DAS are divided into three clusters. The Verbal cluster measures the child's ability to define words and to perform verbal reasoning tasks. The Nonverbal Reasoning cluster measures the child's inductive and sequential reasoning abilities. The Spatial cluster measures visuospatial constructive abilities, spatial memory, and spatial reasoning. Visuospatial construction is known to be the area of greatest weakness for individuals with WS (e.g., Bellugi, Wang, & Jernigan 1994; Mervis, Morris, Bertrand, & Robinson 1999). As indicated in Table 1, mean GCA (General Conceptual Ability; similar to IQ) is 58.14 (in the range of mild MR). As illustrated in Figure 1, however, the mean GCA is misleading. Mean standard scores on both the Verbal Cluster and the Nonverbal Reasoning Cluster are considerably higher than the GCA. In contrast, 50% of the individuals tested performed at floor on the Spatial Cluster.

## Kaufman Brief Intelligence Test

The negative impact of the extreme weakness in visuospatial construction on IQ is well demonstrated by a comparison of the performance of individuals with WS on the DAS and the K-BIT (Kaufman & Kaufman 1990), an IQ test that measures only verbal ability and nonverbal (reasoning) ability. The mean verbal standard scores on the DAS and K-BIT are within 2 points of each other; similarly, the mean nonverbal reasoning standard scores are only 1 point apart. In contrast, mean KBIT IQ is 9 points higher than mean DAS GCA.

## Mullen Scales of Early Learning

The Mullen (Mullen 1995), like the DAS School Age assessment described above, provides a full scale measure of intelligence, but for toddlers and preschoolers. Our Mullen findings indicate that the pattern of performance evident for school aged children with WS (ages 7–17 years) is present by age 2 years. Performance was weakest on the Fine Motor subtest (measuring primarily visuospatial construction); 79% of the participants scored at floor. Performance was considerably better for the two language subtests (averaging about the same as for the DAS and K-BIT verbal standard scores) and for the Visual Reception subtest (measuring

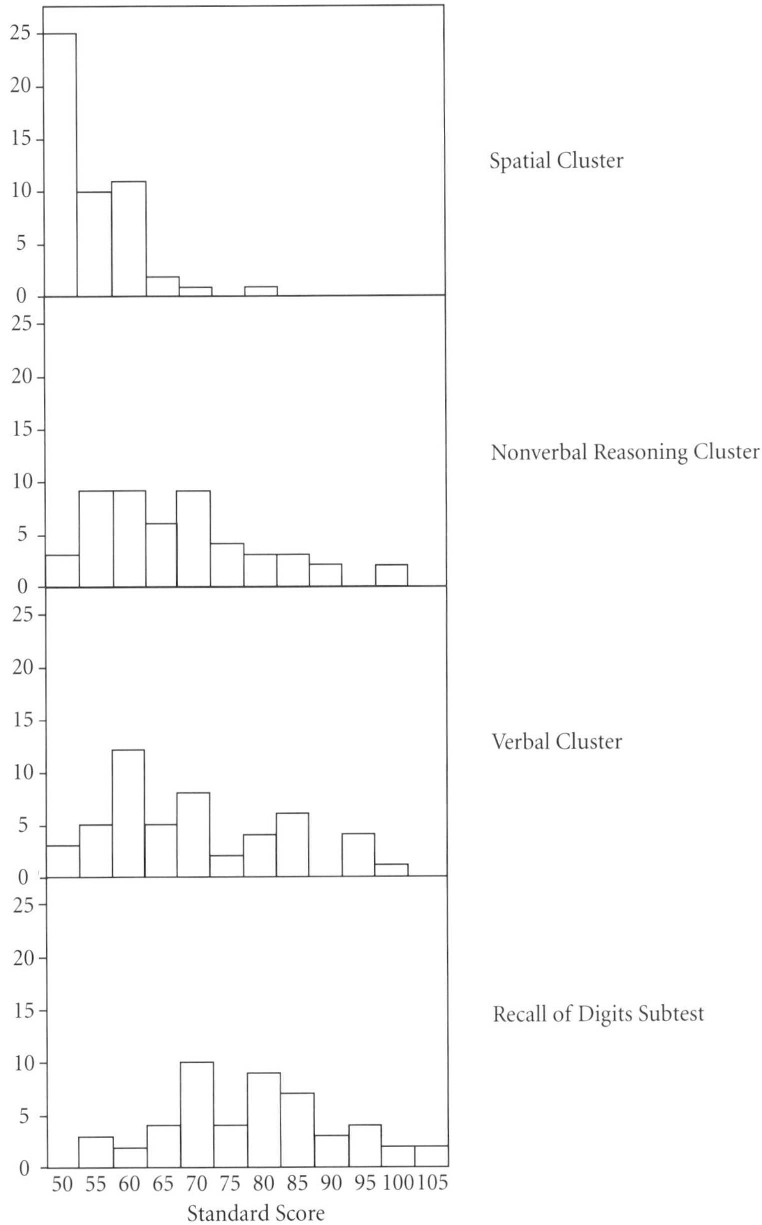


**Figure 1.** Distribution of standard scores for School Age DAS Spatial Cluster, Nonverbal Reasoning Cluster, Verbal Cluster, and Recall of Digit subtest for 50 7–17-year-olds with Williams syndrome. Recall of Digits T score has been converted to the same scale as the Cluster standard scores (mean = 100, SD = 15).

many of the same types of abilities as the nonverbal reasoning sections of the DAS and K-BIT).

Thus, across the three measures of intelligence, a consistent pattern emerges, with the highest standard scores achieved for language abilities. At one level, this pattern of performance is consistent with prior claims that language is a particular strength for individuals with WS. However, the level of performance on these measures does not fit with the claim that language abilities are "excellent"; language standard score means are in the borderline normal to mildly deficient range. Nonverbal reasoning standard scores are only slightly lower. Furthermore, mean IQ is considerably higher than the profound MR range. With this pattern in mind, we turn to standardized assessments that measure specific language abilities.

### Peabody Picture Vocabulary Test (3rd edition) and Expressive Vocabulary Test

The PPVT-III (Dunn & Dunn 1997a) measures receptive single-word vocabulary knowledge. Most words are names for objects, actions, or attributes, although some label more abstract concepts. On average, individuals with WS earn their highest standard score on this measure. Mean performance was in the borderline normal range; 9% scored at least 100 (the mean for the general population).

The Expressive Vocabulary Test (EVT; Williams 1997) measures expressive single word vocabulary. Early items require that the participant names a picture or an attribute of a picture. Later items involve the researcher providing a word that names a picture or some aspect of a picture and the participant providing a synonym. Like the PPVT-III, most target words are labels for objects, actions, or attributes, although some name more abstract concepts. Although the EVT was co-normed with the PPVT-III, individuals with WS typically have considerably more difficulty on the EVT. This difficulty may be due to the conceptual requirement of providing a synonym rather than simply naming the picture.

### Test of Relational Concepts

The TRC (Edmonston & Litchfield Thane 1988) measures comprehension of abstract relational concepts. Five types of concepts are included: temporal (e.g., before/after), quantitative (e.g., most/least), dimensional (e.g., tall/short); spatial (under/over, beginning/end); other (e.g., same/different). We have administered the TRC to 40 5–7-year-olds with WS (Mervis et al., in press), who earned a mean score of 87.03 on the PPVT-III. In contrast, the mean score on the TRC was 58.45.[1] Percent correct for each of the five types of relational concepts was similar to that for a group of typically developing (TD) children matched for raw score on the TRC. Performance on the TRC was the weakest of any language measure.

### Test for Reception of Grammar

The TROG (Bishop 1989) measures receptive understanding of grammar. Constructions range in difficulty from single words to simple sentences, comparatives, passives, and sentences with relative or embedded clauses. Mean performance on this measure was in the borderline normal range. The pattern of performance on the different grammatical constructions was similar to that found by Karmiloff-Smith et al. (1997) in their study of a considerably smaller British sample. In that study, particular difficulty was identified for embedded clauses. For example, if asked to choose the picture matching a sentence such as, "The box the dog is jumping over is brown," the participant typically chose a picture of a brown dog jumping over a black box, rather than the correct picture of a black dog jumping over a brown box. Zukowski (2001, in press) reported the same difficulty in an elicited production task when individuals with Williams syndrome were prompted to describe a picture using embedded clause constructions. For example, if the target sentence was, "The box (that) the dog is jumping over is brown," the participant would be likely to say, "The dog that is jumping over the box is brown."

In summary, across all the language measures administered, average performance is consistently in the mildly deficient to borderline normal range. This level is considerably below that expected for individuals of the same CA in the general population, indicating that both lexical and grammatical abilities of individuals with WS typically are well below the level expected for "excellent" language ability. As is clear from the standard deviations provided in Table 1, there is a great deal of variability in language ability across the WS population. In the next section, we consider the question of whether variability in language ability is related to variability in cognitive ability.

## Correlations between language abilities and cognitive abilities

The pattern of performance we have documented for standardized assessments of language and of visuospatial construction often has been argued to provide strong evidence of the modularity of language – that is, that language is largely decoupled from cognition (e.g., Bellugi et al. 1994; Bellugi, Bihrle, Jernigan, Trauner, & Doherty, S. 1990; Bellugi, Klima, & Wang 1996; Bellugi, Lichtenberger, Jones, Lai, & St. George 2000; Bellugi, Marks, Bihrle, & Sabo 1988; Damasio & Damasio 1992). The presence of a consistent pattern of strengths and weaknesses, however, does not rule out the possibility that WS may provide strong evidence for the centrality of *g* (general intelligence) or central control processes (such as verbal working memory or analytic reasoning ability) to the intellectual abilities of individuals with MR or borderline normal intelligence. To address this possibility, we consider the performance of 50 individuals with WS on a variety of measures of cognitive and language ability (Mervis 1999). We begin by describing group performance on these measures. We then present the pattern of partial correlations among individual performance on these measures. Third, we consider the amount of variance in the language measures that may be accounted for by individual differences in verbal short-term memory, verbal working memory, and reasoning ability.

The sample of 50 individuals included in these analyses includes 26 children (mean CA: 10.76 years, SD: 3.66 years, range: 5–17 years) and 24 adults (mean: CA 30.84 years, SD: 7.80 years, range: 18–47 years). These are all the individuals in our sample who have completed the full set of assessments included in the correlational analyses. The language measures included the verbal subscale from the K-BIT, which assesses expressive vocabulary; the PPVT-R (Dunn & Dunn 1981), which like its successor the PPVT-III measures receptive vocabulary; and the TROG, which measures receptive grammar. Cognitive measures included the nonverbal subscale (Matrices) from the K-BIT, which assesses nonverbal reasoning ability; the DAS Pattern Construction subtest, which measures visuospatial construction; verbal short-term memory as assessed by measures of forward digit span with items administered at a rate of one item per second; and verbal working memory as measured by backward digit span with items administered at a rate of one item per second. Descriptive statistics for the standard scores for most of these measures are provided in Table 2. Because separate standard scores were not available for forward digit performance and backward digit performance, standard scores were not computed for the memory measures. The mean standard score for the measure of visuospatial construction was significantly lower than for any of the other measures ($p < .001$).

## Interrelations among language and cognitive abilities: Partial correlations

The consistent pattern of intellectual strengths and weaknesses associated with WS is unusual among groups with MR or borderline normal intelligence (Mervis et al. 2000). The existence of a consistent pattern across individuals with WS, however, does not necessarily mean that different types of intellectual abilities are dissociated from one another. To address the possibility that *g* may play a role in the abilities of individuals with WS, examination of the pattern of individual differences on these intellectual measures is critical. If ability levels on some or all of the language measures are not significantly related to the cognitive measures, then the case for independence of language abilities is enhanced. In contrast, the finding that ability levels on some or all of the language measures are significantly correlated with some or all of the cognitive measures would provide support for the position that language and cognition are not completely independent.

**Table 2.** Descriptive statistics for reasoning, language, and visuospatial construction assessments included in the correlational analyses (N = 50)

| Measure | Mean | SD | Range |
|---|---|---|---|
| K-BIT IQ | 67.04 | 15.27 | 40–104 |
| K-BIT Matrices | 66.68 | 15.10 | 40–107 |
| K-BIT Vocabulary | 73.28 | 15.94 | 40–105 |
| PPVT-R | 69.18 | 18.37 | 30–110 |
| TROG | 76.20 | 16.32 | 55–112 |
| DAS Pattern Construction | 23.72 | 4.79 | 20–36 |

*Note.* For each of the assessments except DAS Pattern Construction, the population mean is 100, with a standard deviation of 15. The lowest possible standard score is 40 for the K-BIT, 20 for the PPVT-R, and 55 for the TROG. For DAS Pattern Construction, the population mean is 50, with a standard deviation of 10 and a minimum score of 20. PPVT-R standard scores are artificially low for individuals with below average intelligence because the standardization sample did not adequately represent the full range of the general population (Dunn & Dunn 1997b). This problem was corrected in the norming of the PPVT-III. In addition, the minimum score on the PPVT-R is 20 points lower than the minimum score on the PPVT-III.

To consider these possibilities, we began by computing the simple correlations among the three language measures and four cognitive measures, using raw scores as the dependent variable for the non-memory measures and span as the dependent variable for the memory measures. All of these correlations were significant at the $p < .001$ level. Given the wide range of CAs in the sample, however, these correlations cannot be interpreted as supporting the interdependence of language and cognitive abilities in WS. An obvious alternative explanation is that the significance of these correlations is due to the wide range in participants' CAs. To address this possibility, we computed the partial correlations among the seven measures, while controlling for CA. These correlations are presented in Table 3. As indicated in the table, all of the correlations remained significant even after the variance due to CA was partialled out.

This finding suggests that the cognitive and language abilities we measured are not independent of each other, despite clear differences in overall level of performance. Perhaps the most interesting relations from a theoretical perspective are those between the language measures and the measure of visuospatial construction. Previous arguments in favor of the independence of language and cognition in WS have focused on visuospatial construction as the measure of cognition. Given that language abilities are not independent of visuospatial constructive ability in WS, it is likely that measures of central processing (or *g*) mediate between them. If so, correlations between the language measures and visuospatial construction should be greatly weakened when measures of central processing or *g* are partialled out. The

**Table 3.** Partial correlations (controlling for CA) among measures of verbal memory, language, visuospatial construction, and reasoning (N = 50, df = 47)

| | Span F | Span B | K-Voc | PPVT-R | TROG | Pattern |
|---|---|---|---|---|---|---|
| Span F | | | | | | |
| Span B | .42*** | | | | | |
| K-Voc | .48**** | .67**** | | | | |
| PPVT-R | .47**** | .71**** | .82**** | | | |
| TROG | .60**** | .48**** | .72**** | .62**** | | |
| Pattern | .30* | .48**** | .59**** | .46**** | .47**** | |
| K-Matrices | .42*** | .68**** | .77**** | .68**** | .47**** | .57**** |

*Note.* *$p = .03$. ***$p < .005$. ****$p < .001$.

**Table 4.** Partial correlations (controlling for CA and Span B) among measures of verbal short-term memory, language, visuospatial construction, and reasoning (N = 50, df = 46)

| | Span F | K-Voc | PPVT-R | TROG | Pattern |
|---|---|---|---|---|---|
| Span F | | | | | |
| K-Voc | .30* | | | | |
| PPVT-R | .27 | .66**** | | | |
| TROG | .50**** | .60**** | .45**** | | |
| Pattern | .12 | .41*** | .20 | .32* | |
| K-Matrices | .21 | .57**** | .39** | .22 | .38** |

*Note.* *$p < .05$. **$p < .01$. ***$p < .005$. ****$p < .001$.

two best measures of central processing/*g* that we have are backward digit span (a measure of verbal working memory) and K-BIT Matrices (a measure of nonverbal reasoning ability, the ability most closely related to *g*).[2] Backward digit span is the more basic of these measures; reasoning ability clearly requires working memory.

To determine the extent to which verbal working memory may be mediating the relation between language ability and visuospatial construction ability, we computed another set of partial correlations, this time controlling for both CA and backward digit span. The results are shown in Table 4. All of the correlations were reduced substantially below the values found when only CA was controlled. Most importantly, the partial correlation between PPVT-R and DAS pattern construction is no longer significant, suggesting that verbal working memory may be responsible for the significant relation between receptive single-word vocabulary and visuospatial construction. The partial correlations between TROG and DAS pattern construction and between K-BIT vocabulary and DAS pattern construction, although considerably weakened, remained significant.

**Table 5.** Partial correlations (controlling for CA, verbal working memory, and reasoning) among measures of verbal short-term memory, language, and visuospatial construction (N = 50, df = 45)

| | Span F | K-Voc | PPVT-R | TROG |
|---|---|---|---|---|
| Span-F | | | | |
| K-Voc | .22 | | | |
| PPVT-R | .21 | .58**** | | |
| TROG | .48**** | .60**** | .41*** | |
| Pattern | .05 | .25 | .06 | .26 |

*Note.* ***$p = .005$. ****$p < .001$.

To consider the extent to which analytic ability may be mediating the relation between language ability and visuospatial construction ability beyond the impact of verbal working memory, we computed a third set of partial correlations, controlling for CA, backward digit span, and raw score on the K-BIT matrices. The resulting correlations are presented in Table 5. The partial correlations between TROG and DAS pattern construction and between K-BIT vocabulary and DAS pattern construction were no longer significant, suggesting that analytic ability may also mediate between language ability and visuospatial construction ability. For receptive grammar, the role of analytic ability (beyond the role of verbal working memory) is likely most important for syntactically complex utterances, especially ones that have two or more possible meanings (e.g., garden-path sentences; see Frazier 1987). For expressive vocabulary, analytic ability may be useful for determining if the word retrieved from memory is correct.

Even after partialing out the effects of CA, verbal working memory, and analytic ability, the correlations among the language measures remained significant. To consider the possibility that these correlations were mediated by another basic process that was not involved in the relations between language and visuospatial construction, we calculated a final set of partial correlations, controlling for verbal short-term memory (forward digit span) as well as the three variables controlled for in previous analyses. These correlations are shown in Table 6. All of these correlations remained significant, suggesting that one or more language-specific variables may also play a role in the relation between vocabulary (semantics) and grammar.

## Contribution of central processes/g to lexical and grammatical abilities

The results of the previous analyses indicated that there was a substantial amount of shared variance between lexical, grammatical, and visuospatial abilities. Furthermore, most of the shared variance could be accounted for by measures of central

**Table 6.** Partial correlations (controlling for CA, verbal working memory, reasoning, and verbal short-term memory) among measures of language and visuospatial construction (N = 50, df = 44)

| | K-Voc | PPVT-R | TROG |
|---|---|---|---|
| K-Voc | | | |
| PPVT-R | .56**** | | |
| TROG | .57**** | .36* | |
| Pattern | .25 | .06 | .26 |

*Note.* *$p = .02$. ****$p < .001$.

processing/*g*. In this section, we consider a related question: How much of the variance in lexical ability and grammatical ability may be accounted for by verbal working memory, reasoning ability, and verbal short-term memory? To address this question, we conducted three multiple regression analyses, one for each of the three language measures. For each analysis, the independent variables were CA, backward digit span, K-BIT matrices raw score, and forward digit span.

Results suggested an important role for central processes for both lexical and grammatical ability, with a greater role for lexical ability than for grammatical ability. The multiple regression analysis for PPVT-R yielded a multiple R of .91 and an adjusted $R^2$ of .81, indicating that central processes account for most of the variance in receptive lexical ability. The multiple regression analysis for K-BIT vocabulary resulted in almost identical values: a multiple R of .90 and an adjusted $R^2$ of .80, indicating that central processes also account for most of the variance in expressive language ability. The multiple regression analysis for TROG yielded a multiple R of .80 and an adjusted $R^2$ of .61. This analysis suggests an important role for central processes in grammatical ability. At the same time, 39% of the variance remains to be accounted for. It is possible that much of this variance may be attributed to processes specific to language.

## Relations between language and cognition during early language acquisition

In the first section of this chapter, we described converging results from two full-scale measures of intelligence: the School Age form of the DAS (ages 7–17 years) and the Mullen Scales of Early Learning (ages 2–5 years). On both assessments, individuals with WS evidenced a relative strength in language and an extreme weakness in visuospatial construction. We also have considered the relation between language and cognition in a small sample of even younger children with WS, using the mental scale of the first edition of the Bayley Scales of Infant Development (BSID; Bayley 1969). The mental scale of this edition of the BSID is particularly appropriate for differentiating between language and other cognitive abilities because the language items on this assessment tap specifically linguistic skills rather than cognitive and linguistic skills simultaneously (as do many of the items on the second edition of the BSID and on most of the IQ tests designed for older children). We considered items involving syllable production, linguistic imitation, comprehension of single words or multiword utterances, and production of single words or multiword utterances to be language items. The remaining items were considered to be nonlanguage (cognitive). These included measures of nonverbal reasoning (e.g., object permanence, means-ends relations), visual-motor integration (e.g., form boards, peg boards, block construction, drawing), and nonlinguistic imitation.

The participants in this study were 6 children with WS, 6 children with DS, and 6 TD children. The TD children entered the study at age 9 months; children in the other two groups began the study at about age 18 months. Participants were followed longitudinally for at least 13 months, and completed the Bayley 3–5 times, at intervals of about 6 months. To compare a child's performance on the language and nonlanguage items, we considered all of the items from his or her basal (the last 10 items passed before the first item that was failed) through the last item the child passed. For each assessment, we determined the proportion of language items passed (# language items passed / # language items attempted) and the proportion of nonlanguage items passed (# nonlanguage items passed / # nonlanguage items attempted). We then determined the mean difference between the language proportion and the nonlanguage proportion for each child across the 3–5 times he or she completed the BSID. Finally, we computed the mean difference between language and nonlanguage proportions for each group of participants. These proportions are illustrated in Figure 2. For the WS group, the mean difference between the proportion of language items passed and the proportion of nonlanguage items passed was +.239, indicating that general language abilities exceeded general cognitive abilities. The proportion for each of the six children was positive. For the DS group, the mean difference between proportions was –.210, indicating that general cognitive abilities exceeded general language abilities. The proportion for five of the six children was negative. For the TD group, the mean difference between proportions was +.005, indicating that general cognitive abilities tended to be at about the same level as general language abilities. The proportions for most of the children were close to 0. These results, in conjunction with previous findings for older children, adolescents, and adults, indicate that the intellectual profiles for children with WS and children with DS differ from each other and are consistent from very early childhood through adulthood. Furthermore, on average, both groups differ from TD children.

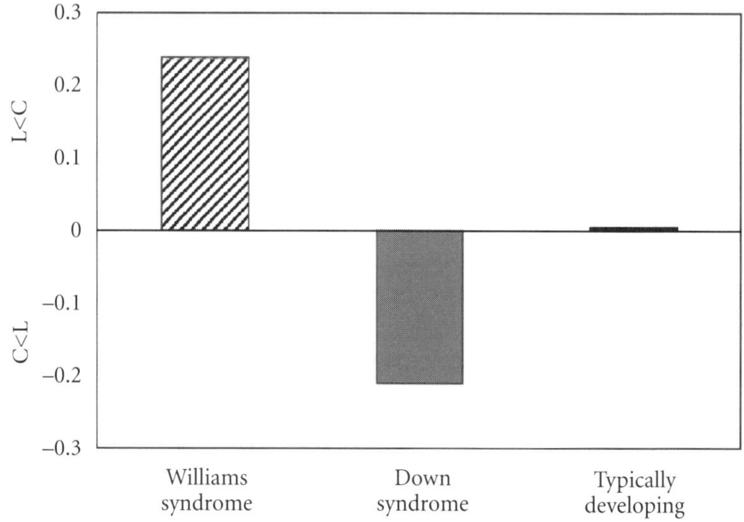


**Figure 2.** Relative strengths of general cognitive (C) abilities and language (L) abilities as measured by the BSID for children with Williams syndrome, children with Down syndrome, and TD children

## Specific relations between early lexical development and cognitive development

The data we have just reviewed indicate that even during the period of very early language acquisition, children with DS evidence a weakness in general language ability relative to general cognitive ability. In contrast, during this same period, children with WS evidence a weakness in general cognitive ability relative to general language ability. Given these contrasting patterns, very young children with these two syndromes provide especially important test cases for consideration of universals and alternate paths to early lexical competence.

Based on studies of TD children and children who have DS, a number of specific relations between particular aspects of early lexical acquisition and hypothetically linked aspects of early nonverbal cognitive development have been identified (see review in Mervis & Bertrand 1997). As we have just shown, on average, TD children have equivalent levels of language abilities and nonverbal cognitive abilities (including nonverbal reasoning and spatial cognition). Thus, findings of specific links between lexical and nonverbal cognitive development for children with typical development are not surprising. That children with DS also evidence these same links is more noteworthy, as these children's general level of nonverbal cognitive ability is usually more advanced than their general level of verbal ability. It would be even more impressive to find that these same links also hold for children whose general level of language ability is more advanced than their general level of nonverbal cognitive ability. To address this possibility, we present data from 10 children with WS who were followed longitudinally for 3–5 years beginning at ages 4–26 months. These children participated in monthly play sessions, after which their parents completed the MacArthur Communicative Development Inventories (CDI; Fenson et al. 1993). If children with WS evidence the same links between specific aspects of lexical development and particular aspects of nonverbal cognitive development, then the case for the universality of these links becomes much stronger. Conversely, if these links do not hold for children with WS but they still acquire the relevant lexical abilities, study of these children will be especially useful for identifying alternate paths to lexical competence. In this section, we consider several specific links that previously had been found to hold for both TD children and children who have DS. These hypothesized links are listed in Table 7. Additional details are provided in Mervis and Bertrand (1997).

### *Canonical babbling and rhythmic banging*

Cobo-Lewis, Oller, Lynch, and Levine (1995) have argued that rhythmic (canonical or reduplicated) babble and rhythmic hand banging should begin at about the same time because they reflect parallel manifestations of rhythmic behaviors. Canonical or reduplicated babble involves repetition of the same consonant-vowel syllable two or more times (e.g., "dada" or "mamama" but not "ga"). Both canonical babble and rhythmic hand banging appear before the onset of lexical comprehension or production. Because the rhythm of canonical babble fits the syllable patterns of mature speech, this type of babble is considered a very important step in the language acquisition process. Parents typically change the way they talk to their infants once canonical babble begins, and these changes likely facilitate the child's acquisition of an initial vocabulary.

At the time they entered the study, 8 of the 10 children with WS already were producing both canonical babble and rhythmic hand banging. Thus, data relevant to this proposed universal were available from only two children, who entered the study at ages 4 and 5 months. Both children first produced canonical babble in the same play session in which they first produced rhythmic banging. Furthermore, the parents of both children reported that their children had begun producing both canonical babble and rhythmic hand banging in the interval between that play session and the previous one. Thus, the limited data available from this study are consistent with the putative universal link between these two abilities. More recently Masataka (2001), in a longitudinal study of 8 infants with WS acquiring Japanese as their native language, also found a strong temporal link between the onsets of canonical babble and rhythmic hand banging.

Table 7. Putative universal cross-domain relations between cognition and language

| Underlying Ability or Realization | Cognitive Manifestation | Lexical Manifestation | Order of Acquisition |
|---|---|---|---|
| Production of deliberately rhythmic sounds | Rhythmic hand banging | Canonical or reduplicated babble | Onset at about the same time |
| Establishment of reference | Onset of production of referential pointing gestures | Onset of production of referential labels for objects or actions | Cognitive prior to lexical |
| Priority of categories based on salient form-function correlations | Initial categories are at the (child-) basic level | Initial object labels refer to (child-) basic categories | Not applicable |
| Parallel realizations:<br>1. All objects belong to a category<br>2. All objects have a name | Onset of spontaneous exhaustive sorting of objects | Onset of vocabulary spurt<br>Onset of ability to fast-map novel object label to object (and other members of the same basic-level category) for which the child did not previously have a name, even when the speaker did not provide an explicit connection (e.g., pointing gesture) between word and object | Onset at about the same time |

*Pointing and the onset of referential production of object names*

The second potential universal link involves the acquisition of the ability to refer. The cognitive manifestation of this link (referential pointing) is expected to precede the lexical manifestation (referential productive language, e.g., object labels). This sequential ordering of referential pointing and referential labeling is one of the most robust findings regarding the transition to language. Infants express communicative intentions nonverbally, by pointing, prior to expressing them verbally, by labeling (e.g., Adamson 1995). This link presumably obtains because the cognitive manifestation of reference (pointing) provides the child with an especially useful way to determine the reference of the words he or she hears. Adults use pointing gestures to indicate reference. Until the child is able to follow these gestures, he or she is likely to have difficulty determining the reference of the adult's words. At the same time, children use pointing gestures to elicit labels from adults.

To determine the relation between the onset of referential pointing and referential word use, we had available data from the videotaped play sessions and also from parental report on the CDI, which includes a question regarding the child's use of referential pointing as well as a vocabulary checklist. For all children, the data from the play session were consistent with parental report, and indicated a very different pattern from that for either TD children or children with MR due to other causes. Only one child with WS, the most delayed in the sample, began to comprehend and produce referential pointing gestures prior to the onset of referential language. The interval between the onsets of the two abilities was only 3 weeks, which is much shorter than the interval that has been found in previous studies of children who do not have WS. The remaining children with WS began to produce referential labels for objects several months (mean: 6 months) before the onset of either comprehension or production of referential pointing gestures. These data make it clear that referential pointing skills are not necessary for the onset of referential language.

Nevertheless, comprehension and subsequent production of referential object labels almost certainly require that the child and adult be engaged in joint attention to an object at the time that the adult labels it. In positing that referential pointing should precede the onset of referential productive language, researchers likely were centering on the attention-focusing function of pointing. Thus, pointing may have been intended as a proxy for participation in episodes of joint attention regarding an object. The data from the children with WS serve as a reminder that there are other ways to establish joint attention to objects. Mervis and Bertrand (1997) identified three alternative methods for establishing such joint attention used by parents of children with WS. First, the adult followed in to the child's focus of attention and then labeled that object. This method has been shown to be especially effective even for TD children (Dunham, Dunham, & Curwin 1993; Tomasello & Farrar 1986). Second, the adult picked up the object to which he or she wanted the child to attend, put it in the place where the child already was looking, and then labeled it. This, the adult directed the child's attention to an object by tapping it. Once the child was looking at the object, the adult labeled it. These methods were successful in inducing children with WS to comprehend and produce object labels referentially.

### *Priority of basic-level categories: Labels and play patterns*

Objects can be categorized at a variety of hierarchical levels. For example, the same object can be a beach ball (subordinate level), a ball (basic level), or a toy (superordinate level). The basic level is more fundamental than the other levels (Rosch,

Mervis, Johnson, Gray, & Boyes-Braem 1976). This is the most general level at which category members have similar overall shapes and at which a person uses similar motor actions for interacting with category members. Although categories at all hierarchical levels are based on form-function correlations, these correlations are most apparent at the basic level. Because of the salience of basic level categories, they should be acquired first. Thus, children's initial functional play patterns (cognitive manifestation of categorization) and the initial extensions of the object labels that they comprehend and produce (linguistic manifestation of categorization) should converge at the (child-) basic level.[3] Longitudinal research on TD children and children with DS has confirmed this relation between initial play patterns and initial object labels for the two categories for which it has been addressed: *ball* and *car*. Although for many categories, nonverbal play patterns are difficult to observe, especially in the laboratory, extensive data are available concerning children's first words from diary studies of TD children acquiring a wide range of native languages. Results of these studies indicate that basic level labels are consistently acquired before subordinate or superordinate level labels.

Data from the monthly play sessions, parental responses on the CDI, and a specially constructed subordinate category checklist indicated that basic level categories had the same priority for the children with WS as for TD children and children with DS. The children with WS played with all the spherical objects (e.g., balls, spherical candles, sleigh bells) in the same manner, by rolling them. In contrast, they did not try to roll any of the nonspherical objects. The children's lexical behavior also indicated that they had formed a child-basic *ball* category; "ball" was comprehended in reference to a wide range of spherical objects, whether or not an adult would have considered them to be balls, but not in relation to objects of other shapes. Eight of the 10 children also produced the word "ball." These children showed the same pattern in production as they had in comprehension. A parallel set of findings was obtained for the *car* category, with all four-wheeled vehicles (but not boats or airplanes) being pushed along, often accompanied by motor noises, and the word "car" comprehended and produced in reference to the same set of vehicles.

Examination of the data from the checklists completed by the parents indicated that in 96% of the cases, the basic level name for an object was comprehended prior to the subordinate level name; in 3% of the cases, the order of acquisition was unclear (both the basic level label and the label for a subordinate category subsumed under that basic level category were first acquired in the same month). The subordinate level name was comprehended before the basic level name in only 1% of the cases. These involved two words: "toothbrush" and "school bus," both of which are atypical of their basic level categories. None of the children comprehended or produced any superordinate level labels prior to comprehending at least one basic level label for an object subsumed under that superordinate.

*Spontaneous exhaustive sorting, the vocabulary spurt, and fast mapping*
Gopnik and Meltzoff (e.g., 1987, 1992) have argued that spontaneous exhaustive sorting and the vocabulary spurt should occur at about the same time because they reflect parallel insights: all objects belong to some category (cognitive insight) and all objects have a name (linguistic insight). Mervis and Bertrand (1993, 1994) have argued that a better linguistic manifestation of this insight is the ability to fast map, that is, the ability to use the Novel Name – Nameless Category (N3C) principle. According to this principle, the child should assume that novel words map to categories for which the child does not yet have a name. Before children have this principle, they must rely on other people to provide an explicit connection between a new word and its referent (e.g., by showing an object to a child and then labeling it, or by labeling an object to which the child was already attending). Once children acquire the N3C principle, however, they no longer need to depend on someone else to make an explicit connection between a label and its referent. The indirect connection provided by hearing a novel word in the presence of an object for which the child does not yet have a name is sufficient for mapping to take place. For both TD children and children with DS, the onsets of spontaneous exhaustive sorting, the vocabulary spurt, and fast mapping have been found to occur at about the same time.

Much of this pattern does not hold for children with WS. In particular, none of the children with WS evidenced a temporal link between the onset of spontaneous exhaustive sorting and the vocabulary spurt or between the onset of the vocabulary spurt and fast mapping. One child evidenced spontaneous exhaustive sorting and the ability to fast map 5 months before she began her vocabulary spurt. The other 9 children had a vocabulary spurt 6–12 + months before the onset of spontaneous exhaustive sorting or fast mapping ability. Some of the children with WS had more than 500 words in their productive vocabularies before they were able to fast map. These data indicate the presence of a viable alternate path to rapid vocabulary acquisition. Although fast mapping is an excellent facilitator of rapid acquisition of new words, other ways must be possible. For individuals with WS, an increase in verbal short-term memory provides a likely alternate path. This possibility is consistent with Bates and Carnevale's (1993) position that the onset of the vocabulary spurt and subsequent rapid accumulation of new words probably result from the child's increasing efficiency at acquiring words using the same procedures as before the vocabulary spurt.

The data from the children with WS did support the universality of a specific link between the onsets of spontaneous exhaustive sorting and the ability to fast map. Eight children demonstrated the onset of both abilities in the same session. The two remaining children demonstrated fast mapping at the session before the one at which they evidenced spontaneous exhaustive sorting.

## Grammatical ability and its relation to cognitive abilities

Grammatical ability often has been considered a particular strength of individuals with WS. In fact, the ability of individuals with WS to comprehend and produce complex syntax was the primary basis for Bellugi et al.'s claim (e.g., Bellugi et al. 1988, 1994, 2000) that WS provides a compelling case for the independence of language from cognition. In this section, we briefly review prior findings on the grammatical abilities of individuals with WS relative to their level of cognitive development and/or their mean length of utterance (MLU). We then describe a study we have conducted on the relation between receptive grammar knowledge and verbal memory ability for school age children and adolescents with WS.

### Relations between level of cognitive ability, MLU, and grammatical complexity

Initial studies of the grammatical abilities of individuals with WS (e.g., Bellugi et al. 1988, 1994) were all based on very small samples of adolescents; comparison groups, when included, were composed of CA- and IQ-matched individuals with DS. Results of these studies indicated that individuals with WS had excellent syntactic abilities; furthermore, Bellugi and her colleagues argued that the grammatical abilities evidenced were much more advanced that would be expected given the significant level of MR associated with WS (e.g., Bellugi et al. 1988, 1990, 1994; see Bellugi et al. 2000 for a summary including results from more recent studies). This conclusion was based on the fact that the WS group performed dramatically better than the DS group on all of the grammatical measures. We have compared the performance of 9- and 10-year-olds with WS and DS (Klein & Mervis 1999) and replicated Bellugi and her colleagues' finding that on average, the spontaneous spoken language of individuals with WS is more complex than that of CA- and IQ-matched individuals with DS. We also have found that children with WS are significantly more advanced at marking tense (third person singular present, regular past tense, BE) than younger children with specific language impairment (SLI) matched for MLU (Mervis & Klein-Tasman 2000; Rice 1999).

Individuals with DS and individuals with SLI are well known to have inordinate difficulty with morphosyntax (e.g., Chapman 1997; Leonard 1998; Rice & Wexler 1996). Thus, excellent performance relative to these two contrast groups does not provide convincing evidence that the grammatical abilities of individuals with WS exceed those that would be expected for overall cognitive level of functioning or MLU. To address this issue, comparisons to other contrast groups are necessary. Studies comparing the spontaneous expressive language abilities of children with WS to those of CA- and IQ-matched children with MR of mixed or unknown etiology have found that MLU and syntactic abilities are equivalent for the two groups, for children acquiring either English (Udwin & Yule 1990) or German (Gosch, Städing, & Pankau 1994). Volterra, Capirci, Pezzini, Sabbadini, and Vicari (1996) compared the spontaneous expressive language of Italian children with WS to younger MA-matched TD children and found that MLU and syntactic abilities were similar for the two groups. In the only study that has considered the production of grammatical constructions as complex as those discussed by Bellugi and her colleagues, Zukowski (2001, in press) used an elicited production task to compare the performance of a group of older children and adolescents with WS to an MA-matched TD group on tasks measuring the ability to form noun-noun compounds, embedded relative clauses, and affirmative and negative questions. Consistent with Bellugi et al.'s findings, most of the participants with WS in Zukowski's study were able to produce these constructions at least once. However, overall level of performance was similar to or somewhat weaker than that of the MA control group, suggesting that the ability to produce these grammatical constructions was to be expected given the overall cognitive level of the participants with WS.

## Relations between memory ability and grammatical ability

In TD populations, verbal working memory is associated with the acquisition of both vocabulary (Gathercole & Baddeley 1989, 1993) and syntax (Kemper et al. 1989; Norman, Kemper, & Kynette 1992). Similarly, the nonword repetition task has been proposed as a phenotypic marker for SLI (Bishop, North, & Donlan 1996). These and other studies suggest that verbal working memory plays an active role in the acquisition and learning of words and grammatical structures in a number of diverse populations. We would therefore expect to find similar relations between language and working memory in individuals with WS. Indeed, given the WS cognitive profile, we hypothesized that verbal working memory may play a *more important* role in the language acquisition of these children than in language acquisition by TD children (Robinson, Mervis, & Robinson 2003). To address this possibility, we compared the relations between verbal short-term memory (forward digit span), verbal working memory (backward digit span), phonological short-term memory (Montgomery's 1996, nonword repetition task), and receptive grammatical abilities (TROG raw score) for a WS group (N = 39, mean CA 10.24 years, range 4.5–16.7 years) to those of a younger TD group (N = 32, mean CA 6.01 years, range 4.08–10.26 years) closely matched for TROG raw score.

As expected, the correlations between the memory measures and the raw scores on the TROG (i.e., number of blocks passed) were significant for the children with WS. Forward digit-span, nonword repetition, and backward digit-span shared partial correlations (controlling for CA) of .33, .48, and .52 with TROG respectively. Taken together, the memory variables accounted for 26% of the variance in the WS

TROG raw scores above and beyond CA. However, regression analysis indicated that forward-digit span alone did not uniquely contribute to variance in the scores once CA, nonword repetition, and backward digit span were taken into account. Nonword repetition, on the other hand, did account for additional unique variance even after CA and the other memory measures were controlled. Thus, it appears that phonological memory may account, in part, for the grammatical skills of children with WS. This finding fits with those of Grant et al. (1997), who reported that nonword repetition scores were significantly related to receptive vocabulary. We would therefore expect that the ability to encode and store small speech units, such as bound morphemes and function words, would similarly be related to grammatical ability. The measure of verbal *working* memory (backward-digit span) accounted for the largest proportion of variance in TROG scores. Even after controlling for CA, forward-digit span, and nonword repetition, backward-digit span accounted for an additional 10% of variance. Thus, the ability to manipulate verbal items, not just store them, seems to be important to grammatical ability.

After controlling for CA, there were no significant differences between the WS group and the TD group in the strength of relation between either forward-digit span and TROG raw scores or nonword repetition and TROG raw scores. The WS group, however, showed a significantly stronger relation between the working memory measure and receptive grammar (partial $r$ = .52) than did the TD group (partial $r$ = .27). Therefore, it is possible that the children with WS may have to rely more heavily than TD children on verbal working memory abilities in order to puzzle out complex grammatical structures. Comprehending phrases, and, presumably, learning grammatical constructions, requires more than the storage of linguistic items in short-term memory. A child must extract the meaning of a phrase from the context of the utterance and then associate it with the linguistic item that is stored in short-term memory. The interpretation of nonlinguistic cues to meaning would involve perceptual, social, and cognitive analysis. For a TD child much of the process of extracting meaning from context would be effortless and not limited by working memory capacity. For a child with deficits in one or more of the domains necessary to the processing and integration of the nonlinguistic cues, however, more effort and time would be required for the meaning extraction and therefore working memory capacity might be more important for language acquisition.

## Summary and conclusion

In 1990, when the research program described in this paper was begun, the prevailing view was that WS provided a paradigmatic example of the independence of language from cognition. In particular, WS was argued to provide strong evidence that excellent language abilities could exist side-by-side with severe MR (e.g., Bellugi et al. 1998, 1990, 1992). Jackendoff (1994: 117) stated that despite significant MR, the language of individuals with WS "is if anything more fluent and advanced than that of their age-mates." The research we have conducted presents a more nuanced picture. The language abilities of individuals with WS are indeed a relative strength. Both vocabulary and grammar are considerably more advanced than would be expected for level of nonverbal cognition as measured by tests of visuospatial construction. Furthermore, both receptive vocabulary and finite verb morphology are more advanced than for children with SLI matched for MLU, and both MLU and grammatical ability are more advanced than for children with DS matched for CA and MA. These findings are consistent with Bellugi et al.'s position.

However, individuals with WS who have language abilities at the level expected for their CA are rare. Mean levels of performance by individuals with WS on a variety of standardized assessments of language are consistently in the borderline to mild deficit range. Grammatical ability as measured by spontaneous language (MLU, IPSyn, noun and verb morphology) is below that of TD peers matched for CA. Instead, for individuals acquiring English as a native language, grammatical ability is at the same level as that of younger TD children matched for general level of cognitive ability. For individuals with WS acquiring native languages with more complex morphology, some aspects of morphological ability are typically below the level expected for general level of cognitive ability (e.g., for French, Karmiloff-Smith et al. 1997; for Hebrew, Levy, & Hermon 2003). Language abilities are only slightly more advanced than nonverbal reasoning abilities. Non-concrete language ability is considerably weaker than concrete language ability. For example, abstract relational vocabulary ability, as measured by the TRC, is considerably below the level expected for concrete vocabulary ability. Finally, not only are language abilities less impressive than previously claimed, IQ is considerably higher than expected based on initial reports. Mean IQ for individuals with WS is in the range of mild MR, not the severe-to-profound MR range reported in Bates' (1990) presentation of Bellugi's research. Therefore, the language abilities of individuals with WS are much more in line with what would be expected given their IQ.

In many important ways, acquisition of language by individuals with WS is best characterized as normal but delayed. For example, although both the onset of vocabulary acquisition and the onset of grammatical acquisition are delayed, the relation between expressive vocabulary size and grammatical complexity is the same as for the general population. Grammatical ability is at the level expected for overall level of cognitive ability. Many of the specific links between particular linguistic abilities and theoretically linked cognitive abilities that hold for TD children and children with DS also are shown by children with WS. For example, canonical babble, a critical step in the beginning of language acquisition, begins at the same time as rhythmic hand banging, the same pattern as found for TD children and children with DS. The early object labels of children with WS name the same child-basic level categories as for TD children and children with DS. Basic level categories and category names are acquired before subordinate or superordinate level categories and category names. The onsets of spontaneous exhaustive sorting and the ability to fast map new words whose referents were not explicitly identified by the speaker occur at about the same time, the same pattern as for TD children and children with DS.

At the same time, several putative links between specific aspects of language development and particular aspects of cognitive development that are evidenced by both TD children and children with DS do not hold for children with WS. In particular, unlike TD children, children with DS, and children with severe MR of a variety of etiologies, children with WS do not comprehend and produce referential pointing gestures prior to beginning to produce referential language. Onset of referential language typically precedes onset of comprehension and production of pointing gestures by 6 months or more. Despite the delay in pointing, parents of children with WS are able to establish joint attention by other communicative methods such as labeling the object that is already the focus of the child's attention or tapping the object on which the speaker wishes the child to focus. Such interactions allow children with WS to begin to acquire language without the ability to comprehend or produce referential pointing gestures.

The finding that for children with WS, the onset of referential language usually precedes the onset of comprehension and production of pointing gestures has important implications for language intervention. The onset of referential communicative gestures often is used as an indicator that children are ready to acquire language; at this point, speech therapy and/or developmental therapy is likely to begin to focus on vocabulary acquisition. Similarly, if children do not come to the attention of intervention agencies until after acquisition of a basic vocabulary, it is assumed that these children have already mastered the referential gesture system. Both of these assumptions are incorrect for children with WS. Children with WS are ready for language intervention focused on vocabulary acquisition long before they begin to produce referential communicative gestures. And many young children with WS who have 200 or more words in their productive vocabularies still have difficulty both comprehending and producing referential communicative gestures and would benefit from therapy directed at improving their nonverbal communicative abilities.

Another set of specific links that holds for TD children and children with DS, but not for children with WS, involves the onset of the vocabulary spurt. For children with WS, the onset of the vocabulary spurt precedes the onsets of both spontaneous exhaustive sorting and fast mapping, typically by 6 months or more. These three abilities, which have previously been claimed to be linked to the related conceptual realizations that all objects belong to a category and that all objects have basic-level names, are evidenced at about the same time for both TD children and children with DS. We have argued that the onset of the vocabulary spurt may well not indicate the realization that all objects have names. Instead, the vocabulary spurt may simply reflect increasing efficiency in applying vocabulary acquisition strategies that the child already had. Given that individuals with WS evidence a relative strength in verbal short-term memory, and that 4-year-olds with WS who evidence logistic vocabulary growth have considerably stronger verbal short-term memory abilities than those with slow linear vocabulary growth (Mervis et al. 2003), it is quite possible that increases in verbal memory ability facilitate the vocabulary spurt for children with WS. Grant et al. (1997) and Lukács, Racsmány, and Pléh (2001) have shown that verbal or phonological memory is strongly related to vocabulary size for older children with WS.

Strong verbal memory abilities, however, while effective at enhancing concrete vocabulary acquisition, are not nearly as helpful for facilitating acquisition of more abstract vocabulary. Thus, although there is a strong correlation between concrete vocabulary size and abstract vocabulary size (Mervis et al. 2003), the abstract relational vocabularies of children with WS are considerably smaller than expected given their concrete vocabulary size. Similarly, adolescents' and adults' understanding of figurative language, although highly correlated with their understanding of concrete language using the same grammatical constructions, is much more limited (Mervis et al. 2003). The end result is that for individuals with WS, the acquisition of abstract language is substantially more delayed than acquisition of concrete language ability, with large discrepancies remaining even in adulthood. Most children with WS, even if their receptive concrete vocabulary is at CA level, would benefit from speech or cognitive therapy focused on relational language and, at older ages, on figurative language. In both cases, it is important that the therapy be designed to ensure that the individual is able to generalize the language that has been taught to novel settings outside of the therapeutic context.

The relation between vocabulary size and verbal short-term memory ability is not the only link between memory ability and language ability evidenced by individuals with WS. At age 4 years, the ability to produce multiword utterances also is strongly related to verbal short-term memory ability (see Mervis et al. 2003). For older children and adolescents, verbal short-term memory, phonological short-term memory, and verbal working memory are all related to grammatical ability. This pattern of relations between memory abilities and grammatical ability also is shown by TD children. However, the strength of the relation between verbal working memory and grammatical ability is significantly greater for children with WS than for TD children matched for receptive grammatical level. This finding suggests that individuals with WS may need to depend more than TD individuals on verbal working memory to figure out complex grammatical structures. In particular, TD children may rely on more advanced conceptual abilities to learn grammar that place fewer demands on working memory, whereas children with WS, who are not able to apply some of these strategies, place a higher demand on verbal working memory to acquire the same grammatical constructions.

In conclusion, language ability is a relative strength for individuals with WS. In many important ways, the acquisition of language by these individuals proceeds in the same manner as for individuals in the general population. There is increasing evidence, however, that verbal memory – often the strongest ability of individuals with WS – is more important for the acquisition of language by these individuals than for their TD peers. The importance of verbal short-term memory to the acquisition of vocabulary by children with WS and the importance of verbal working memory to their grammatical development highlight basic differences between how children with WS and TD children acquire language. It is an open question as to whether these differences are a matter of extremes, or if children with WS acquire language using significantly different mechanisms from TD children.

## Notes

1. Standard scores on the TRC usually are expressed as T scores with a mean of 50, a standard deviation of 10, and a range from 1–90. To make it easier to compare performance on the PPVT-III and the TRC, we have converted the TRC standard scores to the same scale as the PPVT-III (mean = 100, standard deviation = 15) and set the minimum standard score on the TRC at 40, the same as on the PPVT-III.

2. In principle, it is possible that a measure of spatial working memory would have been more appropriate than a measure of verbal working memory, given that the pattern construction assessment is clearly a spatial task and matrices may be solved nonverbally. However, observations of individuals with WS in prior studies as they attempted to solve the pattern construction and matrices tasks suggested that verbal mediation was an important component of their attempts to some both tasks.

3. Although young children are expected to use the same principles (e.g., form-function correlation) to form basic level categories, membership in these categories would not be expected to be identical to that for adult-basic level categories labeled by the same name. The actual categories formed on the basis of these principles will vary because different groups attend to different attributes of the same object, as a function of different experiences or different levels of expertise (Mervis 1987). Because very young children may not share adults' knowledge of culturally appropriate functions of particular objects and the form attributes correlated with those functions, these children may de-emphasize attributes that are important from an adult perspective. At the same time, very young children may notice a function (and its correlated form attributes) for that object that adults ignore, leading the children to emphasize features that are unimportant to adults. In these situations, although there will be

significant overlap in membership between the child-basic and adult-basic categories labeled by the same word, the child-basic category will differ systematically from the corresponding adult-basic category.

## References

Adamson, L. B. (1995). *Communication Development during Infancy.* Madison, WI: Brown and Benchmark.

Bates, E. (1990, April). *Early Language Development: How things come together and how they come apart.* Montreal, Quebec: International Conference on Infant Studies.

Bates, E. & Carnevale, G. F. (1993). "New directions in research on language development". *Developmental Review, 13*, 446–470.

Bayley, N. (1969). *Bayley Scales of Infant Development.* New York, NY: Psychological Corporation.

Bellugi, U., Marks, S., Bihrle, A., & Sabo, H. (1988). "Dissociation between language and cognitive functions in Williams syndrome". In D. Bishop & K. Mogford (Eds.), *Language Development in Exceptional Circumstances* (pp. 177–189). London: Churchill Livingstone.

Bellugi, U., Bihrle, A., Jernigan, T., Trauner, D., & Doherty, S. (1990). "Neuropsychological and neuroanatomical profile of Williams syndrome". *American Journal of Medical Genetics, 6*, 115–125.

Bellugi, U., Bihrle, A., Neville, H., & Doherty, S. (1992). "Language, cognition, and brain organization in a neurodevelopmental disorder". In M. Gunnar & C. Nelson (Eds.), *Developmental Behavioral Neuroscience: The Minnesota symposium* (pp. 201–232). Hillsdale, NJ: LEA.

Bellugi, U., Klima, E. S., & Wang, P. P. (1996). "Cognitive and neural development: Clues from genetically based syndromes". In D. Magnusson (Ed.), *The Lifespan Development of Individuals: Behavioral, neurobiological, and psychosocial perspectives* (pp. 223–243). Cambridge: CUP.

Bellugi, U., Lichtenberger, L., Jones, W., Lai, Z., & St. George, M. (2000). "The neurocognitive profile of Williams syndrome: A complex pattern of strengths and weaknesses". *Journal of Cognitive Neuroscience, 12* (Supplement 1): 7–29.

Bellugi, U., Wang, P., Jernigan, T. L. (1994). "Williams syndrome: An unusual neuropsychological profile". In S. H. Broman & J. Grafman (Eds.), *Atypical Cognitive Deficits in Developmental Disorders: Implications for brain function* (pp. 23–56). Hillsdale, NJ: LEA.

Bishop, D. V. M. (1989). *Test for the Reception of Grammar 2nd ed.* Manchester, UK: Chapel Press.

Bishop, D. V. M., North, T., & Dolan, C. (1996). "Nonword repetition as a behavioural marker for inherited language impairment: Evidence from a twin study". *Journal of Child Psychology and Psychiatry, 37*, 391–403.

Chapman, R. (1997). "Language development in children and adolescents with Down syndrome". *Mental Retardation and Developmental Disabilities Research Reviews, 3*, 307–312.

Cobo-Lewis, A. B., Oller, D. K., Lynch, M. P., & Levine, S. L. (1995, March). "Relationships among motor and vocal milestones in normally developing infants and infants with Down syndrome". Gatlinburg Conference on Research and Theory in Mental Retardation and Developmental Disabilities, Gatlinburg, TN.

Damasio, A. R. & Damasio, H. (1992). "Brain and language". *Scientific American, 267*(3), 88–95.

Dunham, P. J., Dunham, F., & Curwin, A. (1993). "Joint-attentional states and lexical acquisition at 18 months". *Developmental Psychology, 29*, 827–831.

Dunn, L. M. & Dunn, L. M. (1981). *Peabody Picture Vocabulary Test-Revised*. Circle Pines, MN: American Guidance Service.

Dunn, L. E. & Dunn, L. E. (1997a). *Peabody Picture Vocabulary Test 3rd ed.* Circle Pines, MN: American Guidance Service.

Dunn, L. E. & Dunn, L. E. (1997b). *Technical References to the Peabody Picture Vocabulary Test 3rd ed.* Circle Pines, MN: American Guidance Service.

Edmonston, N. K. & Litchfield Thane, N. (1988). *TRC: Test of Relational Concepts*. Austin, TX: PRO-ED.

Elliott, C. D. (1990). *Differential Ability Scales*. San Antonio, TX: Psychological Corporation.

Ewart, A. K., Morris, C. A., Atkinson, D., Jin, W., Sternes, K., Spallone, P., Stock, A. D., Leppert, M., & Keating, M. T. (1993). "Hemizygosity at the elastin locus in a developmental disorder, Williams syndrome". *Nature Genetics, 5*, 11–16.

Fenson, L., Dale, P. S., Reznick, J. S., Thal, D., Bates, E., Hartung, J. P., Pethick, S., & Reilly, J. S. (1993). *MacArthur Communicative Development Inventories: User's guide and technical manual*. San Diego, CA: Singular.

Frazier, L. (1987). "Sentence processing: A tutorial review". In M. Coltheart (Ed.), *Attention and performance: Vol. XII* (pp. 559–586). Hillsdale, NJ: LEA.

Gathercole, S. E. & Baddeley, A. D. (1989). "Evaluation of the role of phonological STM in the development of vocabulary in children: A longitudinal study". *Journal of Memory and Language, 28*, 200–213.

Gathercole, S. E. & Baddeley, A. D. (1993). *Working Memory and Language*. Hillsdale, NJ: LEA.

Gopnik, A. & Meltzoff, A. N. (1987). "The development of categorization in the second year and its relation to other cognitive and linguistic developments". *Child Development, 58*, 1523–1531.

Gopnik, A. & Meltzoff, A. N. (1992). "Categorization and naming: Basic level sorting in eighteen-month-olds and its relation to language". *Child Development, 63*, 1091–1103.

Gosch, A., Städing, G., & Pankau, R. (1994). "Linguistic abilities in children with Williams-Beuren syndrome". *American Journal of Medical Genetics, 52*, 291–296.

Grant, J., Karmiloff-Smith, A., Gathercole, S. A., Paterson, S., Howlin, P., Davies, M., & Udwin, O. (1997). "Phonological short-term memory and its relationship to language in Williams syndrome". *Cognitive Neuropsychiatry, 2*, 81–99.

Jackendoff, R. (1994). *Patterns in the Mind: Language and human nature*. New York: Basic.

Karmiloff-Smith, A., Grant, J., Berthoud, I., Davies, M., Howlin, P., & Udwin, O. (1997). "Language and Williams syndrome: How intact is 'intact'." *Child Development, 68*, 274–290.

Kaufman, A. S. & Kaufman, N. L. (1990). *Kaufman Brief Intelligence Test.* Pines, MN: American Guidance Services.

Kemper, S., Kynette, D., Rash, S., & O'Brien, K. (1989). "Life span changes to adults' language: Effects of memory and genre". *Applied Psycholinguistics, 10*, 49–66.

Klein, B. P. & Mervis, C. B. (1999). "Cognitive strengths and weaknesses of 9- and 10-year-olds with Williams syndrome or Down syndrome". *Developmental Neuropsychology, 16*, 177–196.

Leonard, L. B. (1998). *Children with Specific Language Impairment.* Cambridge, MA: The MIT Press.

Levy, Y. & Hermon, S. (2003). "Morphological abilities of Hebrew-speaking adolescents". *Developmental Neuropsychology, 23*, 61–85.

Lukács, A., Racsmány, M., & Pléh, C. (2001). "Vocabulary and morphological patterns in Hungarian children with Williams syndrome: A preliminary report". *Acta Linguistica Hungarica, 48*, 243–269.

Masataka, N. (2001). "Why early linguistic milestones are delayed in children with Williams syndrome: Late onset of hand banging as a possible rate-limiting constraint on the emergence of canonical babbling". *Developmental Science, 4*, 158–164.

Mervis, C. B. (1987). "Child-basic object categories and early lexical development". In U. Neisser (Ed.), *Concepts and conceptual development: Ecological and intellectual factors in categorization* (pp. 201–233). Cambridge: CUP.

Mervis, C. B. (1999). "The Williams syndrome cognitive profile: Strengths, weaknesses, and interrelations among auditory short-term memory, language, and visuospatial constructive cognition". In E. Winograd, R. Fivush, & W. Hirst (Eds.), *Ecological approaches to cognition: Essays in honor of Ulric Neisser* (pp. 193–227). Mahwah, NJ: LEA.

Mervis, C. B. & Bertrand, J. (1993). "Acquisition of early object labels: The roles of operating principles and input". In A. P. Kaiser & D. B. Gray (Eds.), *Enhancing children's communication: Research foundations for intervention* (pp. 281–316). Baltimore, MD: Brookes.

Mervis, C. B. & Bertrand, J. (1994). "Acquisition of the Novel Name – Nameless Category (N3C) principle". *Child Development, 65*, 1646–1662.

Mervis, C. B. & Bertrand, J. (1997). "Developmental relations between cognition and language: Evidence from Williams syndrome". In L. B. Adamson & M. A. Romski (Eds.), *Communication and Language Acquisition: Discoveries from atypical development* (pp. 75–106). Baltimore, MD: Brookes.

Mervis, C. B. & Klein-Tasman, B. P. (2000). "Williams syndrome: Cognition, personality, and adaptive behavior". *Mental Retardation and Developmental Disabilities Research Reviews, 6*, 148–158.

Mervis, C. B., Morris, C. A., Bertrand, J., & Robinson, B. F. (1999). "Williams syndrome: Findings from an integrated program of research". In H. Tager-Flusberg (Ed.), *Neurodevelopmental disorders* (pp. 65–110). Cambridge, MA: The MIT Press.

Mervis, C. B., Robinson, B. F., Bertrand, J., Morris, C. A., Klein-Tasman, B. P., & Armstrong, S. C. (2000). "The Williams syndrome cognitive profile". *Brain and Cognition, 44*, 604–628.

Mervis, C. B., Robinson, B. F., Rowe, M. L., Becerra, A. M., & Klein-Tasman, B. P. (2003). "Language abilities of individuals with Williams syndrome". In L. Abbeduto (Ed.), *International Review of Research in Mental Retardation: Vol. 27* (pp. 35–81). Orlando, FL: Academic Press.

Montgomery, J. A. (1996). "Examination of phonological working memory in specifically language-impaired children". *Applied Psycholinguistics, 16*, 355–378.

Morris, C. A. & Mervis, C. B. (2000). "Williams syndrome and related disorders". *Annual Review of Genomics and Human Genetics, 1*, 461–484.

Mullen, E. M. (1995). *Mullen Scales of Early Learning*. Circle Pines, MN: American Guidance Service.

Norman, S., Kemper, S., & Kynette, D. (1992). "Adult reading comprehension: Effects of syntactic complexity and working memory". *Journals of Gerontology, 47*, 258–265.

Osborne, L. R., Li M., Pober, B., Chitayat, D., Bodurtha, J., Mandel, A., Costa, T., Grebe, T., Cox, S., Tsui, L. C., & Scherer, S. W. (2001). "A 1.5 million-base pair inversion polymorphism in families with Williams-Beuren syndrome". *Nature Genetics, 29*, 321–325.

Rice, M. L. (1999). "Specific grammatical limitations in children with specific language impairment". In H. Tager-Flusberg (Ed.), *Neurodevelopmental Disorders* (pp. 331–359). Cambridge, MA: The MIT Press.

Rice, M. L. & Wexler, K. (1996). "A phenotype of specific language impairment: Extended optional infinitives". In M. L. Rice (Ed.), *Toward a Genetics of Language* (pp. 215–237). Mahwah, NJ: LEA.

Robinson, B. F., Mervis, C. B., & Robinson, B. W. (2003). "Roles of verbal short-term memory and working memory in the acquisition of grammar by children with Williams syndrome". *Developmental Neuropsychology, 23*, 13–31.

Rosch, E., Mervis, C. B., Gray, W. D., Johnson, D. M., & Boyes-Braem, P. (1976). "Basic objects in natural categories". *Cognitive Psychology, 8*, 382–439.

Tomasello, M. & Farrar, M. J. (1986). "Joint attention and early language". *Child Development, 57*, 1454–1463.

Udwin, O. & Yule W. (1990). "Expressive language of children with Williams syndrome". *American Journal of Medical Genetics Supplement, 6*, 108–114.

Volterra, V., Capirci, O., Pezzini, G., Sabbadini, L., & Vicari, S. (1996). "Linguistic abilities in Italian children with Williams syndrome". *Cortex, 32*, 663–677.

Williams, K. T. (1997). *Expressive Vocabulary Test*. Circle Pines, MN: American Guidance Service.

Zukowski, A. (2001). Uncovering Grammatical Competence in Children with Williams Syndrome. Unpublished doctoral dissertation, Boston University.

Zukowski, A. (in press). "Investigating Knowledge of Complex Syntax: Insights from experimental studies of Williams syndrome". In M. Rice & S. Warren (Eds.), *Developmental Language Disorders: From phenotypes to etiologies*. Mahwah, NJ: LEA.

# Spared domain-specific cognitive capacities?

## Syntax and morphology in Williams syndrome and Down syndrome

Chris Schaner-Wolles
University of Vienna

This paper compares Williams syndrome (a case study) and Down syndrome (large cross-sectional study). The paper focuses both on the particular linguistic deficits and on the spared areas of linguistic competence on the level of the interactive subsystems involved in language processing.

Compared to an unimpaired development, the causes of the syndrome-specific deficits are retardations of specific subsystems. Due to the modular interactive organization of linguistic capacities, local asynchronic retardations produce globally deviant patterns and thereby mask the spared subsystems. This approach requires analyzing data in terms of the responsible subsystems. Mere inductive inspection and juxtaposition of data of the two syndromes would be insufficient and misleading.

Main claim: Spared subsystems exist in both syndromes and provide evidence for a domain specific cognitive capacity.

## 1. Introduction

In present day language acquisition research, the answer to the following question is a topic of intense controversies: Is language acquisition guided by domain-specific or domain-general cognitive capacities?

Domain-general theorists (cf. strong emergentist approaches, see MacWhinney 1999) deny the existence of domain-specific innate abilities and their alleged role in processes by which language is acquired, used, and represented in the brain. In the light of constructivism, their advocates emphasize (1) the importance of learning from a rich linguistic environment and (2) the domain-general nature of those (innate) cognitive capacities involved in the process of language learning. Of course, there is no doubt that attention, memory, auditory processing, pattern detection, association, and other domain-general cognitive tools are important for language development, and that they contribute to the process in non-trivial ways. (cf. e.g. Sabbagh & Gelman 2000). It ought not to be difficult to find evidence in developmental data for their contribution. Evidence to this extent, however, does not warrant the conclusion that domain-specific abilities play no role at all, contrary to what extreme emergentists seem to be convinced of. So, the crucial question is not whether domain-general processes play a role in language acquisition (they do), but whether domain-general tools ALONE are sufficient for language acquisition.

Domain-general theorists seem to be at a loss with cases of dissociations, for example with children who master formal properties of grammar at a high level, while other aspects of cognition are extremely impaired. In this light, the study of Williams syndrome (WS) has recently attracted considerable attention because of its uneven cognitive-linguistic profile, with a remarkable preservation of linguistic abilities in the context of otherwise widespread general cognitive deficits. In early reports on the syndrome, the impression prevailed that the language of individuals with Williams syndrome is totally intact. In the meantime, the generally accepted view of WS is that language abilities are spared, but that this sparing is relative rather than absolute. Moreover, there is growing evidence that WS is characterized by within-domain dissociations of language as well. Recent studies attested deficits and a number of atypical features in the lexical development and in the semantic processing in WS (cf. Bellugi, Bihrle, Neville, Doherty, & Jernigan 1992; Bellugi, Wang, & Jernigan 1994; Rossen, Klima, Bellugi, Bihrle, & Jones 1996; Stevens & Karmiloff-Smith 1997; Tyler, Karmiloff-Smith, Voice, Stevens, Grant, Udwin, Davies, & Howlin 1997). As for the structural and rule-based aspects of grammar, there is little agreement in the literature till now. On the contrary, it seems as if positions have become more entrenched during the last years. Those researchers who defend an innate modular account of the grammar faculty report an intact computational competence in WS (cf. Bellugi et al. 1994; Bromberg, Ullman, Marcus, Kelly, & Coppola 1994; Clahsen & Almazan 1998, 2001; Krause & Penke 2001; Schaner-Wolles 2000a; Zukowski 2001; among others). Opponents of this account, on the other hand, are arguing against the intactness of aspects of grammar in WS, as there are regular morphology (Thomas, Grant, Barham, Gsödl, Laing, Lakusta, Tyler, Grice, Paterson, & Karmiloff-Smith 2001), morphosyntax (Pezzini, Volterra, Ossella, & Sabbadini 1994; Volterra, Capirci, Pezzini, Sabbadini, & Vicari 1996), and syntax (Karmiloff-Smith, Tyler, Voice, Sims, Udwin, Howlin, & Davies 1998; Grant, Valian, & Karmiloff-Smith 2002). Grant, Valian and Karmiloff-Smith (2002) hold the opinion that "*the strong claims made about the intactness of morphosyntax are sometimes supported by weak evidence*" (404), and that "[...] *the syndrome should no longer be used to bolster claims about the existence of independently functioning, innately specified modules in the human brain*" (403).

Critics of domain-specific cognitive capacities for grammar primarily fail to acknowledge dissociations between grammar and general cognitive abilities in WS because they tend to focus on those aspects of grammar that are driven by lexical knowledge (see also Schaner-Wolles 2000a, b for more detailed discussions). In these areas of grammar, correlations with general cognitive impairments are not surprising, given that lexical-semantic knowledge is the interface to the cognitive conceptual system. But this fact is not relevant for an argument against a selectively spared computational system for language. The crucial question in this connection is this: Are there genuine formal, especially syntactic, aspects of the grammatical competence that are spared by general cognitive impairment? If these spared grammatical capacities exist, then this is the relevant piece of evidence for the dissociation controversy. Contrary to the suppositions of Grant et al. (2002:415), it is NOT the case, that "*claims about syntactic modularity require intact syntactic performance or a complete dissociation between syntax and mental age*". Poor performance does not reflect poor competence per se, and is no argument against spared grammatical capacities. Poor performance may reflect for example task-dependent effects and therefore lead to underestimating linguistic competence. On the other hand, poor development or performance may also be a function of how different domain-general cognitive capacities affect the process of language development or language processing. For instance, syndrome-specific cognitive limitations may deprive the language faculty of necessary resources for getting a tight grasp on grammar. As a consequence, the submodules of grammar will start to develop later than in typically developing children, and perhaps they may develop in an asynchronously retarded way, or reach a developmental plateau at a certain point. Auditory short-term memory, for example, is discussed as playing an important role in the development of aspects of language, and in vocabulary acquisition in particular (Gathercole & Baddeley 1990; see Baddeley, Gathercole, & Papagno 1998 for a review of the literature in this connection).

In sum, there is no denying that the grammatical performance of individuals with WS is not intact in an absolute sense. On the other hand, there is enough evidence for relatively spared computational subsystems of grammar in individuals with WS as well. The data to be discussed below from a case study of a twelve-year old German-speaking girl with WS follow this pattern.

Additional support for relatively spared computational subsystems of grammar is gained from other syndromes associated with intellectual disabilities as well, – even from Down syndrome (DS), for which severe, selective impairments of grammar are reported in general (cf. Bates & Goodman 1999; Chapman 1995; Miller 1988, 1996; Fowler 1988, 1990; among others). This notwithstanding, there are exceptions among individuals with DS as well. Rondal (1995) documented two adults with DS, Françoise and Paul. Their grammatical abilities were characterized as normal or quasi-normal at an adult level, in spite of a non-verbal IQ of about 60 and a mental age of about five or six years. And Vallar and Papagno (1993) report the case of a 23-year old Italian woman with DS, who was fluent in three languages

(Italian, English, and French). She showed a remarkably good acquisition of the Italian language and vocabulary. In addition, she was able to learn English and French, although with less proficiency. She was impaired in tasks assessing verbal and non-verbal reasoning, visuo-spatial perception and memory, and verbal long-term memory. However, she had a perfectly normal verbal short-term memory. These findings prompted the authors to support the view that phonological short-term memory, which may occur in the presence of substantial deficits of general intelligence, plays an important role in the development of aspects of language, and in vocabulary acquisition in particular (cf. Gathercole & Baddeley 1990). Apart from this exceptional trilingual DS woman, there is considerable evidence that DS is associated with a specific deficit in verbal short-term memory. Conversely WS has been linked with a deficit in visuo-spatial short-term memory whereas verbal short-term memory is a particular strength (cf. e.g. Jarrold, Baddeley, & Hewes 1999; Jarrold & Baddeley 2001). It has been suggested that the differences in short-term memory deficits might potentially explain the specific patterns of language learning observed in DS and WS (cf. Jarrold et al. 1999; Vicari, Carlesimo, Brizzolara, & Pezzini 1996; Wang & Bellugi 1994; among others). Future work will clearly be needed to understand possible interrelations of this kind. Françoise, for example, the DS woman reported by Rondal (1995) had a relatively superior vocabulary and adult-like language skills but a poor verbal short-term memory. As mentioned before, there is no doubt that specific memory functions may influence aspects of language. However, neither specific verbal short-term memory deficits nor another domain-general cognitive function can explain or be responsible for the spared syntactic skills in DS, which I will report on here.

In a large experimental study on the language of eighty-two German-speaking children, adolescents and adults with DS, we gained strong evidence for spared syntactic abilities in DS as well (cf. Schaner-Wolles 1994, 2000a). As it was attested for other languages before, our German-speaking DS subjects, too, had severe problems with morphology in general and were doing even worse on morphosyntax. This could indeed have been caused by "*a selective impairment in one or more aspects of auditory processing, a deficit that is superimposed on their more general cognitive delay*", as Bates and Goodman (1999:62) argue for DS, supporting an emergentist account. What is more interesting in our German data, however, is that the individuals with DS were able to successfully master complex syntactic principles, e.g. those that govern the clause structure.

This paper is organized as follows. Section 2 elaborates on the grammatical phenomena of German dealt with in the experimental data (verb second property, morphological case marking, pronominal dependency relations). Section 3 reports on the case of a German-speaking girl with Williams syndrome. In particular, her performance data on two sentence-picture matching tasks (a passive-active test and a pronominal dependency test) are presented, and compared with those of typically developing children. Section 4 introduces into the syntactic and morphosyntactic results of sentence repetition tasks from an experimental study on DS referred to in the preceding paragraph. Section 5, finally, compares the WS and DS results, and presents general conclusions.

## 2. The modularity of grammar – exemplified for German

Generative linguistics characterizes the human language processing capacity as a highly modular system. Syntax is one of the modules of grammar, and syntax itself consists of submodules, too. Given that these submodules of the overall grammar processing capacity form cognitively autonomous processing units, they may be impaired or spared selectively. The modular units are autonomous in the sense that modular interaction takes place at the level of input-output relations between the modules and not among processing units of the various subsystems. The system that determines grammatical well-formedness is the combinatorial result of the interaction of all the relevant subsystems. Details aside, at least three main components have to be distinguished, namely the *lexicon*, the *syntactic structure component*, and the component that determines the *antecedent-dependent relations*.

The *lexicon* is the store of the individual grammatical properties of the lexical elements. The lexical item is a local interface between various types of information, namely phonological, morphological, syntactic, and conceptual. An informal example is given in (1).

(1) types of lexical information:

| | | |
|---|---|---|
| phonological: | [li:v] | (=leave) |
| morphological: | 'left' | (=irregular participle morphology) |
| syntactic: | V: A1 (A2) | (=verb with two arguments; one being optional) |
| conceptual: | "X go away (from Y)" | |

The phonological part specifies the information relevant for its articulatory realization; the morphological part contains information about various word forms and stores irregular forms (e.g. irregular participle forms); the syntactic part specifies the categorical and combinatorial properties; and the conceptual part specifies the semantic properties. One crucial aspect needs to be added to this simplified example: the mapping relation between the conceptual information and the combinatorial properties. It is obvious that the variables X and Y must be uniquely associated with their syntactic argument counterparts. This aspect of lexical structure is usually referred to as argument structure. The argument structure expresses the mapping relation between conceptual structure and syntactic structure.

The following example illustrates the function of the *syntactic structure component*. German and English differ with respect to the structure of the main clause. German is a verb second language. This means that the main clause provides an initial position for an arbitrary, single constituent, followed by the finite verb. In generative grammar, the verb second position and the clause-initial position are understood as derived positions. The co-indexed *e*-positions in (2) are the base positions. These are the positions in which the fronted elements would occur if they were not fronted.

(2) [XP$_i$ [V$_j$ [ …e$_i$ … e$_j$]]]

The basic position of the verb is clause final, that is the position of the finite verb in embedded clauses with a complementizer (e.g. *hat* 'has' in (3a)), and of non-finite verbal elements in non embedded clauses (e.g. the past participle *angerufen*, 'phoned' in (3b))

| | | | | | | | | |
|---|---|---|---|---|---|---|---|---|
| (3) | a. | daß | | [er | sie | gestern | *angerufen* | *hat*] |
| | | that | | he | her | yesterday | up-phoned | has |
| | | 'that he has phoned her up yesterday' | | | | | | |
| | b. | [er$_i$ | [*hat*$_j$ | [e$_i$ | sie | gestern | angerufen | e$_j$]]] |
| | | he | has | | her | yesterday | up-phoned | |
| | | 'he has phoned her up yesterday' | | | | | | |
| | c. | [er$_i$ | [*rief*$_j$ | [e$_i$ | sie | gestern | an-e$_j$]]] | |
| | | he | phoned | | her | yesterday | up | |
| | | 'he phoned her up yesterday' | | | | | | |

Declarative clauses – like the examples in (3b), (3c) and (4) – are verb second, which means the finite verb follows a single arbitrary constituent. The variants in (4) differ pragmatically, in terms of the information structure.

| | | | | | | | | |
|---|---|---|---|---|---|---|---|---|
| (4) | a. | [er$_i$ | [*hat*$_j$ | [e$_i$ | sie | gestern | angerufen | e$_j$]]] (= 3b) |
| | b. | [sie$_i$ | [*hat*$_j$ | [er | e$_i$ | gestern | angerufen | e$_j$]]] |
| | c. | [gestern$_i$ | [*hat*$_j$ | [er | sie | e$_i$ | angerufen | e$_j$]]] |
| | d. | [angerufen$_i$ | [*hat*$_j$ | [er | sie | gestern | e$_i$ | e$_j$]]] |

Morphological case marking rather than serialization is the clue for the identification of the grammatical relation of an NP, as illustrated in the examples in (5).

| | | | | | | |
|---|---|---|---|---|---|---|
| (5) | a. | sie:ACC | hat | er:NOM | gestern | angerufen |
| | | her | has | he | yesterday | up-phoned |
| | | 'he has phoned her up yesterday' | | | | |
| | b. | sie:NOM | hat | ihn:ACC | gestern | angerufen |
| | | she | has | him | yesterday | up-phoned |
| | | 'she has phoned him up yesterday' | | | | |

| c. | ihn:ACC | hat | er:NOM | gestern | angerufen |
|---|---|---|---|---|---|
| | him | has | he | yesterday | up-phoned |

'he has phoned him up yesterday'

German has a morphological case system with four cases (nominative, accusative, dative, and genitive). Case is marked on the head noun/pronoun, the attribute, and the determiner. Because of syncretisms and defective paradigms, case morphology does not always uniquely identify the grammatical relations: In (5a, b), '*sie*' (nominative or accusative) is disambiguated once the uniquely identifiable forms '*er*' (nominative, (5a)) or '*ihn*' (accusative, (5b)) is encountered. However, in (5c), case uniquely identifies the subject and the object respectively.

As indicated in (2), the verb second property involves two antecedent gap relations. The phrasal constituent in the first position is the antecedent of a phrasal gap position ($e_i$) and the finite verb is the antecedent of an empty verbal head position ($e_j$).

The formal grammatical relations that constrain the antecedent gap relations are of a format that is found with all sorts of genuine *grammatical dependency relations*. Koster (1987: 105) introduced the term *configurational matrix* for this invariant set of properties (cf. Neeleman & van de Koot 2002). These relations are defined by the following four properties:

(6) B depends on A,

a. obligatorily
b. uniquely
c. locally (i.e. within the same, single, minimal domain)
d. with A as structurally prominent element.

Linguistic implementations of this core relation are manifold. Prototypical cases are: *agreement* (esp. subject-verb agreement; reflexive-antecedent agreement) and *filler-gap relations* (e.g. the relation between a fronted constituent and its base position).

The agreement relation between the finite verb and the subject in German (a language with a richer morphological system than English) is the crucial cue for identifying the subject. The verbal paradigms distinguish number and person (as in (7)), tense (present, preterit) and modality (indicative, subjunctive).

(7)

| | | sein '*be*' | haben '*have*' | lieben '*love*' | sehen '*see*' |
|---|---|---|---|---|---|
| a. | 1.sg. | bin | habe | liebe | sehe |
| b. | 2.sg. | bist | hast | liebst | siehst |
| c. | 3.sg. | ist | hat | liebt | sieht |
| d. | 1.pl. | sind | haben | lieben | sehen |

e. 2.pl. seid habt liebt seht
f. 3.pl. sind haben lieben sehen

Another case is the dependency between a reflexive and its antecedent. German reflexives are clause bound, that is, the antecedent of the reflexive must be a clause mate of the reflexive. In infinitival complements, the antecedent of the reflexive is the phonetically silent subject of the infinitival (PRO), whose own antecedent – the so-called controller – is in the matrix clause. The choice of the controller is verb-specific, i.e. determined by the semantics of the matrix verb. So, in (8a), the controller is the matrix subject, in (8b) the controller is the matrix object. Notice that the reflexive is not marked for gender in German.

(8) a. sie$_i$:NOM hat ihm:DAT versprochen [PRO$_i$ sich$_i$ zu frisieren]
she$_i$ has promised him [PRO$_i$ to comb herself$_i$/*himself$_i$]
b. sie:NOM hat ihm$_i$:DAT geraten [PRO$_i$ sich$_i$ zu frisieren]
she has advised him$_i$ [PRO$_i$ to comb himself$_i$/*herself$_i$]

In German, it is easy to see that the reflexive is only indirectly construed with the NP in the matrix clause, because a reflexive does not accept a dative object as antecedent. In (8b) the dative NP '*ihm*' serves as the antecedent for the silent subject of the infinitival clause, which in turn serves as the required antecedent for the reflexive. The direct antecedent of the reflexive is the subject of the infinitival (PRO), and not the dative.

The control properties interact with the complementary distribution of reflexives and personal pronouns. Clause internal coreference requires a reflexive (8), clause external coreference a personal pronoun (9b). Therefore, in (9a), the pronoun in the infinitival clause cannot be coreferent with the matrix subject, since it controls the infinitive subject. As a consequence, the pronoun in the infinitival clause would incorrectly end up as coreferent with a clause mate antecedent. In (9b), control does not interfere. So, the personal pronoun '*sie*', 'her' in (9a) can only refer to an external referent in the discourse.

(9) a. sie$_i$ hat ihm versprochen [PRO$_i$ sie$^{*}{}_{i}$ zu frisieren]
she$_i$ has promised him [PRO$_i$ to comb her$_{*i}$]
b. sie$_i$ hat ihm$_j$ verboten [PRO$_j$ sie$_i$ zu frisieren]
she$_i$ has forbidden him$_j$ [PRO$_j$ to comb her$_i$]

A third case of unique, local and obligatory dependency relations is the filler-gap relation between a displaced element and its gap at the base position. For each displaced element – as exemplified in the case of German verb second structures in (2)–(4) – there must be a unique, local base position (the gap signified by a coindexed 'e'), for which the displaced element serves as the structurally prominent antecedent element. In these cases, the dependent element is a phonetically silent syntactic entity. The dependency relation links the displaced element to its original position. Note that any German declarative clause instantiates this dependency relation for the clause-initial phrase and for the fronted finite verb. If a child has mastered these core characteristics of a German clause, she has mastered a complex antecedent-gap pattern.

## 3. Williams syndrome – a case report

### 3.1 Method

*Participant*
Kathy is a twelve-year old girl with WS. Her clinical features are typical of WS. Diagnosis was confirmed by positive results for the genetic deletion implicated in WS. At the age of 10;2 years, her IQ (Hamburg-Wechsler Intelligence Scale for Children – Revised HAWIK-R, Tewes 1983) indicated a full scale IQ of 46, a verbal IQ of 53, and a performance IQ of 51. At the age of 12, mental age on the German version of the Stanford-Binet Intelligence Test S-I-T (Terman & Merrill 1965) was 5;8. Her digit span was 3. She did not pass tests of conservation. At the same age as the syntactic abilities presented in this study have been examined, Kathy's morphological and lexical skills show the following interesting characteristics:

First, asymmetries between regular and irregular morphological abilities were neither attested for past participles nor for plurals in Kathy's data. Her correctness rate for existing past participles was nearly 100%. On a 42 items task (half regular, and half irregular forms), she committed a single mistake: *geleget* instead of *gelegt*, 'laid'. So, Kathy's morphological behavior does not show a prevalence of regulars over irregulars, as Clahsen and Almazan (1998, 2001) report for English adolescents with WS. Kathy's good performance on past participles rather matches the results of Pléh and his colleagues, who found in their Hungarian data, that only younger WS children (under ten years of age) with a low verbal memory span were prone to overgeneralize (cf. Lukács, Racsmány, & Pléh 2001; Pléh, Lukács, & Racsmány 2003).

Noun plurals were correct in two thirds of the 45 items on a balanced task.[1] She was performing at the level of four- to five-year old typically developing children. She was using all the different German plural markers. There were no wrong plural forms in the sense of overgeneralized or overregularized forms. All incorrect answers were of one single type, namely a combination of a plural numeral and the test noun in its non marked (=singular) form, e.g. *zwei Auto, zwei Radio, viele Tasche* ('two car, two radio, many bag'), instead of *zwei Auto-s, zwei Radio-s, viele Tasche-n* ('two cars, two radios, many bags').

The fact that Kathy did not overgeneralize any plural forms is not surprising, given that German plural morphology is highly idiosyncratic and dependent on lexical information for the correct choice among the various plural allomorphs (*-e*, *-er*, *-en*, *-s*, and Umlaut). There is no simple rule that could be overgeneralized.[2] Therefore, this finding does not per se contradict Clahsen and Almazan's (1998, 2001) dissociated dual route proposal for WS. They assume an intact rule system, but limited access to lexical information. Since there is no default plural morphology for German, Kathy has no chance to overgeneralize it.

Second, her performance on an expressive language test on local prepositional phrases showed severe semantic problems with spatial prepositions on the one hand, but intact abilities in morphosyntactic agreement marking of gender and case governed by the prepositions. Kathy used only the prepositions *in*, *auf*, and *unter* ('in, on, under'). As for more elaborated spatial conditions and prepositions like *hinter*, *vor*, *neben*, *zwischen* ('behind, in front of, next to, in between') were concerned, she failed totally and did not react at all or inappropriately (e.g. *draußen*, 'outside' instead of *neben dem Sessel*, 'next to the chair'). These preliminary data match the findings on spatial relations in Hungarian-speaking WS individuals as well (cf. Racsmány, Lukács, Pléh, & Király 2001).

*Materials*

Kathy was tested with two sentence-picture-matching tasks. Both were designed for, and used in, previous studies with typically developing children. More detailed information is available elsewhere (Schaner-Wolles 1989; Schaner-Wolles & Haider 1987).

*Passive-active test.* This test, first used in Schaner-Wolles (1989), explores children's ability to understand German reversible passive and active sentences. The test includes a total of twenty sentences with agentive verbs, i.e. six full passives, six agentless passives, and eight active sentences with an 'object:ANIMATE < verb < subject:ANIMATE' order (cf. 5a, c) and unambiguous argument status.[3] For each test sentence, three pictures were presented (as exemplified in Figure A in the Appendix): one picture shows the action as described by the test sentence (e.g. *picture a* for the test sentence "*das Mädchen wird von der Mutter frisiert*", 'the girl is combed by the mother'); a second one shows the same action with the protagonists reversed (reverse role distractor, *picture b*); and the third picture serves as a lexical distractor, showing either another protagonist as in the test sentence (*picture c*) or another action.

As in English, the reduction of the active subject in the passive construction is coded in the verbal morphology, namely by combination of the auxiliary *werden* with the past participle. So, the mastering of passive consists of two tasks. First, the function of the auxiliary in combination with the past participle must be understood as the signal for the missing subject argument. Only then, the shift of the object to the subject position (in English), or to subject case, i.e. nominative (in German) can become transparent to the child. Notice that – unlike in English – there is no fixed subject position in German, as exemplified in (4), (5), and in (11).

*Pronominal dependency test.* The second test was adopted from Schaner-Wolles and Haider (1987). It tests the grammatical constraints on coreference relations between pronouns and their antecedents in eight simple clauses and in twelve clauses with infinitival complements: In simple clauses, a reflexive is used for coreference and a pronoun for disjoint reference (example: *Kevin introduced him* vs. *himself*). In an infinitival complement (see examples (8) and (9)), the interpretation of the silent subject of the infinitival clause, i.e. PRO, interacts with the coreference relation of a pronoun of the infinitival clause (example: *John promised/asked Kevin* PRO *to introduce him/himself*): If the intended coreferent is the controller of the silent subject ('*ask*'), the silent subject necessarily is coreferent, too. So a reflexive is required, otherwise ('*promise*') the personal pronoun is needed. In order to master the coreference relations for pronouns in infinitival clauses, the child must be able to combine two sets of conditions, namely (i) the coreference relations for pronouns and reflexives and (ii) the construal of the silent subject. It must be able to apply (i) in the context of (ii). In this task, the child has to select from four pictures. For the test sentence in (10), for example, *pictures a, b, d*, and *e* of Figure A in the Appendix are offered, with *picture d* as the appropriate one, *picture a* as a distractor for the reflexive/pronoun alternation (i.e. *the mother$_i$ has promised Susi$_j$* [PRO$_i$ *to comb her$_j$*]), *picture e* as a distractor for the silent subject PRO interpretation (i.e. *the mother has asked Susi$_i$* [PRO$_i$ *to comb herself$_i$*]), and *picture b* as the most distant distractor.

(10) die Mutter$_i$:NOM hat der Susi:DAT versprochen [PRO$_i$ sich$_i$ zu frisieren]
the mother$_i$ has promised Susi [PRO$_i$ to comb herself$_i$]

*Procedure*

Kathy was tested individually in her school. The two tests reported here were done at different sessions within one month. Sentences and pictures were randomly ordered within each test. The pictures were displayed in front of the child, who was asked to watch them carefully. Then the child heard the test sentence. Her task consisted of choosing one of the three/four pictures that matches the sentence best. If the child hesitated or indicated that she had not understood the sentence, it was repeated once more. The child was given as much time as she wanted. However, Kathy was usually making her choice immediately. As the results will

**Table 1.** Passive-active test: percentages of correct reactions as a function of sentence types

| | Kathy | Typically Controls (Schaner-Wolles 1989) | |
|---|---|---|---|
| | | 4-year-olds | 5-years-olds |
| reversible full passives | 100.0% | 77.8% | 86.2% |
| reversible agentless passives | 100.0% | 83.3% | 96.3% |
| OVS-actives (with unambiguously marked O and S) | 60.0% | 61.1% | 88.9% |
| OVS-actives (with ambiguously marked O but unambiguously marked S) | 33.3% | 50.0% | 50.0% |

confirm, Kathy did not give the impression that she had specific problems with the procedure of picture-based comprehension tasks.

## 3.2 Results and discussion

*Passive-active test*

Kathy did not make a single mistake in the interpretation of the reversible passive sentences. It seems safe, therefore, to claim that she knows how to handle the grammar of the passive construction. She was even better than the five-year old typically developing children, who were successful in 86.2% only, as Table 1 shows.

For children acquiring English, the passive construction is difficult for quite some time, because they apply a strict word order strategy, i.e. a 'first noun as agent'-strategy, which results in a misinterpretation of the derived subject as agent (cf. Bever 1970). In German, the effect of word order can be tested systematically – in active sentences as well –, since any phrase may be topicalized and can appear in sentence-initial position. As for the active test sentences, Kathy was mistaken in two thirds of all cases. Here, all errors were systematically based on a word order bias. They occurred especially in those OVS test sentences, in which the first NP could have been a potential subject as well, i.e. an animate NP, ambiguously marked for accusative/nominative as in (11a), contrary to (11b) (cf. Table A in the Appendix for the paradigm of the German definite article):

(11) a. das:ACC (=NOM) Mädchen frisiert der:NOM Bub
the:ACC (=NOM) girl combs the:NOM boy
*'it is the girl, the boy is combing'*

b. den:ACC Vater fotografiert der:NOM Bub
the:ACC father photographs the:NOM boy
*'it is the father, the boy is photographing'*

In the comprehension of German passives, however, the role of a word order strategy turned out to be insignificant, both for our typically developing children and for Kathy. The verb second property of German (cf. (3)–(5) above) proved to be the crucial cue which blocks a word order strategy in German. As soon as a child has mastered the principles governing the distribution of the finite verb, she has recognized that the sentence-initial position is not a functionally unique one, i.e. not the subject position. Typically developing children are able to handle the distribution of the finite verb properly at the age of three. So, already the four-year old children were successful in about 80% of the reversible passive test sentences.

In languages like English, word order is a direct reflex of the structural coding of grammatical relations. This situation must be distinguished strictly from the tendency of the subject to occur in sentence-initial position in free order languages. In German, this is just one variant among other grammatically equivalent variants (cf. (4a) vs. (4b–d)). However, it is the preferred variant in an unmarked situation like the one in the test, in which each of the test clauses was presented out of context. This preference is the combinatorial result of various factors, including pragmatic ones. The many mistakes with the active test sentences seem to result from this preference. The oldest control children at the age of four and five behaved much like Kathy, as Table 1 shows. They achieve their poorest results with active sentences like (11a) by misinterpreting the first NP as the subject in 50% of these cases. So, it seems that the expectation to find the subject in a pragmatically unmarked position, namely in the sentence-initial position, overrides conflicting cues, i.e. the presence of a NOM-marked clause internal noun phrase (e.g. *der Bub* in (11)), which necessitate a revision of the preliminary interpretation. This shows that pragmatic factors like marked patterns of word order provoke more mistakes than unmarked ones. Obviously, the specific test situation is equally responsible for the bad results with these marked active sentences, since test sentences are presented in isolation and therefore the unmarked order is expected (since there is no context that legitimates the marked information structure). Even in German-speaking adults, an increased tendency to accidentally misinterpret an unmarked noun phrase in initial position as subject can be observed under circumstances like these (cf. Bayer, de Bleser, & Dronsek 1987).

*Pronominal dependency test*

Kathy's results were generally poor, both for simple sentences and sentences with infinitival complements, with a ratio of correct answers less than 35%, in each case. Quantitatively her scores were far behind those of the youngest group of six-year old typically developing children tested in the original investigation of Schaner-Wolles and Haider (1987). Although they had problems with the tasks as well, they were successful in at least 60%. The 80% level of correct answers was not reached before the age of seven. It turns out that Kathy's main difficulties concerned the interpretation of reflexives vs. personal pronouns. She was not able to apply the grammatical constraints on coreference relations between pronouns and their antecedents yet – neither in clauses with infinitival complements, nor in simple clauses.

A qualitative analysis shows that she does not apply a minimal distance strategy for the interpretation of the PRO subject, as it is known from children acquiring English. In English, a language with strict word order, children tend to choose the nearest NP as the controller of the silent subject of the infinitival clause (cf. Sherman & Lust 1986) and thereby overgeneralize the pattern of object control verbs. This strategy is known as the *minimal distance principle* (MDP). According to the MDP, English-speaking children will systematically misinterpret subject control contexts (cf. (12b)), and at the same time, they will be successful in object control contexts (cf. (12a)). For example, they will decide on *Mary* to be the controller of PRO in both contexts (12a) and (12b).

(12) a. Paul told Mary [PRO to leave]
b. Paul promised Mary [PRO to leave]

Since German is a verb second language with free word order, MDP would not be a reliable strategy, and German does not mislead a learner to assume a positional strategy. German-speaking children do not apply this strategy, nor does Kathy. What this indicates at least is that she does not overgeneralize a positional strategy but follows the same pattern as typically developing children.

### 3.3 Interim conclusions of the WS case study

Two aspects of Kathy's linguistic profile are worth re-emphasizing. First, her command of passive is perfect. Since this was tested with a sentence-picture matching task, this shows that sentence-picture matching does not imply specific inherent difficulties per se for WS individuals, contrary to what Karmiloff-Smith et al. (1998) hypothesize.[4]

Second, the results of binding and control in the pronominal dependency test are clearly behind age equivalent typically developing children. Since, in the study by Clahsen and Almazan (1998), syntactic binding was no problem for two English-speaking WS girls with nearly the same chronological and mental age as Kathy, it is not sufficiently clear yet whether Kathy's results reflect a particular difficulty of the test or a difficulty of the tested linguistic phenomenon, or both. A difficulty of the test could be the length and complexity of the test sentences. A difficulty of the phenomena may be the computing of the interaction of a rule of interpretation on the one hand (interpretation of pronouns and of PRO) and an obligatory (for reflexives) or conditioned (for pronouns) grammatical dependency relation on the other hand.

Further research will be necessary here.

## 4. The Vienna Down syndrome project[5]

The results reported here are part of a cross-sectional study on the language abilities of German-speaking children, adolescents and adults with Down syndrome (DS) that started some fifteen years ago. A comprehensive language test battery consisting of 24 subtests was assembled. The subtests cover the relevant language components namely phonology, morphology, syntax, semantics, lexicon and the textual level. Moreover, the components are tested in different modalities, in the sense that there are subtests on comprehension, imitation and spontaneous production. In the next sections, I will refer to results of the sentence repetition tasks only. For various reasons it seems justified to concentrate exclusively on imitative productions here. First of all, it turned out that for the grammatical aspects under consideration, imitative and spontaneous productions do not differ. Moreover, the data base of the sentence repetition tasks is larger and suitably arranged for comparison among subjects. The data of spontaneous sentence productions are less homogeneous, for obvious reasons.

But before going into detailed results of the sentence repetition tasks, it seems worthwhile to summarize some of the main general findings of the study:

1. No *qualitative* differences in terms of the linguistic inventory and processes were established between the DS and the typically developing groups, in looking at each subtest type separately. The development per linguistic subcomponent is delayed in DS, but not deviant.
2. However, comparisons of the results from different subtests with each other demonstrated asynchronies in the acquisition of various components of the language system. It turned out that delays are not uniform across domains, but greater in some domains than in others. What we have found in DS is therefore best characterized as an asynchronous or disharmonious language delay. So, the overall language of an individual with DS will never be fully parallel to the language of one particular typically developing child, even not of a younger one.
3. As it was attested for other languages in other studies too, it turned out that morphological and morphosyntactic skills are the most deficient ones in our

German-speaking DS subjects. This supports the hypothesis "*that the vast majority of persons with Down syndrome suffer from a specific deficit that interferes more with the acquisition of grammatical morphemes than with the mastery of basic sentence structures*" (Rosenberg & Abbeduto 1993:91–92).

This is exactly what our data show: the individuals with DS have a lot of problems with morphology in general and they are doing worse on morphosyntax. As was attested in individuals with WS (cf. Clahsen & Almazan 1998), there is a discrepancy between regular and irregular morphology in DS as well. For example, they are doing much better on the regular comparative marking of adjectives than on the fairly irregular plural marking of nouns in German – despite of the inverse cognitive complexity of comparative and plurality.

Highly relevant in this respect are the data concerning verbal morphology, subject-verb agreement and verb placement, on which I will focus in the following.

### 4.1 Method – Sentence repetition tasks

*Participants*

Eighty-two individuals with Down syndrome of the standard trisomy 21 type participated in this study. There were forty-five male and thirty-seven female participants. Their chronological age ranged from 7;3 to 41;10 years (M = 17;0, SD = 9;3). Their full scale mental age measured by the German version of the Stanford-Binet Intelligence Test S-I-T (Terman & Merrill 1965), ranged from 2;5 to 7;4 years (M = 4;11, SD = 1;3). Four mental age groups with approximately the same number of individuals have been assembled: MA1 (n = 21) 2;5–3;11 years, MA2 (n = 19) 4;0–4;11 years, MA3 (n = 23) 5;0–5;11 years, and MA4 (n = 19) 6;0–7;4 years. Forty typically developing children (twenty males, twenty females) aged between 2;3 and 6;6 years (M = 4;1, SD = 1;3) formed the control group. They have been grouped into the following four age groups: A1 (n = 10) 2;3–2;11 years, A2 (n = 10) 3;0–3;11 years, A3 (n = 10) 4;0–4;11 years, and A4 (n = 10) 5;0–6;6 years. All the control children attended a kindergarten. The DS children went to special schools for intellectually disabled children; the adults spent the day in special workshops. All participants, both DS and controls, were monolingual speakers of German and lived at home with their own families.

*Materials*

The language test battery included four sentence imitation subtests which examine the ability to repeat sentences of different length and complexity. Participants had to repeat a total amount of fifty-two sentences, ranging from very short, simple sentence like those under (13a–d) to quite long, more complex ones, as under (13e–f).

| (13) | a. | Mama schläft | mommy sleeps | *'mommy is sleeping'* |
|---|---|---|---|---|
| | b. | der Bub läuft | the boy runs | *'the boy is running'* |
| | c. | Papa hat Hunger | daddy has hunger | *'daddy is hungry'* |
| | d. | sie ist müde | she is tired | *'she is tired'* |

e. die Mutter schenkt der Tochter
the:FEM:NOM mother gives the:FEM:DAT daughter
eine Puppe
a:FEM:ACC doll

f. im Park kauft die Mutter dem Kind
in the:MASC:DAT park buys the:FEM:NOM mother the:NEUT:DAT
ein Eis
a:NEUT:ACC ice-cream
*'in the park, the mother buys the child an ice-cream'*

*Procedure*

The language testing took place in the kindergarten, the school or the workshop which the subjects were visiting, i.e. in a familiar environment. All participants were tested individually in a quiet room. Administration of the four subtests was done in four sessions of about half an hour each in the course of one week as part of the comprehensive language test battery. Subtests as well as test sentences were presented in a fixed order, with increasing sentence complexity within each test session. The test procedure was the same for each participant. The experimenter introduced the repetition tasks as a kind of parrot game, saying something like 'Listen very carefully. I will say something and when I am ready you have to repeat just what I said. Say everything what I say. Can you say ...'. Most participants had no problem to understand the task, but some of them were hardly to be talked out of shadowing immediately. Reactions of this kind were excluded as not analyzable. All responses were audio taped, transcribed and double-checked before they were analysed.

## 4.2 Results and discussion

*Global characterization of the reactions*

It seems worthwhile to have a brief look at the global reaction patterns first. Three main types of imitations have been differentiated: (a) *verbatim imitation* of the test sentence, (b) *imitation with changes*, i.e. non-verbatim repetitions with omissions and/or all sorts of changes or mistakes (including ungrammatical serializations, missing or wrong agreement, etc.), and (c) *no answer* (also including repetitions of the last syllable or last word of the test sentence only, shadowed imitations, and

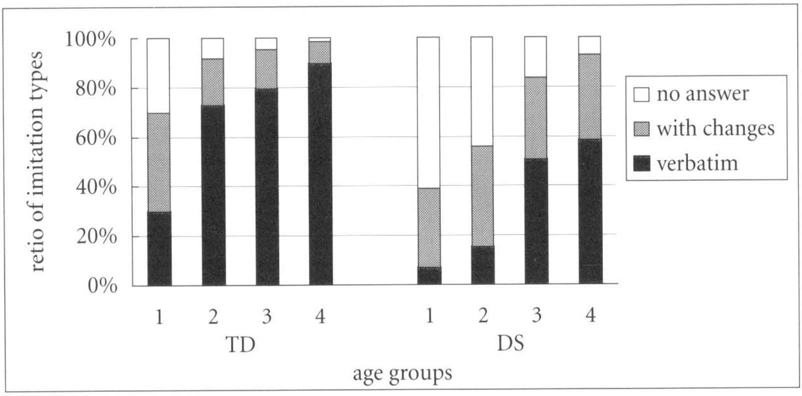


**Figure 1.** Distribution of participant's types of imitation, by group TD (typically developing children) – DS (Down syndrome), and (mental) age group

unintelligible reactions). Figure 1 shows the distribution of these types of imitation for each of the (mental) age groups in the typically developing group (TD) and the Down syndrome group (DS).

In general, the ratio of verbatim repetitions is significantly lower in DS than in TD. t-Tests indicated that the DS and TD groups differed at each age (for all t-tests $p < .05$). Especially DS subjects of the first mental age group often failed completely, and were repeating only the last syllable or the last word of the test sentence – especially with longer sentences. Within DS the two lower age groups were significantly behind age groups 3 and 4 with respect to correct verbatim repetitions (t-tests $p < .05$). The ratio of repetitions with changes, on the other hand, stays nearly constant across the age groups in DS (t-tests $p > .05$). Even in the higher age groups, more than one third of the answers were of this category. In the group of typically developing children, non-verbatim repetitions are diminishing with age.

In further analysis, the non-verbatim repetitions were scanned for different types of changes. In the next sections, I will deal with some types of omissions, ungrammatical serializations, and missing or wrong agreement markers more closely. Different mistakes of this kind may, of course, co-occur in one answer.

Viewed from the vantage point of modular organization of grammar, the general impression of the poor behavior of the DS group might be misleading. It does not necessarily reflect an equally general deficit in each of the components of grammar. It is much more plausible to assume that the overall picture reflects the combinatorial effects of the interaction of components of grammar, some of which are more and some of which are less developed, according to the general patterns of development in language acquisition. Since the overall language output depends on successful interaction among the components, small differences in one of the components multiplied into apparently gross differences on the surface. These have not to correspond to gross differences in any of the components per se. The next sections will illustrate these issues on the basis of an analysis of (a) the subject-verb agreement and verb placement data, and (b) the omission patterns.

Moreover, it is likely that domain-general cognitive abilities may have affected the results as well. In a comparative study, Marcell, Ridgeway, Sewell and Whelan (1995) compared the sentence imitation performance of adolescents and young adults with DS with that of age- and IQ-matched non-DS individuals with other causes of intellectual disability (ID). It turned out, that the DS sentence repetition accuracy was equivalent to the ID group only for two-word sentences and was poorer for every other sentence length. Sentence imitation was related to grammatical comprehension, auditory short-term memory and IQ in both groups. In our data, the DS group with the lowest mental age showed more severe difficulties with sentences longer than two or three words as well. The prevalence of the category 'no answer' in this group is the result of the fact that they often failed completely with longer, and more complex sentences. In comparing the results according to the complexity of the test sentences, it became clear that only individuals with a lower mental age (i.e. in the MA1 and MA2 groups with MA < 5 years) are concerned. Table B in the appendix displays the mean percentages of 'no answer' according to sentence complexity and mental age groups. Indeed our subjects did much better in dealing with the repetition of even longer sentences than expected on the basis of the low auditory short-term memory spans.

*Verbal morphology, subject-verb agreement, and verb placement*

As discussed earlier, German is a verb second language with great superficial freedom of clause internal word order. The verb second position is a derived position. As for the acquisition of these properties, German is a root infinitive language. Notwithstanding massive counterevidence from different children (e.g. Clahsen & Penke 1992; Fritzenschaft, Gawlitzek-Maiwald, Tracy, & Winkler 1990; Schaner-Wolles 1994), it is nevertheless a widely accepted view that children during the so-called root infinitive stage place non-finite verbs at the end of the clause and finite verbs into the verb second position. It has been claimed that the finiteness morphology is the trigger for verb movement (cf. e.g. Poeppel & Wexler 1993). However, there is an indisputable case of a verb second language that does not display any finiteness morphology on the verb al all. This is Afrikaans. In this language, verb second cannot be ascribed to a property that distinguishes between morphological identifiable verbal elements. Hence, on the level of grammar theory, the verb second property can be captured in purely structural terms. This property must be acquired by Afrikaans-speaking children on purely structural grounds without any morphological cues.

Table 2. Subtests 'sentence repetition': verb positions and verb forms

| | | Down syndrome | | Controls | |
|---|---|---|---|---|---|
| *Vfinal | [marked finite] | 13 | (0.7) | 5 | (0.3) |
| Vfinal | [marked non-finite] | 15 | (0.9) | 1 | (0.1) |
| *V2 | [marked non-finite] | **138** | **(7.8)** | 15 | (1.0) |
| V2 | [marked finite] | 1600 | (90.6) | 1436 | (98.6) |
| Total | | 1766 | (100.0) | 1457 | (100.0) |

This is precisely what some of the DS subjects do. In Table 2, the data of the sentence repetition task have been classified according to the four patterns: (1) finite verb in final position; (2) verb in final position without finiteness/agreement marking; (3) verb in second position without finiteness/agreement marking; and (4) finite verb in second position. In adult German, pattern (1) is typical for embedded clauses, and pattern (4) is the declarative main clause pattern. In the unimpaired acquisition of German, pattern (2) is claimed to be typical at the root infinitive stage. Contrary to prevalent claims in the literature (cf. e.g. Poeppel & Wexler 1993), pattern (3) is attested in the data of individual typically developing German children at this stage as well, as mentioned before (cf. e.g. Schaner-Wolles 1994).

Only unambiguous verb second utterances have been counted as verb second structures here. Undecidable utterances, that is, simple sentences consisting of just the verb and a single preceding constituent have been omitted here. Such structures would simultaneously qualify as possible verb second and verb final structures.

What is most remarkable in Table 2 is the high frequency of the verb second pattern in the DS data. They perform as well as the controls: The proportions of verb second structures out of all unambiguous answers are 98.4% for the DS group and 99.6% for the control group. The second remarkable result in Table 2 is the relatively high frequency of non-finite marked verbs in second position in the DS data. Typically developing children demonstrate this pattern only in 15 cases – all of these are from six two-year old children at a syntactically less advanced level (cf. examples in (14)).

(14) a. Papa fahren weg papa drive:INF away *'papa is driving away'*
b. Bub haben Ball boy have:INF ball *'the boy has a ball'*
c. Mama geh weg mom go:STEM away *'mom is going away'*

DS subjects are not only using this pattern more frequently (cf. examples in (15)). They are using it in syntactically more complex answers as well, as (15c, d) show.

(15) a. Mama gehen weg mom go:INF away
b. Vogel flieg weg bird fly:STEM away

| | | |
|---|---|---|
| c. | die Mutter schenken Tochter die Puppe | the mother give:INF daughter the puppet |
| d. | die Puppe sitz auf dem Sessel | the puppet sit:STEM on the chair |

It is worth emphasizing that the pattern in (14) and (15) is a correct serialization pattern with respect to verb placement in main clauses in German. What is missing in the examples in (14) and (15) is just the verbal ending that is the finiteness/agreement marker. Given the persistent problems with morphology and morphosyntax in DS, these non marked verb forms do not wonder. Figure 2 shows this distribution of finite and non-finite marked verb forms across the four age groups in the typically developing children and in the individuals with Down syndrome. It is striking how parallel they are. Since wrong serializations of the verb, like placing it in non-second position, do not occur in any significant number in the DS material either, this indicates that DS subjects are able to master the rule for verb placement without having access to or using the morphological distinctions.

Clear evidence for the fact that DS subjects manage the two complementary positions for the verb comes from utterances with verb-participle combinations, like the examples (15a–b). Lexically, the particle is a prefixed part of the verb. In the syntactic structure, however, the particle is stranded when the verb is fronted (cf. (3c)). The fact that verb particles are stranded precisely when the verb is in second position clearly shows that the individuals with DS are able to master some of the intricacies of the German verb second rule without being aware of the concomitant morphological distinctions. Hence the morphological distinctions cannot be seen as the exclusive trigger of the verb second structure. Data from omissions discussed in the next section support this point.

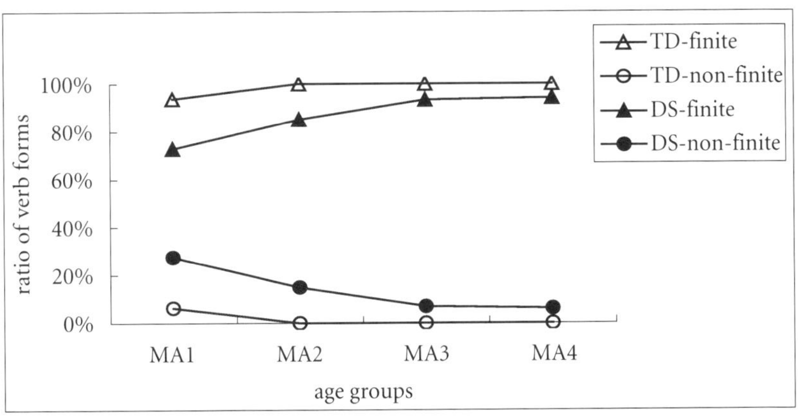


**Figure 2.** Distribution of verb forms by age groups for DS and TD

*Omissions*
That individuals with DS are aware of structural properties of a clause is demonstrated in their omission patterns, too. In repeating the test sentences, the participants with DS as well as the typically developing children made a lot of omissions. There is no qualitative difference in the omission patterns of the two populations. Function words like articles, auxiliaries, prepositions and pronouns tend to be omitted frequently – both in the younger control children and in the individuals with DS. Figure 3 shows the percentages of dropped arguments in both populations. For obvious reasons, obligatory arguments (i.e. subjects and part of the accusative objects) and optional arguments (i.e. some accusative objects and all dative objects) are separated in Figure 3. In fact, there are neither statistically significant differences (all $p > .05$) nor qualitative differences between both populations.

Figure 4 shows the mean percentages of imitated phrases (nominative, accusative, and dative phrases) across the different age groups for typically developing children (TD) and individuals with DS. The developmental paths are parallel for both populations. The results of the individuals with DS are staying behind the typically developing children in the first two mental age groups only. From MA3 on, i.e. from a mental age of five years on, the DS have caught up with the typically developing children for the most part. Exclusively for the dative phrases, they are still lagging behind. The same pattern shows up in the younger TD children as well. It need not surprise that the datives turned out to be the most popular candidates for omission: the dative phrases in the test were exclusively optional arguments, which moreover occurred only in the longer test sentences.

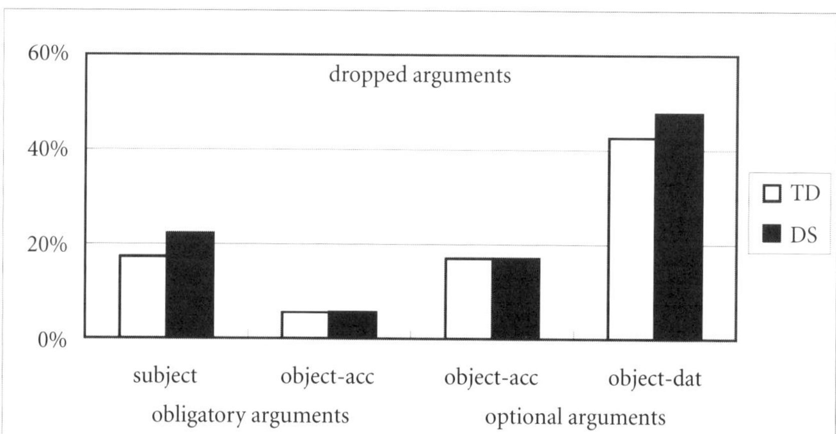


**Figure 3.** Percentages of dropped arguments for typically developing children (TD) and individuals with Down syndrome (DS)

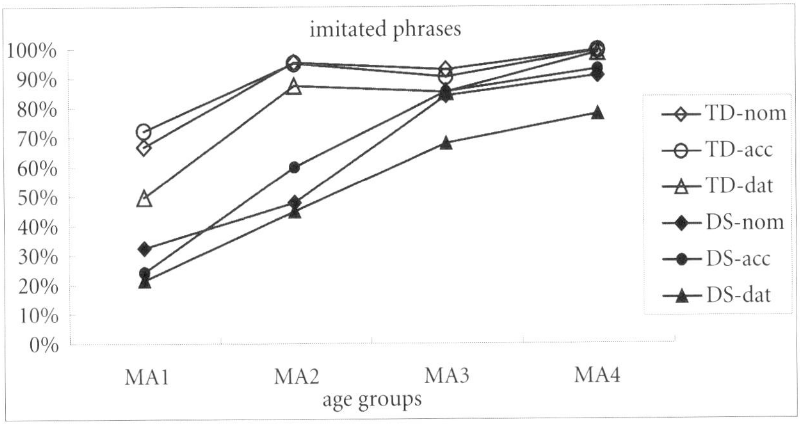


**Figure 4.** Mean percentages of imitated phrases (nominative, accusative, and dative phrases) across age groups for typically developing children (TD) and individuals with DS

A remarkable feature of the omission patterns in the DS data is the fact that omissions of whole phrases lead to restructuring in order to restore the serialization restrictions. If the initial constituent of the sentence was omitted, it was in most cases replaced by another constituent of the clause in order to restore the verb second requirement. Examples of restructuring out of the DS data are given under (16). For comparison, an ungrammatical answer without restructuring of a control child aged 2;10 is given in (17).

(16) a. das Mädchen holt einen Teller → Teller holt sie
the:NEUT:NOM girl takes a:MASC:ACC plate — plate takes she (correct in German)
'*the girl is taking a plate*'
b. Heute bleibt der Bub zu Hause → der Bub bleibt zu Hause
today stays the:MASC:NOM boy at home — the boy stays at home
'*today, the boy is staying at home*'

(17) Heute bleibt der Bub zu Hause → *bleibt der Bub zu Hause
today stays the:MASC:NOM boy at home — stays the boy at home
'*today, the boy is staying at home*'

If the DSs are able to restore the grammatical pattern, this reflects the mastering of some of the essential syntactic principles that govern the well-formedness of a German clause.

### 4.3 Interim conclusions of the DS study

Inflection and verb placement in German reflect the modular interaction between syntax and morphology. However, contrary to a widespread belief, there is good evidence that the acquisition of verb second is not necessarily dependent on morphological features attached to functional positions in the sentence structures. The morphological distinction reflects a structural relation. It identifies the structurally most prominent verbal element. The morphological distinctions provide cues for the identification of the relevant element, but they cannot be the unique trigger of the verb second phenomenon in the acquisition process, as the DS data show.

The data from DS provide clear evidence for a discrepancy between the acquisition of the morphological distinctions – and consequently of the subject-verb agreement marking – on the one hand, and the distributional regularities of verb placement on the other. The verb placement regularity is mastered despite severe limitations in the acquisition of the finiteness morphology and in the morphosyntactic abilities.

The results are in line with the view that individuals with DS have specific difficulties with grammatical morphology and morphosyntax, and fewer problems with the mastering of basic sentence structures (Chapman et al. 1992; Rosenberg & Abbeduto 1993). They contradict Fowler's (1990) assumption that there is a primary deficit in syntax and a ceiling on rudimentary syntactic development in DS. Our study shows that the vast majority of individuals with DS is quite successful in mastering the basic sentence structures and argument structures. Moreover, even the adults with DS showed continuing syntactic development. This did not only turn out in the analyses of our data according to chronological age, but also in the tailor-made language training programs that were carried out in the course of the project. For space reasons, I cannot go into detail here. It turned out that especially the adolescents and adults with DS benefited a lot from this language training.

To put it in a nutshell, the primary deficits in the expressive language of DS are most likely located in the morphological and morphosyntactic subcomponents. The apparently deviant grammatical behavior in DS is the result of the modular interaction of non-deviant developmental patterns in each of the interacting modules. It is the *asynchronous* acquisition of morphological and distributional regularities that produces results that look deviant in comparison to typical acquisition. Upon closer scrutiny, however, the very same patterns can be found, with much lower frequency though, in the data of typically developing children as well.

## 5. General conclusions

If analysed systematically, DS and WS provide evidence for a relatively spared language faculty within an ensemble of partially low-level non-linguistic cognitive capacities. Moreover, within-language dissociations are characteristic of both syndromes. That means that certain verbal abilities develop at a faster rate than others, possibly with the existence of delays which cannot catch up on.

As for the syntactic and morphosyntactic components of grammar, common patterns became evident in both syndromes, and these patterns are attested for typically developing children as well. The general structure of the within-language dissociations are of the same kind for both syndromes: Once the analysis is focused on the level of the relevant modules rather than on the general overall impressions, differences between the grammatical abilities in DS and in WS turn out to be quantitative rather than qualitative, or relative rather than absolute.

The syntactic structure component, as well as syntactic features of the lexicon and the argument structure, are relatively spared in both DS and WS. But each group has difficulties with grammatical dependency relations: for DS, all types of grammatical dependency relations are clearly difficult. This is not only true for the agreement relation between the finite verb and the subject, but also for NP internal agreement. This gives rise to even more pronounced and persistent problems in German, since determiners and adjectives have to agree with the head noun in gender, number, and case; and as mentioned before, there is a lot of syncretism in the paradigms, as exemplified for the definite article in Table A in the appendix.

Individuals with WS on the other hand seem to handle grammatical dependency relations more easily. However, less pronounced difficulties may nevertheless persist in these areas as well, as some studies have reported before (cf. Karmiloff-Smith, Grant, Berthoud, Davies, Howlin, & Udwin 1997; Pezzini et al. 1994; Volterra et al. 1996; and Schaner-Wolles 2000a for a discussion). The WS girl studied here had the same difficulties with more complex dependency relations (interaction of binding and control) as typically developing children have before the age of about seven.

Both in DS and WS, the patterns of errors in grammar are within the range of the patterns of typical language acquisition: the same types occur, but with higher frequency and longer persistence. In all, these findings suggest that the individual sequence of the grammatical development is fairly uniform for all three groups, DS, WS, and typically developing children. At least from the point of view of the grammatical development, there is no evidence in support for Vicari, Caselli, Gagliardi, Tonucci and Volterra's (2002) assumption that "[...] *the two syndromes develop differently along distinct trajectories*".

This notwithstanding, individuals with DS are more delayed in their overall language development than individuals with WS, and they are more out of step with particular linguistic subcomponents, such as grammatical morphology and morphosyntax, than it is the case in WS. So, having put the emphasis on the relatively spared language faculty in both syndromes so far, a crucial question remains to be answered: *What accounts for the difference between the linguistic behavior in DS and WS?*

This question concerns the influence of other cognitive capacities on the developmental process of language acquisition. As touched upon in the introduction, there is much to be said for the verbal short-term memory as one crucial factor in this connection. Verbal short-term memory is a particular strength in WS, and an area of particular weakness or selective impairment in DS (cf. Wang & Bellugi 1994; Vicari et al. 1996; Karmiloff-Smith et al. 1997; Jarrold et al. 1999, 2001).

Such syndrome-specific cognitive limitations may deprive the language faculty of the necessary support for getting a tight grasp on grammar. As demonstrated above, they may affect specific subcomponents to a different extent. Thus, the submodules of grammar show module-specific, differential delays, and develop at different rates, i.e. in an *asynchronously delayed* way. This results in within-domain dissociations. Given that such limitations prevent the learner from passing a certain stage in one of the submodules of grammar, this has overall consequences for the whole system. The causal effect is local, however. One might want to call this local difference a qualitative difference, in the sense that typically developing children do pass this level at which individuals with DS or WS stagnate. Even if this ceiling effect shows "*that WS language follows a different path to normal acquisition* [...]" (Karmiloff-Smith et al. 1997:258), it does not warrant the conclusion that the underlying system of grammar is qualitatively different. In terms of inventory and processes, the system components have the same features one finds at various stages of typical development. On the local level of components, the patterns of acquisition do not differ from typical development. It is the developmentally asynchronous assembly of components that gives rise to a linguistic profile that appears to be qualitatively different. But the different quality is not significant in itself, once one understands its origin. The asynchrony is not caused by the linguistic system itself. It is an epiphenomenon of the embedding of the linguistic system in an atypical general cognitive environment.

## Acknowledgments

I am very grateful to all the participants who took part in the studies reported here, to their parents, and to the staffs of the schools and kindergartens where the investigations were done. I would also like to thank two anonymous reviewers, the audience of the ISES2 conference in May 2002 at the University of Potsdam, and Hubert Haider for helpful comments and suggestions. The responsibility for remaining shortcomings is of course mine.

## Notes

1. See Schaner-Wolles (2001) for a description of the plural test and results of typically developing children.

2. Cf. Schaner-Wolles (2001) for a more detailed discussion, and arguments against the proposals of Clahsen, Rothweiler, Woest, and Marcus (1992) about the German plural system and its acquisition, who claim *-s* to be a default plural marker.

3. If one of the two arguments is ambiguously case-marked (e.g. *sie* in (5a)), the other one is unambiguously case-marked (*er* in (5a)), guaranteeing an effective inference on the actual case of the ambiguously case-marked one.

4. Cf. Karmiloff-Smith et al. (1998:347): "*The sentence-picture matching task revealed an across-the board impairment.* [...] *In the sentence-picture matching task, for example, the participant has to listen to and decode the sentence, maintain it in their memory (when it is spoken), process the pictures and compare the sentence to each one of the pictures, eventually selecting the one that best matches.* [...] *Because WS individuals have clear cognitive impairments, tasks which rely heavily upon general cognitive abilities may overestimate the extent of the linguistic impairment.*"

5. This project has been funded by grants (no. P3632 and P5517) of the Austrian Science Fund (FWF).

## References


Baddeley, A. D., Gathercole, S. E., & Papagno, C. (1998). "The phonological loop as a language learning device". *Psychological Review, 105*, 158–173.

Bates, E. & Goodman, J. C. (1999). "On the emergence of grammar from the lexicon". In B. MacWhinney (Ed.), *The Emergence of Language* (pp. 29–79). Mahwah, NJ: LEA.

Bayer, J., de Bleser, R., & Dronsek, C. (1987). "Form und Funktion von Kasus bei Agrammatismus". In J. Bayer (Ed.), *Grammatik und Kognition. Psycholinguistische Untersuchungen* (pp. 81–117). Opladen: Westdeutscher Verlag.

Bellugi, U., Bihrle, A., Neville, H., Doherty, S., & Jernigan, T. (1992). "Language, cognition, and brain organization in a neurodevelopmental disorder". In M. R. Gunnar & C. A. Nelson (Eds.), *Developmental Behavioral Neuroscience* [The Minnesota Symposia on Child Psychology, Vol. 24] (pp. 201–232). Hillsdale, NJ: LEA.

Bellugi, U., Wang, P. P., & Jernigan, T. L. (1994). "Williams syndrome: An unusual neuropsychological profile". In S. H. Broman & J. Grafman (Eds.), *Atypical Cognitive Deficits in Developmental Disorders: Implications for brain functions* (pp. 23–56). Hillsdale, NJ: LEA.

Bever, T. G. (1970). "The cognitive basis for linguistic structures". In J. R. Hayes (Ed.), *Cognition and the Development of Language* (pp. 279–362). New York, NY: Wiley.

Bromberg, H., Ullman, M., Marcus, G., Kelly, K., & Coppola, M. (1994). "A Discussion of Memory and Grammar: Evidence from Williams syndrome". Talk at the 18th Annual Boston University Conference on Language Development, Nov. 1994.

Chapman, R. S. (1995). "Language development in children and adolescents with Down Syndrome". In P. Fletcher & B. MacWhinney (Eds.), *The Handbook of Child Language* (pp. 641–663). Oxford: Blackwell.

Chapman, R. S. & Hesketh, L. J. (2001). "Language, cognition, and short-term memory in individuals with Down syndrome". *Down's Syndrome: Research Practice, 7*(1), 1–7.

Clahsen, H., Rothweiler, M., Woest, A., & Marcus, G. F. (1992). "Regular versus irregular inflection in the acquisition of German noun plurals". *Cognition, 45*, 225–255.

Clahsen, H. & Almazan, M. (1998). "Syntax and morphology in Williams syndrome". *Cognition, 68*, 167–198.

Clahsen, H. & Almazan, M. (2001). "Compounding and inflection in language impairment: Evidence from Williams Syndrome (and SLI)". *Lingua, 111*, 729–757.

Clahsen, H. & Penke, M. (1992). "The acquisition of agreement morphology and its syntactic consequences: New evidence on German Child Language from the Simone-corpus". In J. M. Meisel (Ed.), *The Acquisition of Verb Placement: Functional categories and V2 phenomena in language acquisition* (pp. 181–223). Dordrecht: Kluwer.

Fowler, A. (1988). "Determinants of rate of language growth in children with Down syndrome". In Lynn Nadel (Ed.), *The Psychobiology of Down Syndrome* (pp. 217–245). Cambridge, MA: The MIT Press.

Fowler, A. (1990). "Language abilities of children with Down syndrome: Evidence for a specific syntactic delay". In D. Cicchetti & M. Beeghly (Eds.), *Children with Down Syndrome: A developmental perspective* (pp. 302–328). Cambridge: CUP.

Fritzenschaft, A., Gawlitzek-Maiwald, I., Tracy, R., & Winkler, S. (1990). "Wege zur komplexen Syntax". *Zeitschrift für Sprachwissenschaft, 9*, 52–134.

Gathercole, S. E. & Baddeley, A. D. (1990). "Phonological memory deficits in language disordered children: Is there a causal connection?" *Journal of Memory and Language, 29*, 336–360.

Grant, J., Valian, V., & Karmiloff-Smith, A. (2002). "A study of relative clauses in Williams syndrome". *Journal of Child Language, 29*(2), 403–416.

Jarrold, C., Baddeley, A. D., & Hewes, A. K. (1999). "Genetically dissociated components of working memory: Evidence from Down's and Williams syndrome". *Neuropsychologia, 37*(6), 637–651.

Jarrold, C. & Baddeley, A. D. (2001). "Short-term memory in Down syndrome: Applying the working memory model". *Down Syndrome Research and Practice, 7*(1), 17–23.

Karmiloff-Smith, A., Grant, J., Berthoud, I., Davies, M., Howlin, P., & Udwin, O. (1997). "Language and Williams syndrome: How intact is 'intact'?" *Child Development, 68*(2), 246–262.

Karmiloff-Smith, A., Tyler, L. K., Voice, K., Sims, K., Udwin, O., Howlin, P., & Davies, M. (1998). "Linguistic dissociations in Williams syndrome: Evaluating receptive syntax in on-line and off-line tasks". *Neuropsychologia, 36*(4), 343–351.

Koster, J. (1987). *Domains and Dynasties: The radical autonomy of syntax*. Dordrecht: Foris.

Krause, M. & Penke, M. (2001). "Inflectional morphology in German Williams syndrome". *Brain and Cognition, 48*(2–3), 410–413.

Lukács, Á., Racsmány, M., & Pléh, C. (2001). "Vocabulary and morphological patterns in Hungarian children with Williams syndrome: A preliminary report". *Acta Linguistica Hungarica, 48*(1–3), 243–269.

MacWhinney, B. (Ed.). (1999). *The Emergence of Language*. Mahwah, NJ: LEA.

Marcell, M. M, Ridgeway, M. M., Sewell, D. H., & Whelan, M. L. (1995). "Sentence imitation by adolescents and young adults with Down's syndrome and other intellectual disabilities". *Journal of Intellectual Disability Research, 39*(3), 215–232.

Miller, J. F. (1988). "The developmental asynchrony of language development in children with Down syndrome". In L. Nadel (Ed.), *The Psychobiology of Down syndrome* (pp. 167–198). Cambridge, MA: The MIT Press.

Miller, J. F. (1996). "The search for the phenotype of disordered language performance". In M. L. Rice (Ed.), *Toward a Genetics of Language* (pp. 297–314). Mahwah, NJ: LEA.

Neeleman, A. & van de Koot, H. (2002). "The configurational matrix." *Linguistic Inquiry, 33*(4), 529–574.

Pezzini, G., Volterra, V., Ossella, M. T., & Sabbadini, L. (1994). "Le abilità linguistiche". In A. Giannotti & S. Vicari (Eds.), *Il Bambino con sindrome di Williams* (pp. 95–117). Milano: Franco Angeli.

Pléh, C., Lukács, Á., & Racsmány, M. (2003). "Morphological patterns in Hungarian children with Williams syndrome and the rules debates". To appear in *Brain and Language*.

Poeppel, D. & Wexler, K. (1993). "The full competence hypothesis of clause structure in early German". *Language, 69*, 1–33.

Racsmány, M., Lukács, Á., Pléh, C., & Király, I. (2001). "Some cognitive tools for word learning: The role of working memory and goal preference". *Behavioral and Brain Sciences, 24*(6), 1115–1117.

Rondal, J. A. (1995). *Exceptional Language Development in Down Syndrome. Implications for the cognition-language relationship*. Cambridge: CUP.

Rosenberg, S. & Abbeduto, L. (1993). *Language and Communication in Mental Retardation. Development, processes, and intervention*. Hillsdale, NJ: LEA.

Rossen, M. L., Klima, E. S., Bellugi, U., Bihrle, A., & Jones, W. (1996). "Interaction between language and cognition: Evidence from Williams syndrome". In J. H. Beitchman, N. Cohen, M. Konstantareas, & R. Tannock (Eds.), *Language, Learning, and Behavior Disorders: Developmental, biological and clinical perspectives* (pp. 367–392). New York: CUP.

Sabbagh, M. A. & Gelman, S. A. (2000). "Buzzsaws and blueprints: What children need (or don't need) to learn language. Review essay on: Brian MacWhinney (Ed.), (1999). *The emergence of language*. Mahwah, NJ: LEA." *Journal of Child Language, 27*(3), 715–726.

Schaner-Wolles, C. (1989). "Strategies in acquiring grammatical relations in German: Word order or case marking?" *Folia Linguistica, 23*(1–2), 131–156.

Schaner-Wolles, C. (1994). "Intermodular synchronization: On the role of morphology in the normal and impaired acquisition of a verb-second language". In R. Tracy & E. Lattey (Eds.), *How Tolerant is Universal grammar? Essays on language learnability and language variation* (pp. 205–224). Tübingen: Niemeyer.

Schaner-Wolles, C. (2000a). "Within-language dissociations in mental retardation: Williams-Beuren and Down syndrome". In S. C. Howell, S. A. Fish, & T. Keith-Lucas (Eds.), *Proceedings of the 24th Annual Boston University Conference on Language Development*, (pp. 633–644). Somerville, MA: Cascadilla Press.

Schaner-Wolles, C. (2000b). "Sprachentwicklung bei geistiger Retardierung: Williams-Beuren-Syndrom und Down-Syndrom". In Hannelore Grimm (Ed.), *Sprachentwicklung. Enzyklopädie der Psychologie, Vol IIIC3* (pp. 663–685). Göttingen: Hogrefe.

Schaner-Wolles, C. (2001). "On the acquisition of noun plurals in German". In C. Schaner-Wolles, J. Rennison, & F. Neubarth (Eds.), *Naturally! Linguistic studies in honour of Wolfgang Ulrich Dressler presented on the occasion of his 60th birthday* (pp. 451–460). Torino: Rosenberg and Sellier.

Schaner-Wolles, C. & Haider, H. (1987). "Spracherwerb und Kognition – Eine Studie über interpretative Relationen". In J. Bayer (Ed.), *Grammatik und Kognition. Psycholinguistische Untersuchungen* (pp. 41–80). Opladen: Westdeutscher Verlag.

Sherman, C. & Lust, B. (1986). "Syntactic and lexical constraints on the acquisition of control in complement sentences". In B. Lust (Ed.), *Studies in the Acquisition of Anaphora. Volume I: Defining the constraints* (pp. 279–308). Dordrecht: Reidel.

Stevens, T. & Karmiloff-Smith, A. (1997). "Word learning in a special population: Do individuals with Williams syndrome obey lexical constraints?" *Journal of Child Language, 24*(3), 737–765.

Terman, L. M. & Merrill, M. A. (1965). *Stanford-Binet Intelligenz-Test S-I-T*. German version adapted by H.-R. Lückert. Göttingen: Verlag für Psychologie Hogrefe.

Tewes, U. (1983). *Hamburg-Wechsler Intelligenztest für Kinder. HAWIK-R*. Bern: H. Huber.

Thomas, M. S. C., Grant, J., Barham, Z., Gsödl, M., Laing, E., Lakusta, L., Tyler, L. K., Grice, S., Paterson, S., & Karmiloff-Smith, A. (2001). "Past tense formation in Williams syndrome". *Language and Cognitive Processes, 2*(16), 143–176.

Tyler, L. K., Karmiloff-Smith, A., Voice, J. K., Stevens, T., Grant, J., Udwin, O., Davies, M., & Howlin, P. (1997). "Do individuals with Williams syndrome have bizarre semantics? Evidence for lexical organization using an on-line task". *Cortex, 33*, 515–527.

Vallar, G. & Papagno, C. (1993). "Preserved vocabulary acquisition in Down's syndrome. The role of phonological short-term memory". *Cortex, 29*(3), 467–483.

Vicari, S., Carlesimo, G., Brizzolara, D., & Pezzini, G. (1996). "Short-term memory in children with Williams syndrome: A reduced contribution of lexical-semantic knowledge to word span". *Neuropsychologia, 34*(9), 919–925.

Vicari, S., Caselli, M. C., Gagliardi, C., Tonucci, F., & Volterra, V. (2002). "Language acquisition in special populations: A comparison between Down and Williams syndromes". *Neuropsychologia, 40*, 2461–2470.

Volterra, V., Capirci, O., Pezzini, G., Sabbadini, L., & Vicari, S. (1996). "Linguistic abilities in Italian children with Williams syndrome". *Cortex, 32*, 663–677.

Wang, P. P. & Bellugi, U. (1994). "Evidence from two genetic syndromes for a dissociation between verbal and visual-spatial short-term memory". *Journal of Clinical and Experimental Neuropsychology, 2*, 317–322.

Zukowski, A. (2001). Uncovering Grammatical Competence in Children with Williams Syndrome. Unpublished doctoral dissertation, Boston University.

## Appendix

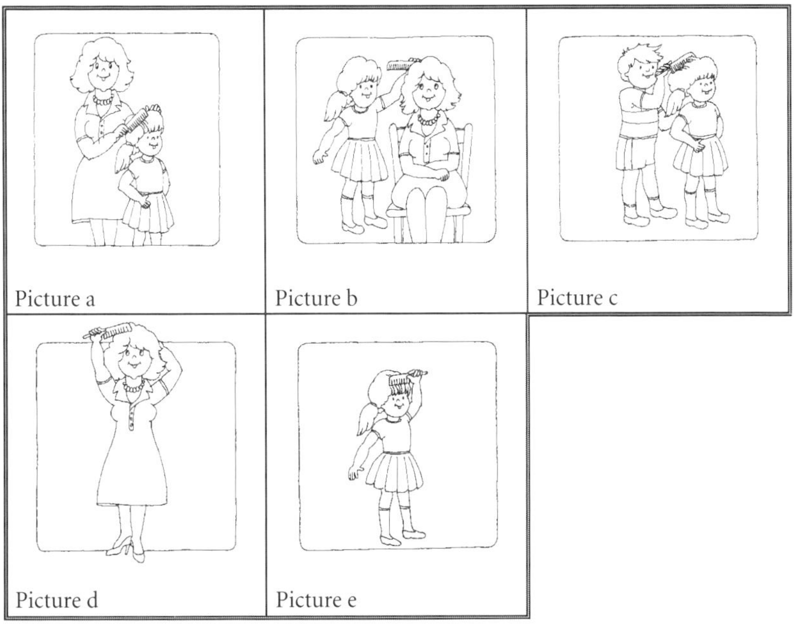


**Figure A.** Pictures a, b, c are examples taken from the *passive-active test* for the test sentence "*das Mädchen wird von der Mutter frisiert*" ('the girl is combed by the mother'). Test pictures a, b, d, e illustrate the *pronominal dependency* test sentence in (10): "*die Mutter hat der Susi versprochen, sich zu frisieren*" ('the mother has promised Susi to comb herself').

**Table A.** Inflection paradigm for the definite article in German

| | NOM | ACC | DAT | GEN |
|---|---|---|---|---|
| masc.sg. | der | den | dem | des |
| neuter.sg. | das | das | dem | des |
| fem.sg. | die | die | der | der |
| plural | die | die | den | der |

**Table B.** Mean percentages of 'no answer' in the individuals with DS by mental age group and by complexity of the test sentences. The complexity types are varying from two-three-word sentences (= complexity 1), to long sentences with two objects and an adverbial phrase (= complexity 6).

| no answer | complex1 | complex2 | complex3 | complex4 | complex5 | complex6 |
|---|---|---|---|---|---|---|
| MA1 | 35.7 | 53.1 | 64.6 | 60.3 | 68.3 | 66.7 |
| MA2 | 30.7 | 34.8 | 36.5 | 31.0 | 43.0 | 48.7 |
| MA3 | 6.5 | 8.0 | 11.1 | 11.6 | 18.1 | 14.1 |
| MA4 | 3.5 | 2.0 | 2.3 | 1.1 | 3.5 | 3.9 |
| F(3,78) | 9.159 | 26.831 | 26.276 | 22.922 | 19.555 | 20.722 |
| | p = .0000 | p = .0000 | p = .0000 | p = .0000 | p = .0000 | p = .0000 |

# Phonological processing in Williams syndrome

Steve Majerus
University of Liège

Phonological processing has been considered as a particular strength in language processing in Williams syndrome (WS). However, in this review, I argue that phonological processing is not completely normal. Although basic phonological processes such as identification, segmentation, short-term storage and articulation of phonological information seem to be at mental age- and chronological age-appropriate levels, other aspects are impaired: (1) performance in metaphonological awareness tasks is very poor; (2) processing of complex nonwords is below verbal mental age levels; (3) performance in these tasks is less affected by sublexical phonological knowledge. Phonological processing seems indeed to be atypical in WS, possibly characterized by the development of overly detailed phonological representations.

## Introduction

The present chapter reviews the 'state of the art' of phonological processing in Williams syndrome (WS). Despite being considered as a particularly well developed component of language processing, the integrity and nature of phonological processing in WS has not yet been extensively explored. Nevertheless, as I will show, the existing data suggest that, contrary to common assumptions, different aspects of phonological processing are not preserved in WS. Furthermore, this chapter will present data on verbal short-term memory (STM) processing which has also been considered as fairly well developed and as representing further evidence for intact phonological processing abilities in WS. I will critically appraise to what extent verbal STM is really preserved in WS and whether good performances in verbal STM tasks can be considered as evidence for good phonological processing abilities. The chapter will conclude by suggesting that phonological representations could be overly specific and organized in an unusual way in WS.

## Phonological processing

Current evidence for preserved phonological processing in WS is largely based on clinical observations and descriptions of children or adults with WS. These descriptions generally report fluent and well-articulated speech in WS without any phonological or phonetic deformations (e.g., Bellugi, Lichtenberger, Jones, Lai, & George 2000; Reilly, Klima, & Bellugi 1991; Volterra, Capirci, Pezzini, Sabbadini, & Vicari 1996). Some subjects might even present quite remarkable abilities to acquire the phonology of foreign languages, as suggested by the case study of the 20-year old WS woman, CS, who was a perfect trilingual, speaking fluently Swiss German, High German and French (Barisnikov, Van der Linden, & Poncelet 1996).

Experimental evidence for a proficiency in phonological processing comes from studies that have used rather indirect measures of phonological processing, such as phonological fluency tasks. In these tasks, the WS individual is asked to produce, during a limited time period, as many lexical exemplars beginning with a given phoneme as possible; these tasks measure the speed of access to the phonological form of words stored in long-term memory and are supposed to require well developed phonological analysis and segmentation abilities. Children and adults with WS generally perform at the same level as mental or even chronological age-matched controls (Barisnikov et al. 1996; Pezzini, Vicari, Volterra, Milani, & Ossella 1999; Volterra et al. 2001; Volterra et al. 1996; Volterra et al. 1999). For example, the case CS, reported by Barisnikov et al. (1996), showed chronological age-appropriate performance for producing words beginning either with /p/, /v/ or /r/ (number of words produced: 15, 15 and 9, respectively; controls: 19.1 ± 10.01, 14.3 ± 5.9, and 13.1 ± 5.8, respectively). However, it must be noted that phonological fluency tasks can also be realized on the basis of an acoustic similarity between the target phoneme and the onset of the words, and normal performance on these tasks does not necessarily demonstrate that phonological analysis and segmentation abilities are intact in WS. Thus, preserved performance on phonological fluency tasks cannot really be considered as a very strong argument in favour of preserved phonological processing in WS.

To my best knowledge, the only study that has more directly assessed basic phonological analysis abilities in WS has been realized recently by Böhning, Campbell and Karmiloff-Smith (2001) who assessed integration of auditory and visual (labial) cues in speech perception. Among other results, these authors showed that individuals with WS performed as well as chronological age-matched controls in perceiving and repeating auditorily presented simple nonsense syllables differing by a single phoneme (e.g., /Schwa ba:/, /Schwa va:/). This study suggests, at least, that low level perceptual analysis for acoustic-phonetic information seems to be preserved in WS. But we still do not know whether higher level phonological processing is also preserved in WS, like perception and segmentation of more complex phonological strings as well as phonological awareness.

This question has been explored in a study by Laing, Hulme, Grant and Karmiloff-Smith (2001), investigating the relationship between phonological awareness abilities and reading development in 15 WS subjects and a control group matched for reading test age, as well as verbal and non-verbal mental age. Laing et al. observed equivalent performance in the WS group and the control group for most measures of phonological awareness (rhyme awareness, spoonerisms) except for phoneme deletion measures, suggesting that phonological awareness abilities might be relatively preserved in WS. However, the verbal age-matched control group (mean age: 6 years 9 months; range: 5 years to 9 years 2 months) was much younger than the WS group (mean age: 15 years 1 month; range: 9 years to 27 years 7 months), due to the matching not only of mental verbal age, but also of reading age and non-verbal mental age which are typically relatively low in WS. This makes a comparison of the means between the WS and the control groups' phonological awareness measures relatively difficult, especially as the control group with an age range of 5 years to 9 years 2 months comprised children for whom phonological awareness abilities were still relatively poor while others had fully developed phonological awareness abilities, leading to a large variance in the scores for the phonological awareness measures. Also we do not know whether phonological awareness abilities are still preserved in WS individuals when compared to a control group matched for verbal mental age only (which is normally better developed in WS than reading ability) and to a control group matched for chronological age.

In a recent study, we investigated phonological awareness abilities in four French-speaking children with WS (age range: 10 years 1 month – 12 years 7 months) compared to a slightly younger control group of normally developing children (age range: 7 years 2 months – 12 years 1 month) matched on verbal age (receptive vocabulary age determined by the French version of the Peabody Picture Vocabulary Test; Dunn, Thériault-Whalen, & Dunn 1993) as well as to a control group matched on chronological age only (age range: 10 years 4 months – 12 years 9 months) (Majerus, Barisnikov, Vuillemin, Poncelet, & Van der Linden 2003). The tasks were (1) minimal pair discrimination task (a word-pair was presented, with the two words being either identical, either differing by a single phoneme), (2) rhyme judgment task (a word-pair was presented, with the two words having similar or dissimilar rhymes), (3) phoneme detection task (a word was presented, followed by a phoneme and the participants were asked to judge whether the target word began with the specified phoneme). In these tasks, the participants had to make explicit judgments about the phonological similarity at the word- (task 1), rhyme- (task 2) and phoneme-level (task 3). Furthermore we also assessed phonological processing in a more implicit way by measuring the influence of phonological lexical and sublexical knowledge on performance in these tasks.[1] The influence of phonological knowledge was assessed by contrasting performance for items having pre-existing lexical or sublexical representations stored in LTM: in each task, we compared performance for words *versus* nonwords, measuring the influence of lexical phonological knowledge on performance by assuming that lexical knowledge would facilitate performance for words. Furthermore, the influence of sublexical phonological knowledge was assessed by comparing performance for nonwords containing phoneme associations which are frequent in French phonology *versus* nonwords containing less frequent phonotactic associations; we assumed that sublexical phonological knowledge would facilitate performance for phonologically more familiar nonwords. The rationale of this experimental design was based on a number of psycholinguistic studies in normal children and adults showing more accurate and faster processing for words *versus* nonwords, and for phonotactically frequent *versus* less frequent nonwords in a variety of language tasks (e.g., Vitevitch & Luce 1998, 1999; Gathercole, Frankish, Pickering, & Peaker 1999).

The results showed that relative to both control groups, the four WS children were impaired on the majority of the phonological awareness tasks, although there was also some degree of variability: while three of the four children were impaired on more than 6 out of a total of nine measures, one child was impaired only on four measures (see Figures 1a, 1b and 1c). However, on the whole, our results show that, when compared to more homogeneous control groups than was the case in the study by Laing et al. (2001), clear difficulties in phonological awareness measures are observed. This suggests that explicit metaphonological judgments such as required in phonological awareness tasks may be not be really preserved in WS. Regarding now the more implicit measures of phonological processing, as measured by the influence of lexical and sublexical phonological knowledge on performance in the phonological awaraness tasks, no consistent advantage was observed for words relative to phonotactically frequent nonwords, nor for phonotactically frequent nonwords relative to phonotactically infrequent nonwords. These results suggest either that sublexical and lexical phonological knowledge is not automatically activated in phonological awaraness tasks in WS, or even that phonological representations are structured in an abnormal way in WS. It must be noted that no lexicality or phonotactic frequency effects were observed in the control groups either; however, this was related to ceiling performance at the phonological awareness tasks for both control groups. Further evidence for a possible atypical organization of phonological representations in WS will be presented in the next section of this chapter.

To sum up this section on phonological processing in WS, the still relatively small literature suggests that (1) basic phonetic-acoustic analysis of phonological information seems to be preserved, (2) complex and explicit meta-phonological processing as required in phonological awareness tasks might not really be preserved, possibly related to difficulties in meta-cognitive processing which is fre-

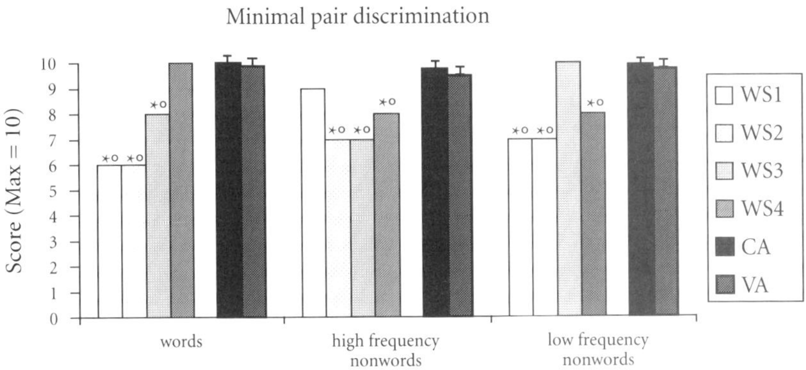


**Figure 1a.** Performance of WS children WS1, WS2, WS3 and WS4 for the minimal pair discrimination task, as a function of stimulus category (words, phonotactically frequent nonwords, phonotactically infrequent nonwords) (adapted from Majerus, Barisnikov, Vuillemin, Poncelet, & Van der Linden 2003). CA: chronological age-matched control group; VA: verbal mental age-matched control group. * difference significant at $p < .05$ compared to mean scores obtained in CA controls (modified t-tests, Crawford & Garthwaite 2002); ° difference significant at $p < .05$ compared to mean scores obtained in VA controls.

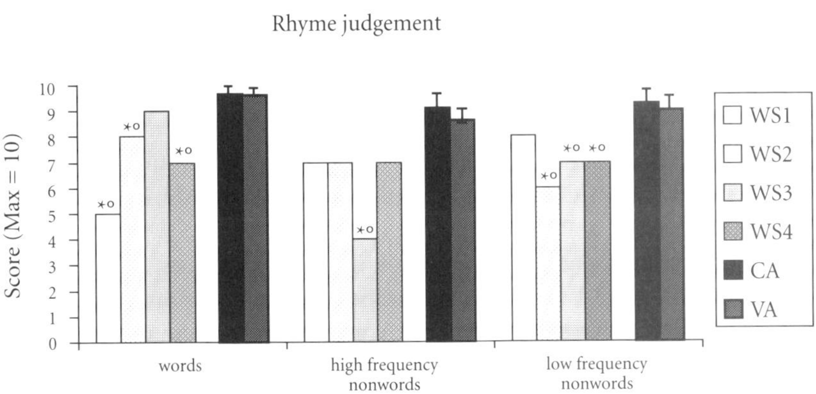


**Figure 1b.** Performance of WS children WS1, WS2, WS3 and WS4 for the rhyme judgement task, as a function of stimulus category (words, phonotactically frequent nonwords, phonotactically infrequent nonwords) (adapted from Majerus, Barisnikov, Vuillemin, Poncelet, & Van der Linden 2003).

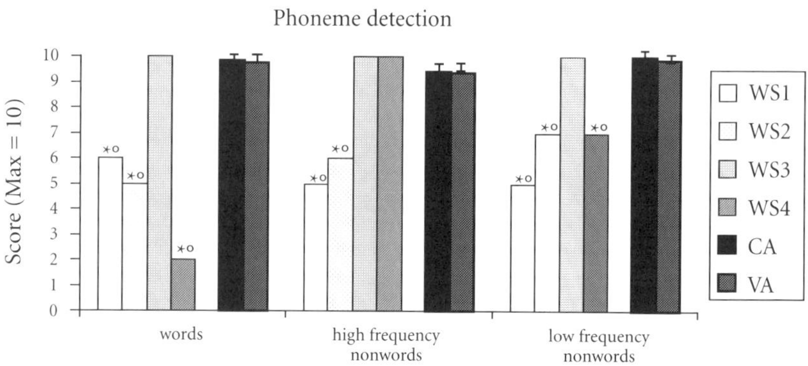


**Figure 1c.** Performance of WS children WS1, WS2, WS3 and WS4 for the phoneme detection task, as a function of stimulus category (words, phonotactically frequent nonwords, phonotactically infrequent nonwords) (adapted from Majerus, Barisnikov, Vuillemin, Poncelet, & Van der Linden 2003).

quently impaired in any population with mental retardation, (3) alternatively, the network of phonological representations might be organized in an unsual way.

## Verbal short-term memory processing

As we have noted in the introduction, preserved verbal STM in WS has been considered as further evidence for preserved phonological processing abilities. Indeed, in verbal STM tasks, verbally presented material of increasing length has to be repeated exactly in the same form and in the same order as it was presented. This necessitates the intervention of a phonologically based short-term memory system that temporarily stores phonological traces of the verbal stimuli that have been presented for immediate serial recall (Baddeley & Hitch 1974; Baddeley 1986; Baddeley, Gathercole, & Papagno 1998). Furthermore, verbal STM tasks require, besides well developed phonological short-term storage capacities, well developed abilities in phonological analysis, identification, segmentation and articulatory planning of the phonological information contained in the auditorily presented verbal stimuli. Given these considerations, we will, firstly, examine to what extent verbal STM processing is preserved in WS. Then we will critically appraise whether preserved performance in verbal STM tasks can really be considered as evidence for preserved phonological processing.

Several studies have shown a proficiency in WS for STM tasks using verbal stimuli. Indeed, subjects with WS present normal performance, relative to mental age-matched or chronological age-matched controls, for immediate serial recall of auditorily presented word or digit sequences (Barisnikov et al. 1996; Jarrold, Baddeley, & Hewes 1999; Vicari, Brizzolara, Carlesimo, Pezzini, & Volterra 1996; Volterra et al. 1999; Wang & Bellugi 1994). This relative strength in verbal STM cannot not be attributed to a more general preservation of STM processing as STM for visuo-spatial material is severely impaired (e.g., Barisnikov et al. 1996; Vicari et al. 1996; Volterra et al. 1999). More precisely, a number of studies have also shown that STM performance in WS individuals is affected by the same phonological variables as in normally developing children: they show an advantage for short-term recall of phonologically similar versus dissimilar words and for long versus short words (Barisnikov et al. 1996; Vicari, Carlesimo, Brizzolara, & Pezzini 1996). Phonologically dissimilar words are thought to be represented by more distinctive traces in STM than phonologically similar words and thus are easier to retrieve (Baddeley & Hitch 1974; Baddeley 1986). The word length effect has also been interpreted as being related to the phonological characteristics of the items to be recalled: longer words contain more phonological information and thus take more time to be rehearsed in STM or lead to more interference between stimuli due to their greater phonological complexity (Baddeley & Hitch 1974; Baddeley 1986; Nairne 1990; Service 1998). These data suggest that STM performance in WS seems to be based on phonological coding to the same extent as in normal controls. However, it must be noted that the phonological similarity and word length effects, although significant at the group level, can be relatively inconsistent when considering individual performance profiles, for both WS and control groups. For example, in our recent study with four WS children, we observed that the word length effect was absent in one subject, and the phonological similarity effect was absent in two WS subjects (Majerus et al. 2003). Similar results have nevertheless also been observed in studies with normal controls: for example, Logie, Della Salla, Laiacona, Chalmers and Wynn (1996) showed that not all normal adults showed phonological similarity and word length effects, even if a majority did, possibly reflecting interindividual differences in the use of alternative non-phonologigal strategies (e.g., mental imagery). Whatever the interpretation of these results may be, these studies show that verbal STM performance in subjects with WS is influenced as consistently or inconsistently as in normal controls by phonological factors such as word length and phonological similarity.

However, the most stringent evidence for a preservation of phonological short-term storage capacities in WS, and, more generally, for a strength in phonological processing, should come from STM tasks measuring specifically short-term storage capacities for phonological information like nonwords. Grant, Karmiloff-Smith, Gathercole, Paterson, Howlin, Davies and Udwin (1997) observed that performance on an English nonword repetition task in a group of WS children was below the performance level expected from their verbal mental age, suggesting that short-term storage of phonological information was not really a strength in this WS group. However, it must be noted that the nonwords used by Grant et al. (1997) and taken from the Nonword Repetition Test (a task developed by Gathercole and Baddeley (1996) and frequently used to test verbal STM capacity in children) were rather complex multisyllabic nonwords containing many grammatical morphemes such as "-ation", "-ually", and "-tory". As individuals with WS have difficulties in generalizing familiar grammatical morphemes to new words (see chapters by Clahsen, Ring, & Temple, and by Penke & Krause, this book), it cannot be excluded that the relatively low performance for nonword repetition in the WS group could be partially explained by these difficulties in grammatical generalization rules that are likely to support performance in normal children. Hence, using less complex nonwords with a simple CVC structure and containing no grammatical morphemes might yield better performance in STM for nonwords in WS. For example, Barisnikov et al. (1996) showed that their WS case CS showed chronological age-appropriate performance in a nonword repetition task that was made up of consonant-vowel and consonant-consonant-vowel nonword syllables containing no grammatical morphemes (Poncelet & Van der Linden 2003).

This also raises the more general question of the influence of phonological knowledge encoded in long-term memory (LTM) on verbal STM performance in WS. Indeed, recent STM models consider that verbal STM is not an independent system, but that it strongly interacts with lexical and sublexical phonological language representations stored in LTM. These models consider that the verbal STM store is connected to phonological and lexical LTM representations which reactivate the temporary STM traces of the stimuli to be recalled and thus prevent excessive decay of the STM traces (see for example, Baddeley 2000; Baddeley, Gathercole, & Papagno 1998; Gupta & MacWhinney 1997; R. Martin, Lesch, & Bartha 1999). Some models go even further and consider that STM is merely the temporary activation of phonological, lexical and semantic LTM representations (see for example, Cowan 1988, 1995, 1999; Gathercole & A. Martin 1996; N. Martin & Saffran 1992; for a review and critical appraisal of these different positions, see also Majerus, Lekeu, Van der Linden, & Salmon 2001; Majerus, Van der Linden, Poncelet, & Metz-Lutz 2003; Miyake & Shah 1999; Nairne 2002). Following these models, performance in verbal STM tasks is not only determined by storage capacity of the verbal STM store, but also by the availability of phonological lexical or sublexical representations stored in LTM. In other words, support of LTM representations in verbal STM tasks is only possible for those verbal stimuli for which corresponding lexical and sublexical representations in LTM exist, such as words or nonwords with a highly familiar phonological structure. Empirical data in normal children and adults have indeed shown that recall of words in STM tasks is better than recall of nonwords (lexicality effect) (e.g., Hulme, Maughan, & Brown 1991; Gathercole et al. 1999; Majerus & Van der Linden 2003). Similarly, STM performance for nonwords has also been shown to be influenced by sublexical phonological LTM representations encoding the statistical characteristics of the structure of the native phonology (phonotactics): Gathercole et al. (1999) and Majerus and Van der Linden (2003) showed that nonwords containing phoneme associations that are frequently associated in the native phonology increase performance in a nonword immediate serial recall task compared to nonwords containing infrequent phoneme associations (phonotactic frequency effect). Similarly, children recall more nonwords that have been rated high in wordlikeness than nonwords with a low wordlikeness rating (Gathercole 1995).

Given these theoretical considerations, the observation of a normal influence of phonological knowledge in nonword STM performance could represent further evidence for the preservation of phonological processing in WS. Grant, Karmiloff-Smith, Berthoud, and Christophe (1996) presented to English-speaking individuals with WS a French and an English nonword repetition task, based on the Nonword Repetition Test described earlier. WS individuals showed better performance for repeating English than French nonwords, suggesting that phonological knowledge about the sound structure of English indeed influenced their STM performance, as was also the case in mental age-matched controls. However, overall level of performance was significantly poorer for repeating both English and French nonwords, relative to controls, suggesting that phonological storage capacities and/or the support of phonological LTM knowledge were nevertheless reduced. Grant et al. (1997) furthermore showed that their WS group showed similar wordlikeness effects in nonword repetition than controls. However, as noted before, the interpretation of these results is somewhat problematic as all these nonwords had a rather complex multisyllabic structure including many grammatical morphemes; hence, it is not clear whether the wordlikeness effect observed in the WS group reflected the intervention of phonological knowledge about word forms or rather the WS children's difficulty with generalization rules for grammatical morphemes that could have had a very low frequency in unwordlike nonwords, further disadvantaging recall of these nonwords in the WS group.

In our study I have already partially described, we also re-examined STM for words and nonwords in four children with WS (Majerus et al. 2003). Furthermore, we investigated more specifically the influence of phonotactic knowledge on nonword STM performance by comparing immediate serial recall for nonwords containing phonotactically frequent or infrequent phoneme associations. The words and nonwords presented had all a very simple consonant-vowel-consonant syllabic structure. The performance of the WS children was compared to both a verbal mental-age matched and a chronological age-matched control group. If STM storage capacities are preserved then we should expect normal performance especially for those nonwords where a contribution from phonological LTM is least likely, i.e. nonwords with low phonotactic frequencies. Moreover, if the influence of sublexical phonological knowledge is normal, then we should expect a normal advantage

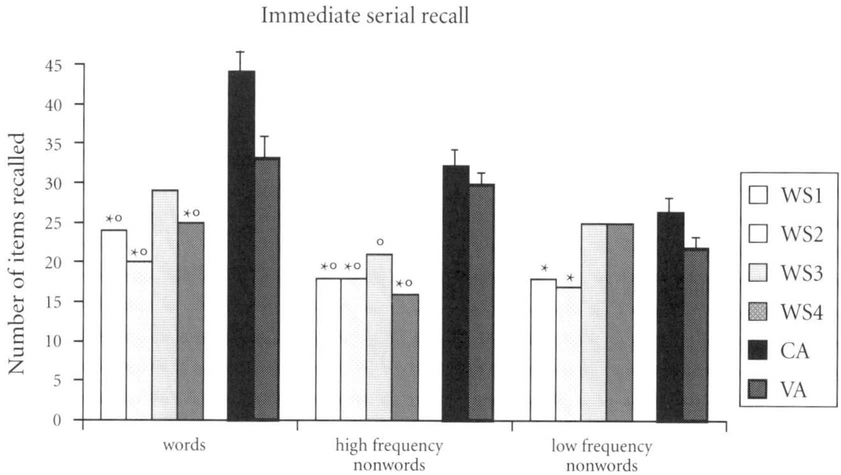


**Figure 2.** Performance of WS children WS1, WS2, WS3 and WS4 on a verbal immediate serial recall task, as a function of stimulus category (words, phonotactically frequent nonwords, phonotactically infrequent nonwords) (adapted from Majerus, Barisnikov, Vuillemin, Poncelet, & Van der Linden 2003). CA: chronological age-matched control group; VA: verbal mental age-matched control group. * difference significant at $p < .05$ compared to mean scores obtained in CA controls; ° difference significant at $p < .05$ compared to mean scores obtained in VA controls.

for high phonotactic frequency *versus* low phonotactic frequency nonwords. Finally, if the influence of lexical phonological knowledge is normal, then we should also observe a normal advantage for words over nonwords. We observed indeed that STM performance for low frequency nonwords was normal for the four children compared to the mental age-matched control group (see Figure 2). However performance was significantly impaired for both high frequency nonwords and words in three of the WS children relative to both control groups. Most importantly, while controls consistently showed an advantage for high frequency over low frequency nonwords as well as for words over nonwords, these effects were either reduced, absent or even inversed in each of the four WS children. Thus our data suggest that (1) phonological STM capacities might indeed be preserved in WS, (2) the influence of phonological lexical and sublexical knowledge is however impaired and deficits in STM tasks will appear for storage of verbal information with strong correspondencies in phonological LTM.

Do these STM data now provide further evidence for preserved phonological processing? The answer to this question depends on the interpretation we give to the reduced lexicality and phonotactic frequency effects we have observed in the STM tasks and that show that phonological lexical and sublexical knowledge did not support STM performance to the same extent as in controls. A possible interpretation is that phonological knowledge is intact, but that there is a problem at the level of the interactions between this knowledge and the information stored in STM; the connections between the STM store and the lexical and sublexical LTM representations could be weaker than is the case in normally developing subjects. This interpretation is reasonable if we assume that the STM store and the representations in LTM are processed in different cognitive systems with interactive links that are optional and can be modulated. The recent studies on LTM influences in STM processing, however, argue for very direct and obligatory interactions between STM and LTM language representations, as evidenced by the fact that the magnitude of the lexicality and phonotactic frequency effects does not change during development and that these effects are present already very early during development (these effects have been observed in children as young as four years) (Majerus & Van der Linden 2003; Majerus, Van der Linden, & Lambert 2003). Furthermore, the interactive links between STM and language LTM representations proposed by recent STM models we have already shortly described are considered to be very strong, obligatory and automatic (e.g., Baddeley, Gathercole, & Papagno 1998; Gupta & MacWhinney 1997; R. Martin, Lesch, & Bartha 1999). As we have also noted, some models even consider that verbal STM directly reflects the temporary activation of LTM representations in the language network and that performance in STM tasks merely depends on the duration of the temporary activation of the LTM representations, and not on storage capacities of a separate STM system (e.g., Cowan 1999; N. Martin & Saffran 1992). Thus a more plausible and direct interpretation of our results would be that the phonological lexical and sublexical language representations themselves are impaired in WS and therefore cannot influence STM performance normally. The network of lexical and sublexical representations might indeed by abnormally structured, a hypothesis that could explain both the reduced lexicality and phonotactic frequency effects observed in the STM tasks, but also in the phonological awareness tasks. The suggestion of an abnormal organization of the phonological network in WS is supported by other data showing that in word fluency tasks, subjects with WS tend to produce a greater number of low frequency words than controls (Bellugi et al. 1994; Jarrold, Hartley, Phillips, & Baddeley 2000; Rossen, Klima, Bellugi, Bihrle, & Jones 1996). Vicari et al. (1996) also observed reduced word frequency effects in immediate serial recall for words in a group of WS participants. A final interpretation of our data is that STM performance in Williams syndrome is not based on a phonological STM system that interacts with the language network, but on a more acoustical non-verbal STM store that stores all kinds of auditory information as an acoustic trace, bypassing the phonological network. Although there are no direct data to support this suggestion and thus it must be considered as rather hypothetical, indirect evidence for this interpretation can be found in reports describing 'hyperverbal' or 'cocktail party speech', where WS children seem to repeat accurately any verbal information they hear, but without organizing this information in any linguistically meaningful way (Gosch, Städing, & Pankau 1994; Udwin & Yule 1990). These aspects will be further discussed in the following conclusion.

## Conclusions and perspectives

Basic phonological processes such as identification, segmentation, short-term storage and articulation of phonological information seem to be at a mental age- and chronological age-appropriate level and thus seem to represent a strength of language processing in WS. However, we also have identified a number of possible weaknesses at the level of (1) metaphonological processes, and (2) the organization of the phonological language network, at both the lexical and sublexical level. Furthermore, although basic speech perception performance seems to be preserved as evidenced by normal analysis and repetition of verbal information, the processes by which this performance is achieved have not yet been explored extensively and might be qualitatively different from those characterizing normally developing children and adults.

Some authors recently argued that phonological representations in WS might indeed be atypical, in the sense that they would be more specific than in normally developing children. For example, Thomas et al. (2001) showed that English-speaking children and adults with WS had difficulties in generalizing the past tense rule "add -ed" to novel verbs; they interpreted this finding as reflecting the existence of overly specific phonological representations that impede generalization of repeatedly occurring segments of these representations (the "-ed" suffix) to novel word forms such as verbs in this case. In other words, children with WS would store the past tense form of each regular verb as a separate instance instead of storing the general rule "add -ed" that could be applied to the stem of each regular verb. Thomas et al. (2001) presented further computational modelling data that captured, among other phenomena, the difficulties for generalizing the past tense rule to novel verbs, by simply augmenting the 'discriminability' of the sounds making up each word. This suggestion is further supported by the heightened sensitivity to auditory information (hyperacusis) as well as the good verbal STM capacities observed in WS which, together, could permit the construction of overly detailed and specific phonological representations. Heightened sensitivity to auditory information and good auditory-verbal STM capacity could however not only lead to very specific phonological representations, but also to overly specific phonemic representations: for example, each subtle acoustic variation /$b_1$/, /$b_2$/ or /$b_3$/ at the level of voice onset time (VOT) for the phoneme /b/ could be represented in the

WS language network as separate phoneme entries /$b_1$/, /$b_2$/ or /$b_3$/ while normal children and adults would generalize each instance to the phoneme entry /b/ without hearing any difference between /$b_1$/, /$b_2$/ or /$b_3$/. Overly specific phonemic and phonological representations could then explain the reduction of phonotactic frequency effects we have observed in our study because normal phonotactic frequency effects rely on the existence of abstract phonotactic representations that encode the regularity of occurrence of different phoneme associations. For a speech perception system with overly detailed phonemic representations, less regularities between phoneme associations will be encoded as for this system, many more different phoneme categories will exist than the 45 phonemes characterizing English, for example, and thus frequency of co-occurrence of two given phonemes will be much poorer. Overly specific phonological representations could also account for poor performance in phonological awareness tasks: lack of more general phonological categories would make it more difficult to understand the phonological concepts of rhyme or phoneme which represent indeed an abstraction of similarities between many different acoustic events. As a result, conscious identification of similarities or dissimilarities at the rhyme- or phoneme-level will be very hard to achieve in WS.

Regarding empirical data for this suggestion of possible abnormalities at the level of early speech perception and phonological processing, promising but still indirect and partial support is provided by some neurophysiological studies exploring cognitive event-related potentials (ERP) to auditory verbal information in WS (Bellugi, Mills, Jernigan, Hickok, & Galaburda 1999; Mills, Neville, & Bellugi 1996). Mills, Neville and Bellugi (1996) showed that ERP's of WS subjects showed indeed an abnormal positive peak 200 msec after presentation of words; this peak was not observed in normal children or adults. Most importantly, this positive peak was apparent mostly over temporal regions underlying phonological processing in normally developing children and adults. Furthermore, neuroanatomical data have revealed disproportionate growth of the posterior superior temporal gyrus normally implicated in speech perception and phonological processing; an exaggerated leftward asymmetry has also been observed in the same region (Hickok et al. 1995a, b). These data suggest possible abnormalities in brain tissue underlying speech perception and phonological processing in WS and that could induce the development of atypical phonemic and phonological representations in WS. For example, in children presenting developmental dyslexia, a relationship has indeed been observed between phonologically based reading deficits and an exaggerated leftward asymmetry of the planum temporale and planum parietale (Leonard et al. 2002). Finally, the commonly reported hyperacusis in WS could also be related to these anatomical differences at the level of the superior temporal gyrus wich includes the primary auditory cortex.

However, more direct psycholinguistic data in favour or against the suggestion of overly detailed phonological representations in WS are still lacking. An important step in this direction would be to investigate more deeply phoneme identification in WS, by studying sensitivity for linguistically relevant acoustic information and by determining whether individuals with WS present similar phoneme categorization functions as a function of variation of different acoustic discriminatory features as normally developing children and adults (for example, the perceptive discrimination of the phonemes /b/ – /p/ as a function of acoustic variations along the VOT continuum). Secondly, processing at the sublexical phonological level, such as the phonotactic level of representation, must also be explored more extensively in speech perception, by using reaction time measures that are much more sensitive to the manipulation of phonotactic frequency patterns in speech perception tasks than only measures of response accuracy.

In sum, the quantitative level of performace for basic phonological processing such as perception and repetition of phonological information can be considered as relatively good in WS. However, this does not mean that the processes underlying phonological processing are preserved. WS might achieve a relatively normal level of performance in basic phonological tasks, and yet use qualitatively different processes to attain this level of performance. The nature of phonological processes and representations in WS clearly needs further research.

## Acknowledgments

This work has been supported by a Research Fellowship grant from the Fonds National de la Recherche Scientifique, Belgium. I would like to thank Susanne Bartke, Marita Böhning and an anonymous reviewer for very helpful and inspiring comments on a previous version of this manuscript.

## Note

1. We consider these measures as more implicit, as the subjects are not necessarily aware of the possible influence of lexical and sublexical phonological knowledge on performance, which is automatically activated at the moment of presentation of the stimuli, especially when comparing phonotactically frequent and infrequent nonwords.

## References

Baddeley, A. D. (2000). "The episodic buffer: A new component of working memory?". *Trends in Cognitive Sciences, 4*, 417–423.

Baddeley, A. D. (1986). *Working memory*. Oxford: Clarendon Press/OUP.

Baddeley, A. D., Gathercole, S., & Papagno, C. (1998). "The phonological loop as a language learning device". *Psychological Review, 105*(1), 158–173.

Baddeley, A. D. & Hitch, G. J. (1974). "Working memory". In G. H. Bower (Ed.), *The Psychology of Learning and Motivation* (pp. 47–90). San Diego, CA: Academic Press.

Barisnikov, K., Van der Linden, M., & Poncelet, M. (1996). "Acquisition of new words and phonological working memory in Williams syndrome: A case study". *Neurocase, 2*, 395–404.

Bellugi, U., Mills, D. L., Jernigan, T. L., Hickok, G., & Galaburda, A. M. (1999). "Linking cognition, brain structure, and brain function in Williams syndrome". In H. Tager-Flusberg (Ed.), *Neurodevelopmental Disorders* (pp. 111–136). Cambridge, MA: The MIT Press.

Bellugi, U., Wang., P., & Jernigan, T. L. (1994). "Williams syndrome: An unusual neuropsychological profile". In S. Broman & J. Grafman (Eds.), *Atypical Cognitive Deficits in Developmental Disorders: Implications for brain functions* (pp. 23–56). Hillsdale, NJ: LEA.

Bellugi, U., Lichtenberger, L., Jones, W., Lai, Z., & St George. M. (2000). "The neurocognitive profile of Williams syndrome: A complex pattern of strengths and weakness". *Journal of Cognitive Neuroscience, 12* (Supplement), 7–29.

Böhning, M., Campbell, R., & Karmiloff-Smith, A. (2001). "Audiovisual speech perception in Williams syndrome". *Neuropsychologia, 39*, 1–11.

Cowan, N. (1999). "An embedded-processes model of working memory". In A. Miyake & P. Shah (Eds.), *Models of Working Memory: Mechanisms of active maintenance and executive control* (pp. 62–101). Cambridge: CUP.

Crawford, J. R. & Garthwaite, P. H. (2002). "Investigation of the single case in neuropsychology: Confidence limits on the abnormality of test scores and test score differences". *Neuropsychologia, 40*, 1196–1208.

Dunn, L. M., Thériault-Whalen, C. M., & Dunn, L. M. (1993). *Echelle de vocabulaire en images Peabody. Adaptation française du Peabody Picture Vocabulary Test.* Toronto, Canada: Psycan.

Gathercole, S. E. (1995). "Is nonword repetition a test of phonological memory or long-term knowledge? It all depends on the nonwords". *Memory and Cognition, 23*, 83–94.

Gathercole, S. E. & Baddeley, A. D. (1996). *The Children's Test of Nonword Repetition*. London: The Psychological Corporation.

Gathercole, S. E., Frankish, C. R., Pickering, S. J., & Peaker, S. (1999). "Phonotactic influences on short-term memory". *Journal of Experimental Psychology: Human Learning and Memory, 25*(1), 84–95.

Gathercole, S. E. & Martin, A. J. (1996). "Interactive processes in phonological memory". In S. E. Gathercole (Ed.), *Models of short-term memory* (pp. 73–100). Hove: Psychology Press.

Gosch, A., Städing, G., & Pankau, R. (1994). "Linguistic abilities in children with Williams-Beuren syndrome". *American Journal of Medical Genetics, 52*, 291–296.

Grant, J., Karmiloff-Smith, A., Gathercole, S. E., Paterson, S., Howlin, P., Davies, M., & Udwin, O. (1997). "Phonological short-term memory and its relationship to language in Williams syndrome". *Cognitive Neuropsychiatry, 2*(2), 81–99.

Grant, J., Karmiloff-Smith, A., Berthoud, I., & Christophe A. (1996). "Is the language of people with Williams syndrome mere mimicry? Phonological short-term memory in a foreign language". *Cahiers de Psychologie Cognitive / Current Psychology of Cognition, 15*(6), 615–628.

Gupta, P. & MacWhinney, B. (1997). "Vocabulary acquisition and verbal short-term memory: computational and neural bases". *Brain and Language, 59*, 267–333.

Hickok, G., Bellugi, U., & Jones, W. (1995). "Asymmetrical abilities letter". *Science, 270*, 219–220.

Hickok, G., Neville, H. J., Mills, D. L., Jones, W., Rossen, M., & Bellugi, U. (1995). "Electrophysiological and quantitative MR analysis of the cortical auditory system in Williams syndrome". *Cognitive Neuroscience Society Abstracts, 2*, 66.

Hulme, C., Maughan, S., & Brown, G. D. (1991). "Memory for familiar and unfamiliar words: Evidence for a long-term memory contribution to short-term memory span". *Journal of Memory and Language, 30*, 685–701.

Jarrold, C., Baddeley, A. D., & Hewes, A. K. (1999). "Genetically dissociated components of working memory: Evidence from Down's and Williams syndrome". *Neuropsychologia, 37*, 637–651.

Jarrold, C., Hartley, S. J., Phillips, C., & Baddeley, A. D. (2000). "Word fluency in Williams syndrome: Evidence for unusual semantic organisation?" *Cognitive Neuropsychiatry, 5*(4), 293–319.

Laing, E., Hulme, C., Grant, J., & Karmiloff-Smith, A. (2001). "Learning to read in Williams syndrome: Looking beneath the surface of atypical reading development". *Journal of Child Psychology and Psychiatry, 42*(6), 729–739.

Leonard, C. M., Lombardino, L. J., Eckert, M. A., Mockler, J. L., Rowe, L. A., Williams, S., & DeBose, C. B. (2002). "Anatomical risk factors that distinguish dyslexia from SLI predict reading skill in normal children". *Journal of Communication Disorders, 35*, 501–531.

Logie, R. H., Della Salla, S., Laiacona, M., Chalmers, P., & Wynn, V. (1996). "Group aggregates and individual reliability: The case of verbal short-term memory". *Memory and Cognition, 24*(3), 305–321.

Majerus, S., Barisnikov, K., Vuillemin, I., Poncelet, M., & Van der Linden, M. (2003). "An investigation of verbal short-term memory and phonological processing in four children with Williams syndrome". *Neurocase, 9*(5), 390–401.

Majerus, S., Lekeu, F., Van der Linden, M., & Salmon, E. (2001). "Deep dysphasia: Further evidence on the relationship between phonological short-term memory and language processing impairments". *Cognitive Neuropsychology, 18*(5), 385–410.

Majerus, S. & Van der Linden, M (2003). "LTM effects on verbal STM: A replication study". *British Journal of Developmental Psychology, 21*(2), 303–310.

Majerus, S., Van der Linden, M., & Lambert, V. (2003). "STM and vocabulary development in young children: what is the nature of the relationship?" In preparation.

Majerus, S., Van der Linden, M., Poncelet, M., & Metz-Lutz, M.-N. (2003). "Can phonological and semantic STM be dissociated? Further evidence from Landau-Kleffner syndrome". *Cognitive Neuropsychology*. In press.

Martin, N. & Saffran, E. M. (1992). "A computational account of deep dysphasia: Evidence from a single case study". *Brain and Language, 43*, 240–274.

Martin, R. C., Lesch, M. F., & Bartha, M. C. (1999). "Independence of input and output phonology in word processing and short-term memory". *Journal of Memory and Language, 41*, 3–29.

Mills, D. L., Neville, H., & Bellugi, U. (1996). "Cerebral organization for spared cognitive functions in adults with Williams syndrome". *Presented at the Williams Syndrome Association Professional Conference, King of Prussia, PA.*

Miyake, A. & Shah, P. (1999). *Models of Working Memory: Mechanisms of active maintenance and executive control.* Cambridge: CUP.

Nairne, J. S. (2002). "Remembering over the short-term: The case against the standard model". *Psychological Review, 53*, 53–81.

Nairne, J. S. (1990). "A feature model of immediate memory". *Memory and Cognition, 18*, 251–269.

Pezzini, G., Vicari, S., Volterra, V., Milani, L., & Ossella, M. T. (1999). "Children with Williams Syndrome: Is there a single neuropsychological profile?" *Developmental Neuropsychology, 15*, 141–155.

Poncelet, M. & Van der Linden, M. (2003). "Evaluation du stock phonologique de la mémoire de travail: élaboration d'une épreuve de répétition de non-mots pour population francophone." *Revue de Neuropsychologie*. In press.

Reilly, J., Klima, E. S., & Bellugi, U. (1990). "Once more with feeling: Affect and language in atypical populations". *Development and Psychopathology, 2*, 367–391.

Roodenrys, S., Hulme, C., Alban, J., & Ellis, A. W. (1994). "Effects of word frequency and age of acquisition on short-term memory span". *Memory and Cognition, 22*, 695–701.

Rossen, M., Klima, E. S., Bellugi, U., Bihrle, A., & Jones, W. (1996). "Interaction between language and cognition: Evidence from Williams syndrome". In J. H. Beitchman, N. Cohen, M. Konstantareas, & R. Tannock (Eds.), *Language, Learning, and Behavior Disorders: Developmental, biological, and clinical perspectives* (pp. 367–392). New York, NY: CUP.

Service, E. (1998). "The effect of word length on immediate serial recall depends on phonological complexity, not articulatory duration". *The Quarterly Journal of Experimental Psychology, 51A*(2), 283–304.

Thomas, M. S. C., Grant, J., Barham, Z., Gsödl, M. K., Laing, E., Lakusta, L., Tyler, L. K., Grice, S., Paterson, S., & Karmiloff-Smith, A. (2001). "Past tense formation in Williams syndrome". *Language and Cognitive Processes, 16*, 143–176.

Udwin, O. & Yule, W. (1990). "Expressive language of children with Williams syndrome". *American Journal of Medical Genetics, S6*, 108–114.

Vicari, S., Brizzolara, D., Giovanni, A. C., & Pezzini G. (1996). "Memory abilities in children with Williams syndrome". *Cortex, 32*(3), 503–514.

Vicari, S., Carlesimo, G., Brizzolara, D., & Pezzini, G. (1996). "Short-term memory in children with Williams syndrome: A reduced contribution of lexical-semantic knowledge to word span". *Neuropsychologia, 34*(9), 919–925.

Vitevitch, M. S. & Luce, P. A. (1998). "When words compete: Levels of processing in perception of spoken words". *Psychological Science, 9*(4), 325–329.

Vitevitch, M. S. & Luce, P. A. (1999). "Probabilistic phonotactics and neighborhood activation in spoken word recognition". *Journal of Memory and Language, 40*, 374–408.

Volterra, V., Capirci, O., & Caselli, M. C. (2001). "What atypical populations can reveal about language development: The contrast between deafness and Williams syndrome". *Language and Cognitive Processes, 16*(2/3), 219–239.

Volterra, V., Capirci, O., Pezzini, G., & Sabbadini, L. (1996). "Linguistic abilities in Italian children with Williams syndrome". *Cortex, 32*, 663–677.

Volterra, V., Longobardi, E., Pezzini, G., Vicari, S., & Antenore, C. (1999). "Visuo-spatial and linguistic abilities in a twin with Williams syndrome". *Journal of Intellectual Disability Research, 43*, 294–305.

Wang, P. P. & Bellugi, U. (1994). "Evidence from two genetic syndromes for a dissociation between verbal and visual-spatial short-term memory". *Journal of Clinical and Experimental Neuropsychology, 16*(2), 317–322.

# Fast mapping in Williams syndrome

## A single case study

Marita Böhning, Franziska Starke and
Jürgen Weissenborn
University of Potsdam / Humboldt University, Berlin

We investigated fast mapping for non-words of different word classes in a 4;7-year-old child with Williams-Syndrome (WS) and controls matched for chronological, lexical and syntactic age. Performance was tested after a first video presentation (T1), one week later after a second presentation (T2), and another week later without a presentation (T3). Whereas at T1 performance of the WS-individual was better than control performance, controls performed significantly better at T2/T3. We argue that these findings follow from the known hyperacusis of WS-individuals, resulting in over-detailed sub-lexical phonological memory representations, combined with a weakness of LTM. Our results support the view that the mechanisms of linguistic performance in WS-individuals are the same as in unimpaired children except for a difference in their acoustic capacities.

### Introduction

Early language acquisition in individual children with Williams syndrome (WS) has not yet been studied in great detail. Until now most studies have focused on adults, i.e. subjects who have basically finished language acquisition, or are group studies containing both children and adults (Bellugi, Marks, Bihrle, & Sabo 1988; Bellugi, Wang, & Jernigan 1994; Wang & Bellugi 1994; Karmiloff-Smith, Klima, Bellugi, Grant, & Baron-Cohen 1995; Barisnikov, Van der Linden, & Poncelet 1996; Karmiloff-Smith, Klima, Bellugi, Grant, & Baron-Cohen 1997; Stevens & Karmiloff-Smith 1997; Tyler et al. 1997; Clahsen & Almazan 1998; Howlin, Davies, & Udwin 1998; Jarrold, Baddeley, & Hewes 1998; Karmiloff-Smith et al. 1998). These studies therefore do not directly address the issue of the course of language development in single subjects with WS. As Tager-Flusberg (1999: 8) argues, using experimental groups that vary widely in age means "obscuring the role of developmental and experiential factors". This observation holds for all areas of language development in subjects with WS. Thus, studies on the mental lexicon in WS subjects have almost exclusively been concerned with its structural aspects leaving aside developmental aspects. Methodologically, these studies are mostly based on the results of tests such as the BPVS[1]/PPVT[2] (Mac Donald & Roy 1988; Grant, Karmiloff-Smith, Berthoud, & Christophe 1996; Rossen, Klima, Bellugi, Bihrle, & Jones 1996; Volterra, Capirci, Pezzini, Sabbadini, & Vicari 1996; Grant et al. 1997; Karmiloff-Smith et al. 1997; Stevens & Karmiloff-Smith 1997; Clahsen & Almazan 1998, 2001; Karmiloff-Smith et al. 1998; Jarrold, Baddeley, & Hewes 1999; Mervis, Morris, Bertrand, & Robinson 1999; Pezzini, Vicari, Volterra, Milani, & Ossella 1999; Volterra, Longobardi, Pezzini, Vicari, & Antenore 1999; Calamandrei et al. 2000; Jarrold, Hartley, Philips, & Baddeley 2000; Clahsen & Temple 2001; Jarrold, Baddeley, Hewes, & Philips 2001; Stojanovik, Perkins, & Howard 2001; Thomas et al. 2001; Grant, Valian, & Karmiloff-Smith 2002; Temple, Almazan, & Sherwood 2002). The results of these studies are not uniform. Lexical abilities may be above non-verbal mental age (Rossen et al. 1996; Volterra et al. 1996; Karmiloff-Smith et al. 1997; Clahsen & Almazan 1998, 2001; Clahsen & Temple 2001; Thomas et al. 2001), in correspondence with non-verbal mental age (Pezzini et al. 1999; Volterra et al. 1999; Calamandrei et al. 2000), and below non-verbal age, even within the same subjects, depending on the task characteristics as shown in a recent study by Temple et al. (2002). Furthermore, findings suggest a dissociation between productive and receptive lexical knowledge in WS (Volterra et al. 1996), with perception preceding production as in unimpaired language development (e.g. Bates, Dale, & Thal 1995).

With respect to the issue of early lexical development in children with WS little research has been done so far (Capirci, Sabbadini, & Volterra 1996; Singer Harris, Bellugi, Bates, Jones, & Rossen 1997; Masataka 2000; Mervis & Robinson 2000; Nazzi & Karmiloff-Smith 2002; Siegmüller 2003). Methodologically these studies such as the one with older subjects focus on the evaluation of lexical knowledge on the basis of standardized tests like the BPVS and the PPVT. They show that lexical acquisition in children with Williams syndrome is generally delayed when compared to unimpaired children. This means that the size of the vocabulary in children with WS is smaller than the vocabulary of children of the same chronological age.

These studies still leave open the question regarding the learning mechanisms subjects with WS can make use of for the acquisition of linguistic knowledge in general, and of lexical knowledge in particular. With respect to the nature of the learning mechanisms in subjects with WS, the question has been answered differently by different authors. Thus, on the one hand, Clahsen and Almazan (1998, 2001) have argued that the learning mechanisms in WS subjects are the same as in unimpaired subjects but that they may lack specific components. On the other hand Karmiloff-Smith and colleagues (Karmiloff-Smith et al. 1997) have proposed that language learning in subjects with WS may draw on mechanisms qualitatively different from those normally at work in first language acquisition, resembling rather those to be found in second language acquisition.

The only study so far on word learning which has looked into the issue of the lexical learning mechanisms available to subjects with WS is the one by Stevens and Karmiloff-Smith (1997). They investigated whether their subjects (chronological age range 8;7–31;2 years; BPVS age range 4;5–16;4 years; N = 11) were successful in doing fast mappings and whether they used the three constraints on lexical learning, postulated by Markman and her colleagues (Markman & Hutchinson 1984; Markman & Wachtel 1988; Markman 1989, 1992, 1993), i.e. the Whole Object Constraint,[3] the Mutual Exclusivity Constraint[4] and the Taxonomic Assumption[5]. These constraints are considered to be default assumptions that help the child to solve the indeterminacy problem in the mapping from meaning to sound (e.g. Quine 1960). It has been shown in a number of studies, that these learning mechanisms seem to be operative in normally developing children from the age of 19 months onward (e.g. see Markman 1998; for a different view see Akhtar & Tomasello 2000). On the basis of their findings Stevens and Karmiloff-Smith (1997) argue that their subjects were able to do fast mappings, and that they used the Mutual Exclusivity Constraint, but did not use the Whole Object Constraint nor the Taxonomic Constraint successfully. But given the age range of the subjects in the group study by Stevens and Karmiloff-Smith (1997) and the fact that according to Markman (e.g. 1994) the lexical constraints characterize early word learning, the question is whether their results can be generalized to the word learning behavior of younger WS subjects who are still at an initial stage of lexical development.

With respect to fast mapping the study leaves open two further questions. Firstly, we are not told whether the subjects had integrated the new words permanently into their mental lexicon given that no second sufficiently delayed naming or comprehension tests were applied. Secondly, it does not tell us whether the subjects would have been able to fast map also names of properties and events, i.e. adjectives and verbs respectively.

The main aim of the present study has been to investigate the following three questions derived from the findings on lexical acquisition in WS subjects summarized so far:

Firstly, given the generally observed initial delay in lexical development in WS children, what are the fast mapping capacities of WS children at the early stage of word learning as compared to unimpaired controls?

Secondly, if WS children are able to fast map, is the result of the fast mapping integrated permanently into their mental lexicon?

Thirdly, is there a difference in the fast mapping of names for objects, properties and events, i.e. nouns, adjectives and verbs respectively?

Following a study by Monika Rothweiler (1999) in which fast mapping was examined in children with SLI and in normally developing children, we have used a design which allows us to address the role of short-term and long-term memory in the mapping process. This was done by including three test times instead of only one. In order to mimic the normal acquisition process more closely words from three different word classes were included in the set of words to be learned, i.e. nouns, verbs and adjectives.

Although our study is a single case study we assume that our findings will have to be integrated into any account of the acquisition of linguistic knowledge of individuals with WS. They thus also constitute a contribution to reach this goal.

## Method

### Participants

The experiment was carried out with a single female subject with WS and four control groups of unimpaired children.

*The WS subject*
Name: Lina
Age: 4 years; 7 months

Lina was diagnosed with Williams Syndrome at the age of 8 weeks when her parents had to take her to the hospital due to feeding difficulties and heart problems. The early diagnosis of WS was later confirmed by a positive FISH test (fluorescent in situ hybridization). Lina was born at full term following a normal pregnancy. There were no complications during delivery. She has no hearing problems. At the time of testing, Lina had undergone several heart operations.

Lina sat at 10 months and started walking when she was 2;6 years old. At this age she started to go to a kindergarten which had an integration program for learning disabled children. Lina lives with her parents. She has a healthy sister who is five years older than her with whom she has a very close relationship.

Her language development can be summarized as follows: She started babbling at the age of 9 months. At the age of 2;0 she started to repeat words but produced very few words on her own. At age 3;0 Lina started to use two-word-utterances. She was seen by the authors for the first time at age 3;3. At that time, her age of lexical development was below 2;6 years (measured on the productive naming test by De Bleser & Kauschke in prep.). Her age of syntactic development was between age 2;0 and 2;5 according to criteria presented in Penner (1999). At age 4;10 Lina's lexical age was 3;0 and her syntactic age was still between 2;0–2;5. Her non-verbal IQ, as measured at age 6;1 with the *Culture Fair Intelligence Test – 5th revised edition* (CFT1) (Weiß & Osterland 1997), is 65. This value is in correspondence to formerly reported non-verbal IQs in WS. For the experiment Lina was tested at home in a quiet room with a television and a video recorder.

*Controls*

Given the observation that children with Williams syndrome generally show a delay in language acquisition it could not necessarily be assumed that Lina would perform as with chronologically age-matched controls. The following four control groups were therefore included in our study:

1. Children matched for syntactic age (Penner 1999), N = 9, age 2;0–2;5, 4 boys & 5 girls.
2. Children matched for lexical age (De Bleser & Kauschke in prep.), N = 7, age 2;6–2;11, 3 boys & 4 girls.
3. Children matched for chronological age, N = 5, age 4;6–5;1, 3 boys & 2 girls.
4. Children older than the WS child, N = 5, age 6;9–7;5, 2 boys & 3 girls.

The last group was included in order to be able to account for Lina's performance in case she performed better than the age-matched controls. None of the controls suffered from known neurological impairments, developmental delay, learning difficulties or a history of special needs. The lexical development of all the controls was additionally tested with the naming test for nouns and verbs (De Bleser & Kauschke in prep.). Its results showed no delays in vocabulary development.[6]

Control children were tested individually at the kindergarten or at school in a quiet room, using a television and a video recorder.

*Materials*

The test materials consisted of six video taped TV films of a total duration of five minutes. The characters in all the films are a comic mouse and a small comic elephant. When shown on German TV, the films were muted. For the fast mapping experiment, voice-over narration was added to each film. There were six stories, containing 12 target non-words from three word classes, i.e. 4 nouns, 4 verbs, and 4 adjectives. Unlike the fast mapping study by Carey and Bartlett (1978) in which the non-word "chromium" was presented just once, in our study each of the 12 new words was presented four times. This change of procedure was introduced in order to accommodate the task to the higher number of items to be learned.

For the nouns there were two monosyllabic masculine nouns and two disyllabic feminine nouns. The verbs consisted of disyllabic infinitival forms and past participle forms, and monosyllabic inflected 3rd person singular forms. Two of

Table 1. Material

| Material | Meaning |
|---|---|
| **Nouns** | |
| 1. die Kaafe (feminine) | 1. an old-fashioned milk churn |
| 2. die Kosel (feminine) | 2. a belt that attaches the mouse to a balloon |
| 3. der Nelf (masculine) | 3. a pocket in the mouse's fur |
| 4. der Lent (masculine) | 4. a musical instrument |
| **Verbs (all forms used in experiment)** | |
| 1. risten (transitive)<br>3rd form singular: ristet (4x) | 1. the little elephant grabs sth. with his trunk |
| 2. peken (transitive)<br>3rd form singular: pekt (1x)<br>infinitive: peken (1x)<br>past participle: gepekt (2x) | 2. the elephant's trunk is lengthened by the mouse |
| 3. timpern (intransitive)<br>3rd form singular: timpert (3x)<br>infinitive: timpern (1x) | 3. the mouse thrashes about her arms and legs in order to land with the balloon |
| 4. roggeln (intransitive)<br>3rd form singular: roggelt (2x)<br>infinitive: roggeln (2x) | 4. making music using the elephant's trunk |
| **Adjectives** | |
| 1. sarig (attribute) | 1. carrying an object in an inattentive way |
| 2. bakig (attribute) | 2. music that sounds disharmonious |
| 3. fappig (state) | 3. frustrated |
| 4. kirtig (state) | 4. having an idea |

the verbs were transitive, i.e. requiring a direct object in the accusative case, and two were intransitive, i.e. not requiring an object. All the adjectives were disyllabic. Two of the adjectives referred to emotional states and two to attributes. In order to keep the test items phonologically simple none of them contained an initial consonant cluster. With respect to their segmental structure the non-words were constructed in such a way that they displayed typical phonotactic properties of their corresponding word classes. Thus, for example, the final syllable of the feminine nouns contains a schwa-vowel as in 'Nase'/nose. The final syllable of the adjective '*-ig*' is typical for adjectives referring to properties such as 'farbig'/colored. Finally, the verbs are used in the forms mentioned above. All the items used are shown in Table 1. An example of the stories represented in the films can be found in the Appendix.

Similar to the study by Rothweiler (1999), we preferred a video presentation to a picture presentation as a film allowed for a more natural contextualization of the test items. Also, as Rice and Woodsmall (1988) have shown, language learning via

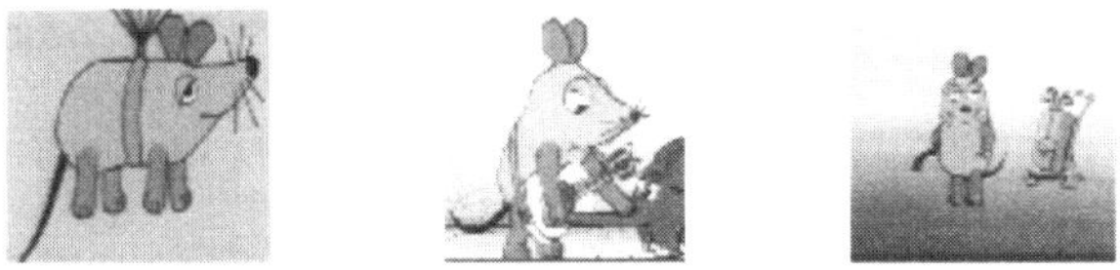

(a) Object (Noun) *Kosel* (b) Action (Verb) *peken* (c) State (Adjective) *fappig*

**Figure 1.** Example pictures from comprehension task (screenshots)

input from television in experiments is a successful method. A color television and a video recorder were used to present the six films. The volume was kept constant at about 55 dB for each participant. Example pictures for each word class used in the experiment are shown in Figure 1.

## Procedure

Each child was tested three times: at T1, T2, and T3. At T1 she watched the film twice. Immediately afterwards a comprehension test was carried out with the 12 test items in order to see how many of them the child could remember. The same procedure was repeated one week later (T2), only this time the films were presented once. Yet another week later (T3) only comprehension was tested. Table 2 summarizes the procedure.

Comprehension was tested with a word-picture matching task. For each of the 12 test items, i.e. novel words, the child was presented with the target picture, i.e. a screenshot from the films, and three foils (see Tables 3–5). The presentation of the test items was preceded by the presentation of three practice items (screenshots from the films) consisting of pictures of objects and their names which were familiar to the child. The function of the practice items was to test whether the child had in fact understood the task. In addition to the test trials, we included four filler trials (also screenshots from the films), i.e. two nouns and two verbs referring to familiar objects and events. The function of the filler items was to make sure that

**Table 2.** Procedure

| Fast mapping experiment | Procedure |
|---|---|
| T1 | 1. presentation of video (twice)<br>2. comprehension task |
| T2 (+ one week) | 1. presentation of the video (once)<br>2. comprehension task |
| T3 (+ one week) | comprehension task |

Table 3. Nouns

| TARGET | Foil 1: another new object; same agent as on target picture |
|---|---|
| Foil 2: existing object; same agent as on target picture | Foil 3: unrelated picture (other agent or showing just an existing object) |

Table 4. Verbs

| TARGET | Foil 1: picture presenting another new verb; same agent as on target picture |
|---|---|
| Foil 2: picture presenting existing verb; same agent as on target picture | Foil 3: unrelated picture (other agent) |

Table 5. Adjectives

| TARGET | Foil 1: picture presenting another new adjective; same agent as on target picture |
|---|---|
| Foil 2: picture presenting existing adjective; same agent as on target picture | Foil 3: unrelated picture (other agent) |

even children with very poor mapping performance would successfully recognize some of the words, thus keeping their level of frustration low.

## Results

The results of the three tests at T1, T2, and T3 for the controls (means, standard deviations, and percentage) and for the WS child Lina are shown in Table 6 and illustrated in Figure 2.

The control groups show a higher level of performance with increasing chronological age, the oldest children being the best performers (Mann-Whitney tests: $p < 0.05$ at all 3 test times for *syntactic group* vs. *older group* and *lexical group* vs. *older group*). All control groups show their best performance at T2. However, mean performance at the different test times did not differ significantly (McNemar Chi Square test). Performance of the WS child Lina was best at T1 (8/12 correct) and then decreased from T2 (3/12 correct) to T3 (2/12 correct). Here too, the differences were not significant (McNemar Chi Square test).

However her performance does differ from that of the control subjects in T-scores. In order to compare the performance of the single WS child with that of

Table 6. Results

| Groups/single case | | Means and Standard Deviations T1 | T2 | T3 |
|---|---|---|---|---|
| Syntactical age group | Mean | 4.22 | 4.89 | 4.11 |
| (2;0–2;5) | (SD) | (1.92) | (0.60) | (1.83) |
| | % correct | 35.2 | 40.8 | 34.3 |
| Lexical age group | Mean | 5.00 | 6.00 | 4.86 |
| (2;6–2;11) | (SD) | (1.63) | (1.63) | (1.46) |
| | % correct | 41.7 | 50.0 | 44.7 |
| Chronological age group | Mean | 4.80 | 6.80 | 5.00 |
| (4;6–5;1) | (SD) | (1.79) | (2.68) | (0.71) |
| | % correct | 40.0 | 56.7 | 41.7 |
| Older children group | Mean | 7.00 | 8.20 | 7.20 |
| (6;9–7;1) | (SD) | (0.71) | (0.84) | (1.10) |
| | % correct | 58.3 | 68.3 | 60.0 |
| Lina (4;7) – single case | Score | 8.00 | 3.00 | 2.00 |
| | % correct | 66.7 | 25.0 | 16.7 |

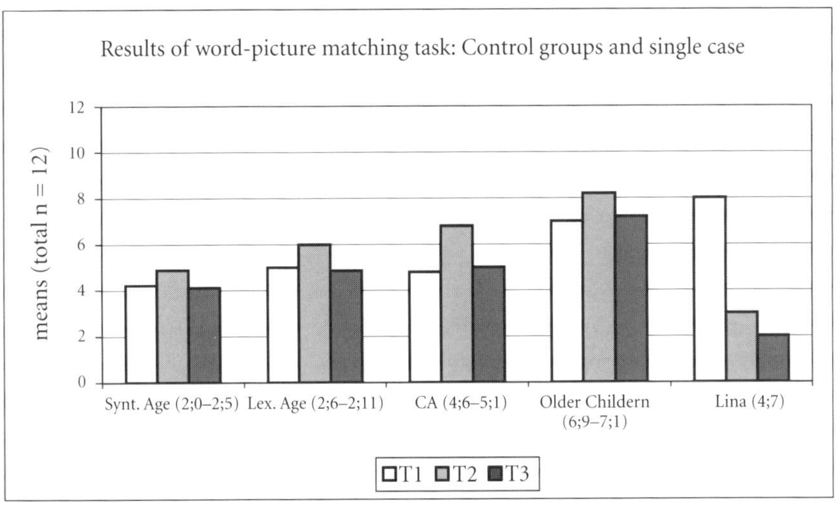


Figure 2. Results

the controls, we transformed Lina's score on the comprehension test into T-scores. In the T-score transformation the group's mean is assumed to be M = 50, while one standard deviation is SD = 10. Thus, if the WS child yields a T-score of 50, her performance is not significantly deviant from the performance of the controls. If she yields a T-score of 60, her performance is 1 SD from the mean, thus her

**Table 7.** T-score transformation

| test times | age of group | > −2 SD T < 30 | −2 SD T = 30–40 | −1 SD T = 40–50 | | +1 SD T = 50–60 | +2 SD T = 60–70 | > +2 SD T > 70 |
|---|---|---|---|---|---|---|---|---|
| T1 | 2;0–2;5 | | | | | | 69,68 | |
| | 2;6–2;11 | | | | mean | | 68,41 | |
| | 4;6–5;1 | | | | of | | 68,88 | |
| | 6;9–7;5 | | | | control | 51,41 | | |
| T2 | 2;0–2;5 | 18,5 | | | group | | | |
| | 2;6–2;11 | | 31,59 | | M = 50 | | | |
| | 4;6–5;1 | | 35,82 | | | | | |
| | 6;9–7;5 | −11,9 | | | | | | |
| T3 | 2;0–2;5 | | 38,47 | | | | | |
| | 2;6–2;11 | | 30,41 | | | | | |
| | 4;6–5;1 | 7,75 | | | | | | |
| | 6;9–7;5 | 2,73 | | | | | | |

performance would be better than the performance of the controls, etc. The result of this transformation procedure is shown in Table 7.

As can be seen in Table 7, the WS child achieved a higher level of performance than the three youngest control groups at T1. At age 4;7 she is in fact performing as the 6;9–7;5-year-olds at T1. Her performance at T2 and T3 also differs from that of the control subjects. At these test times she performs less well than all the control groups, i.e. more than −1 SD. In comparison to the syntactically matched control group and the lexically matched control group she performs within the second SD from the groups' mean. In comparison to the chronologically matched control group, and the control group of older children she performs more than 2 SDs lower than the normally developing children.

As in the controls there were no statistically significant differences in the performance for the different word classes.

To summarize, for the WS child we found, though not significant, inner-subject differences regarding performance at different test times, i.e. she achieved a higher level of performance at T1 than at T2 or T3. To the contrary, there are significant differences between the WS child and the control groups. At T1 the WS child showed a significantly better performance than the three youngest control groups matched for syntactic age, lexical age, and chronological age respectively. She showed performance similar to that of the older control group. At T2 and T3 however, the WS child performed worse (> 1 SD) than all control groups.

## General discussion and conclusion

The results of our study for the control children confirmed prior results concerning the fast mapping capacities of normally developing children. The controls overall were able to fast map 35.2 to 58.3 per cent of the new words after only few exposures during a single learning session (for similar results see Rothweiler 1999). Their performance improved after a second exposure to the new words a week later, i.e. 40.8 to 68.3 per cent. This performance level did not decrease significantly a week later, i.e. 34.3 to 60.0 per cent. That is, the second exposure to the new words must have reinforced their mental representations created during the first exposure, leading to a stable representation in long-term memory as evidenced by the performance at the third test point.

Finally the result that the oldest children (6;9–7;5) were the best performers in the comprehension task at all test times requires some discussion. We would like to suggest three reasons for this finding. Firstly, it has been shown that with increasing age children show higher levels of overall recall (Ornstein & Haden 2001). That is, the capacity for intentional and conscious memorizing increases with chronological age. The highest increase in memory abilities takes place between 6–10 years of age (Schneider & Büttner 1995). This may lead to the observed better performance in our oldest subjects. Secondly, we have to assume that the size of lexical knowledge in the older children is larger than in the younger ones. This means that there should be more unknown words in the films other than the test items for the younger controls than for the older. Thus, the older children should be able to focus more on the target words than the younger ones because most other words in the films should already be known to them. In other words, the older children can rely more on top down lexical processes for identifying and interpreting new words, i.e. for mapping sound onto meaning than younger children. And thirdly, the greater size of the lexicon in older children is also increasing the syntactic bootstrapping capacities for identifying the meaning of unknown words to the extent that the grammatical knowledge of the children is related to the size of their vocabulary (Bates & Goodman 1999).

In the following the results of the WS child will be discussed with respect to the three leading questions of our study repeated here for convenience:

Firstly, given the generally observed initial delay in lexical development in WS children, what are the fast mapping capacities of WS children at the early stage of word learning as compared to unimpaired controls?

Secondly, if WS children are able to fast map, is the result of the fast mapping integrated permanently into their mental lexicon?

Thirdly, is there a difference in the fast mapping of names of objects, properties and events, i.e. nouns, adjectives and verbs respectively?

Concerning the first question the results of our study show that the WS child Lina was able to do fast mappings: At T1 she recognized 66.7 per cent of the new words correctly even surpassing the performance of children two years older. This clearly shows that like unimpaired children matched for chronological and linguistic age Lina must be able to segment the speech input in a way which recognizes the unknown test words, to map them appropriately and efficiently onto the corresponding objects, actions and properties in the visual input, and to store the result of the mapping in short-term memory. With respect to the phonological processes involved these findings corroborate the findings of other authors that these are basically the same as in non-WS children (see Majerus in this volume, for an overview). Two additional comments are in order here: firstly, our findings support the view of Barisnikov (1996; for a different view see Grant et al. 1997) that short-term memory for non-words when phonologically simple, and, more specifically, close to the canonical structure of the child's language, is as good as or even better than in age matched controls. Secondly, if we assume that lexical constraints are an important prerequisite for fast mapping, our findings strongly suggest that the results of Stevens and Karmiloff-Smith (1997) for much older WS subjects which show that they may not use them as do unimpaired children, may not hold for younger WS children who should still be in the initial phase of vocabulary acquisition.

Concerning the second question, however, contrary to the controls, the performance of the WS child decreased dramatically over the following two test points. Apparently she did not build up long-term mental representations for the new words after the first exposure at T1. Consequently the second presentation of the new words a week later could not reinforce already existing lexical representations.

With respect to the third question, no difference between the fast mappings of different word classes were found, neither for the WS child nor for the controls.

These results raise two interesting further questions: Firstly, why does the WS child show a better fast mapping performance at T1 than all the control groups? And secondly, why does she not seem to be able to build up stable lexical representations in long-term memory despite her seemingly intact short-term memory capacities?

With respect to the first question we would like to propose the following answer: It has been suggested (Thomas et al. 2001; Majerus, Barisnikov, Vuillemin, Poncelet, & Van der Linden in press and Majerus in this volume) that possibly related to the known hyperacusis of WS individuals, their sublexical segmental discriminatory capacities are stronger than in non-WS individuals (overly detailed phonology hypothesis). Whereas, as has been argued by the same authors this may keep WS subjects from disregarding allophonic differences between occurrences of the same lexical item, thus preventing them from building up a stable phonological representation. These stronger than usual discriminatory capacities of WS subjects, combined with the above mentioned strength of short-term memory for simple and canonical phonological structures may lead, under the specific conditions of our experiment to the observed good performance at T1. That is, we assume that during the first presentation of the film at T1 the WS child builds up a more detailed short-term sublexical memory representation of the test items than the controls. This representation gets then reinforced under the immediately following second presentation which is acoustically identical to the first one due to the fact that it is recorded material. This last fact may result in an advantage for the WS child over the controls, given her good STM capacities and her greater discriminatory capacities in identifying the test items, leading to a strengthening of the short-term memory trace of more non-words than in the controls. This "more complete" STM representation of the non-words in the WS child then results in better recall of the items in the immediately following comprehension test which does not rely on LTM capacities.

Our results can thus be considered as providing support for the hypothesis put forward by various authors (Thomas et al. 2001; Majerus et al. in press and Majerus in this volume) that WS children may start out with a richer segmental inventory than non-WS children given their greater acoustic discriminatory capacities. This explanation of the good performance of the WS child in the first comprehension test would also predict her bad performance under the second test a week later, given that the non-words to be fast mapped were only presented once, thus no reinforcement in short-term memory could take place, and also given that the WS child assumingly could not rely on long-term memory representations of these items as with the controls.

We will now turn to the crucial second question why the WS child does not seem to succeed in building up LTM representations of the non-words in the same way the controls must be able to given their performance at T3. That the linguistic LTM capacities of individuals with WS may be weaker than in unimpaired individuals has been pointed out by several authors (e.g. Barisnikov et al. 1996; Vicari, Brizzolara, Carlesimo, Pezzini, & Volterra 1996). We would like to suggest that this may equally be the result of the greater sensitivity of the WS individuals to acoustic differences. Differently from the WS children in the unimpaired children, each occurrence of a specific target item reinforces its already existing memory trace given that the children's perceptual mechanisms focus on the similarities between the different occurrences. This means that in our experiment the controls in the first presentations heard each target item possibly eight times more often than the WS child because each occurrence of a target word was identified as a token of the type of this target word which may have been already constituted at the first occurrence of the target word. This leads to lexical LTM representations which are relatively abstract as compared to a given occurrence of this item.

The WS child, to the contrary, according to our assumption, focuses on the differences of the occurrences of the target items. This could result either in as many different lexical LTM representations as there had been acoustically different occurrences of the target item, if, as assumed by various authors possibly already one occurrence of a lexical item had been enough to build up a LTM representation (e.g. Carey & Bartlett 1978), or it may, in the other extreme, result in no LTM representation at all if a necessary critical mass of input had not been reached.

Now, under these assumptions, if the presentation of the target item in the comprehension test at T2 or T3 does not acoustically match the WS child's lexical LTM representations of these items perfectly this child will not be able to identify the target, leading to a result which would not differ from the one if the child had no LTM representation of the target at all.

The fact that in our study the performance of the WS child at T2 and T3 does not differ is compatible with both explanations. Further research will be necessary to decide between these alternatives.

To conclude, with respect to the general issue whether the mechanisms underlying the linguistic performance in children with WS are the same or different from those in unimpaired children our findings support the interpretation that they are the same, except for a difference in the acoustic perceptual capacities of the children which may lead to differences in their lexical representations. These differences in turn may explain the observed performance differences with unimpaired children in particular linguistic processing tasks such as fast mapping, and the differences in linguistic development. Obviously, further research has to determine whether our findings based on one individual with WS hold for children with WS in general.

## Acknowledgements

We are very grateful to Lina and her family who have supported our research for so many years. Thank you to A. Mühlberg for collecting the data and to the control children and their parents for the participation in this study. We also want to thank S. Collins, A. Crocket-Naini, M. Rothweiler, and J. Siegmüller for helpful comments.

An earlier version of this paper has been presented at the International workshop on "Separability of cognitive functions: What can be learned from Williams Syndrome?" University of Massachusetts, Amherst, August 2001.

## Notes

1. British Picture Vocabulary Scale (Dunn, Dunn, Whetton, & Pintilie 1982).

2. Peabody Picture Vocabulary Test (Dunn & Dunn 1981).

3. Definition of the Whole Object Constraint: "…, a child should first hypothesize that the new word refers to an object as an exemplar of a category of similar objects, and not to the object's part, substance, etc." (Markman & Wachtel 1988).

4. Definition of the Mutual Exclusivity Constraint: "The mutual exclusivity assumption leads children to prefer only one label for an object" (Markman 1994:218).

5. Definition of the Taxonomic Assumption: "…the taxonomic assumption .. states that terms refer to entities of the same kind. An object term would refer to objects of the same kind, a color term to colors of the same kind, an action term to actions of the same kind, and so on" (Markman 1994:203).

6. Following this, it is assumed that verbal age, mental age and chronological age do coincide.

## References


Akhtar, N. & Tomasello, M. (2000). "The social nature of word learning". In R. Michnick Golinkoff, K. Hirsh-Pasek, L. Bloom, L. B. Smith, A. Woodward, N. Akhtar, M. Tomasello, & G. Hollich (Eds.), *Becoming a Word Learner: A debate on lexical acquisition* (pp. 115–135). Oxford: OUP.

Barisnikov, K., Van der Linden, M., & Poncelet, M. (1996). "Acquisition of new words and phonological working memory in Williams syndrome: A case study". *Neurocase, 2*, 395–404.

Bates, E., Dale, P. S., & Thal, D. (1995). "Individual differences and their implications for theories of language development". In P. Fletcher & B. MacWhinney (Eds.), *The Handbook of Child Language* (pp. 96–151). Oxford: Blackwell.

Bates, E. & Goodman, J. (1999). "On the emergence of grammar from the lexicon". In B. MacWhinney (Ed.), *The Emergence of Language* (pp. 29–79). Mahwah, NJ: Psychology Press.

Bellugi, U., Marks, S., Bihrle, A., & Sabo, H. (1988). "Dissociation between language and cognitive functions in Williams syndrome". In D. Bishop & K. Mogford (Eds.), *Language Development in Exceptional Circumstances* (pp. 132–149). Hillsdale, NJ: LEA.

Bellugi, U., Wang, P. P., & Jernigan, T. (1994). "Williams syndrome: An unusual neuropsychological profile". In S. H. Broman & J. Grafman (Eds.), *Atypical Cognitive Deficits in Developmental Disorders: Implications for brain functions* (pp. 23–56). Hillsdale, NJ: LEA.

Calamandrei, G., Alleva, E., Cirulli, F., Queyras, A., Volterra, V., Capirci, O., Vicari, S. Giannotti, A., Turrini, P., & Aloe, L. (2000). "Serum NGF levels in children and adolescents with either Williams syndrome of Down syndrome." *Developmental Medicine and Child Neurology, 42*, 746–750.

Capirci, O., Sabbadini, L., & Volterra, V. (1996). "Language development in Williams syndrome: A case study". *Cognitive Neuropsychology, 13*, 1017–1039.

Carey, S. & Bartlett, E. (1978). "Acquiring a single new word". *Papers and Reports in Child Language Development, 15*, 17–29.

Clahsen, H. & Almazan, M. (1998). "Syntax and morphology in Williams syndrome". *Cognition, 68*, 167–198.

Clahsen, H. & Almazan, M. (2001). "Compounding and inflection in language impairment: Evidence from Williams syndrome (and SLI)". *Lingua, 110*, 729–757.

Clahsen, H. & Temple, C. (2001). "Words and rules in children with Williams syndrome". In Y. Levy & J. Schaeffer (Eds.), *Language Competence across Populations* (pp. 1–40). Mahwah, NJ: LEA.

De Bleser, R. & Kauschke, C. (in preparation). *Benenntest für Nomen und Verben*. Potsdam.

Dunn, L. M. & Dunn, L. M. (1981). *Peabody Picture Vocabulary Test – Revised*. Circle Pines, MN: American Guidance Service.

Dunn, L. M., Dunn, L. M., Whetton, C., & Pintilie, D. (1982). *British Picture Vocabulary Scale*. Windsor Berks.: NFER-Nelson.

Grant, J., Karmiloff-Smith, A., Berthoud, I., & Christophe, A. (1996). "Is the language of people with Williams syndrome mere mimicry? Phonological short-term memory in a foreign language". *Cahiers de Psychologie Cognitive, 15*, 615–628.

Grant, J., Karmiloff-Smith, A., Gathercole, S. A., Paterson, S., Howlin, P., Davies, M., & Udwin, O. (1997). "Phonological short-term memory and its relationship to language in Williams syndrome". *Cognitive Neuropsychiatry, 2*, 81–99.

Grant, J., Valian, V., & Karmiloff-Smith, A. (2002). "A study of relative clauses in Williams syndrome". *Journal of Child Language, 29*, 403–416.

Howlin, P., Davies, B., & Udwin, O. (1998). "Cognitive functioning in adults with Williams syndrome". *Journal of Child Psychology and Psychiatry, 39*, 183–189.

Jarrold, C., Baddeley, A. D., & Hewes, A. K. (1998). "Verbal and nonverbal abilities in the Williams syndrome phenotype: Evidence for diverging developmental trajectories". *Journal of Child Psychology and Psychiatry, 39*, 511–523.

Jarrold, C., Baddeley, A. D., & Hewes, A. K. (1999). "Genetically dissociated components of working memory: Evidence from Down´s and Williams syndrome". *Neuropsychologia, 37*, 637–651.

Jarrold, C., Baddeley, A. D., Hewes, A. K., & Philips, C. (2001). "A longitudinal assessment of diverging verbal and non-verbal abilities in the Williams syndrome phenotype". *Cortex, 37*, 423–431.

Jarrold, C., Hartley, S. J., Philips, C., & Baddeley, A. D. (2000). "Word fluency in Williams syndrome: Evidence for unusual semantic organization?" *Cognitive Neuropsychiatry, 5*, 293–319.

Karmiloff-Smith, A., Klima, E., Bellugi, U., Grant, J., & Baron-Cohen, S. (1995). "Is there a social module? Language, face processing, and theory of mind in individuals with Williams syndrome". *Journal of Cognitive Neuroscience, 7*, 196–208.

Karmiloff-Smith, A., Klima, E., Bellugi, U., Grant, J., & Baron-Cohen, S. (1997). "Language and Williams syndrome: How intact is intact?" *Child Development, 68*, 246–262.

Karmiloff-Smith, A., Tyler, K. T., Voice, K., Sims, K., Udwin, O., Howlin, P., & Davies, M. (1998). "Linguistic dissociations in Williams syndrome: Evaluating receptive syntax in on-line and off-line tasks". *Neuropsychologia, 36*, 343–351.

Mac Donald, G. W. & Roy, D. L. (1988). "Williams syndrome: A neuropsychological profile". *Journal of Clinical and Experimental Neuropsychology, 10*, 125–131.

Majerus, S., Barisnikov, K., Vuillemin, I., Poncelet, M., & Van der Linden, M. (in press). "An investigation of verbal short-term memory and phonological processing in four children with Williams syndrome". submitted to *Neurocase*.

Markman, E. (1989). *Categorization and naming in children*. Cambridge, MA: The MIT Press.

Markman, E. (1992). "Constraints on word learning: Speculations about their nature, origins, and domain specificity". In M. Gunnar & M. Maratsos (Eds.), *Modularity and Constraints in Language and Cognition* (pp. 59–103). Hillsdale, NJ: LEA.

Markman, E. (1993). "Constraints children place on word meanings". In P. Bloom (Ed.), *Language Acquisition* (pp. 154–179). New York, NY: Core Readings.

Markman, E. (1998). "Early use of word learning constraints". *Annual Report of Educational Psychology in Japan, 37*, 21–26.

Markman, E. & Hutchinson, J. E. (1984). "Children's sensitivity to constraints on word meaning: Taxonomic versus thematic relations". *Cognitive Psychology, 18*, 1–27.

Markman, E. & Wachtel, G. (1988). "Children's use of mutual exclusivity to constrain the meaning of words". *Cognitive Psychology, 20*, 121–157.

Markman, E. M. (1994). "Constraints on word meaning in early language acquisition". *Lingua, 92*, 199–227.

Masataka, N. (2000). "Information from speech and gesture is integrated when meanings of new words are categorized in normal children but not in children with Williams syndrome". *Cognitive Studies, 7*, 37–51.

Mervis, C., Morris, C. A., Bertrand, J., & Robinson, B. F. (1999). "Williams syndrome: Findings from an integrated program of research". In H. Tager-Flusberg (Ed.), *Neurodevelopmental Disorders: Contributions to a new framework from cognitive neuroscience* (pp. 65–110). Cambridge, MA: The MIT Press.

Mervis, C. B. & Robinson, B. F. (2000). "Expressive vocabulary ability of toddlers with Williams syndrome or Down syndrome: A comparison". *Developmental Neuropsychology, 17*, 111–126.

Nazzi, T. & Karmiloff-Smith, A. (2002). "Early categorization in young children with Williams syndrome". *Neuroreport, 13*, 1–4.

Ornstein, P. A. & Haden, C. A. (2001). "Memory development or the development of memory?" *Current Directions in Psychological Science, 10*, 202–205.

Penner, Z. (1999). *Screeningverfahren zur Feststellung von Störungen in der Grammatik*. Luzern: SZH.

Pezzini, G., Vicari, S., Volterra, V., Milani, L., & Ossella, M. T. (1999). "Children with Williams syndrome: Is there a single neuropsychological profile?" *Developmental Neuropsychology, 15*, 141–155.

Quine, W. V. O. (1960). *Word and Object*. Cambridge, MA: The MIT Press.

Rice, M. L. & Woodsmall, L. (1988). "Lessons from television: children's word learning when viewing". *Child Development, 59*, 420–429.

Rossen, M., Klima, E., Bellugi, U., Bihrle, A., & Jones, W. (1996). "Interaction between language and cognition: Evidence from Williams syndrome". In J. H. Beitchman, N. Cohen, M. Konstantareas, & R. Tannock (Eds.), *Language, Learning and Behavior Disorders: Developmental, biological, and clinical perspectives* (pp. 367–392). New York, NY: CUP.

Rothweiler, M. (1999). "Neue Ergebnisse zum fast mapping bei sprachnormalen und bei sprachentwicklungsgestörten Kindern". In J. Meibauer & M. Rothweiler (Eds.), *Das Lexikon im Spracherwerb* (pp. 252–276). Tübingen: Francke (UTB).

Schneider, W. & Büttner, G. (1995). "Entwicklung des Gedächtnisses". In R. Oerter & L. Montada (Eds.), *Entwicklungspsychologie: Ein Lehrbuch* (pp. 654–704). Weinheim: Psychologie Verlags Union.

Siegmüller, J. (2003). Sprachkompetenz bei Williams-Beuren-Syndrom. Unpublished dissertation, University of Potsdam.

Singer Harris, N. G., Bellugi, U., Bates, E., Jones, W., & Rossen, M. (1997). "Contrasting profiles of language development in children with Williams and Down syndrome". *Developmental Neuropsychology, 13*, 345–370.

Stevens, T. & Karmiloff-Smith, A. (1997). "Word learning in a special population: Do individuals with Williams syndrome obey lexical constraints?" *Journal of Child Language, 24*, 737–765.

Stojanovik, V., Perkins, M., & Howard, S. (2001). "Language and conversational abilities in Williams syndrome: How good is good?" *International Journal of Language and Communication Disorders, 36*, 234–239.

Tager-Flusberg, H. (1999). "An introduction to research on neurodevelopmental disorders from a cognitive neuroscience perspective". In H. Tager-Flusberg (Ed.), *Neurodevelopmental disorders* (pp. 3–24). London: Bradford.

Temple, C., Almazan, M., & Sherwood, S. (2002). "Lexical skills in Williams syndrome: A cognitive neuropsychological analysis". *Journal of Neurolinguistics, 15*, 463–495.

Thomas, M. S. C., Grant, J., Barham, Z., Gsödl, M., Laing, E., Lakusta, L., Tyler, L. K. T., Grice, S., Patterson, S., & Karmiloff-Smith, A. (2001). "Past tense formation in Williams syndrome". *Language and Cognitive Processes, 16*, 143–176.

Tyler, L. K., Karmiloff-Smith, A., Voice, K., Stevens, T., Grant, J., Udwin, O., Davies, M., & Howlin, P. (1997). "Do individuals with Williams syndrome have bizarre semantics? Evidence for lexical organization using an on-line task". *Cortex, 33*, 515–527.

Vicari, S., Brizzolara, D., Carlesimo, G. A., Pezzini, G., & Volterra, V. (1996). "Memory abilities in children with Williams syndrome". *Cortex, 32*, 503–514.

Volterra, V., Capirci, O., Pezzini, G., Sabbadini, L., & Vicari, S. (1996). "Linguistic abilities in italian children with Williams syndrome". *Cortex, 32*, 663–677.

Volterra, V., Longobardi, E., Pezzini, G., Vicari, S., & Antenore, C. (1999). "Visuo-spatial and linguistic abilities in a twin with Williams syndrome". *Journal of Intellectual Disability Research, 43*, 294–305.

Wang, P. P. & Bellugi, U. (1994). "Evidence from two genetic syndromes for a dissociation between verbal and visual-spatial short-term memory". *Journal of Clinical and Experimental Neuropsychology, 16*, 317–322.

Weiß, R. & Osterland, J. (1997). *CFT 1: Culture Fair Intelligence Test, 5th revised edition.* Göttingen: Hogrefe.

## Appendix

### An example story from the fast mapping video

**The Balloon**
Oh, the mouse has got a KOSEL (*N, fem.*) around her belly! The KOSEL holds the mouse to the balloon. The mouse wants to land but she can't! The mouse TIMPERs (*V, third person singular*) with her legs and she also TIMPERs with her tail trying to land. Hmmm... She also TIMPERs with her ears. Now, the mouse is KIRTIG (*emotional state adjective*)! If she TIMPERs very strongly, the balloon will burst, the KOSEL will come down and the mouse will land. Now, there she is with the KOSEL around her belly and she is happy.

**Der Ballon**
Oh, hier hat die Maus eine KOSEL um ihren Bauch. Die Kosel hält die Maus fest an einem Ballon. Die Maus will landen, aber das klappt nicht. Die Maus TIMPERT mit den Beinen und sie TIMPERT auch mit dem Schwanz, um runter zu kommen. Hm, sie TIMPERT sogar mit den Ohren. Jetzt ist die Maus KIRTIG. Sie muss so doll hin und her TIMPERN bis der Ballon platzt, die KOSEL abreißt und sie runterfällt. Nun sitzt sie da, mit der Kosel um ihren Bauch und freut sich.

# Language in preschool Italian children with Williams and Down syndromes

Virginia Volterra, Olga Capirci, and Maria Cristina Caselli
Stefano Vicari
Institute of Cognitive Sciences and Technologies, CNR, Rome /
Children's Hospital Bambino Gesù, Santa Marinella, Italy

In the first section, studies conducted on communicative and linguistic abilities in Italian speaking children with Williams syndrome (WS) and with Down syndrome (DS) are briefly reviewed. These studies were carried out separately on the two populations. In the second section results of more recent studies comparing directly early stages of language development in the two genetically distinct syndromes are reported. Our findings confirm that language is not ahead of mental age in children with WS at an early age and further suggest that the apparently spared linguistic abilities in these children are in part an artifact of comparisons made with DS children, whose morphosyntactic abilities are more compromised relative to their non verbal mental age and to their lexical repertoire.

The best way to study language acquisition and development is to explore all those conditions in which language does not develop or does develop in atypical ways. The study of language acquisition in special populations provides a privileged standpoint, offering particular insight into the relationship between linguistic, perceptual and cognitive abilities. Through a close comparison of data on language development and use in individuals displaying atypical profiles, we can better explore the role played by cognitive and/or perceptual factors.

The Williams syndrome (WS) has received special attention for the particular cognitive and linguistic profile that has been described by some authors. Older children and adolescents with WS were described as exhibiting unusual linguistic abilities despite poor performance in various visuospatial tasks. A facility for language was rarely observed in other populations with the same degree of mental retardation. For this reason, it has been suggested that WS may provide evidence for the independence of language from cognition (Pinker 1994, 1999 and Maratsos

& Matheny 1994 for discussion). The hypothesized dissociation between language and nonverbal cognition seemed to emerge most clearly when performance by children with WS was compared with performance by children with Down syndrome (DS) on the same verbal and non-verbal tasks (Bellugi & St. George 2001, for a recent review).

In the last ten years our Laboratory at CNR, (Institute of Psychology, now Institute of Cognitive Sciences and Technologies) in collaboration with the Children's Hospital Bambino Gesù (Department of Neurology and Rehabilitation at Santa Marinella) has conducted various studies on language in children with atypical development.

In the present chapter we will briefly review the studies conducted on communicative and linguistic abilities in Italian children with WS and in Italian children with Down syndrome (DS). Because until recently our studies were carried on the two syndromes separately, our review will describe first studies conducted on children and adolescents with WS and then studies conducted on children and adolescents with DS. In both cases the review is presented, as much as possible, according to a chronological perspective. Then we will report the first results of a major program for investigating and directly comparing early stages of language development in children with WS and in children with DS.

Our main goal is to investigate whether children with comparable levels of general cognitive impairment, but genetically distinct syndromes, are equivalently delayed in language acquisition, and if and how their linguistic profiles differ early in development in a richly inflected language like Italian.

## Review of previous studies on Italian children with WS and DS

In a first study (Volterra, Capirci, Pezzini, Sabbadini, & Vicari 1996) we decided to investigate linguistic abilities of Italian children with WS in order to answer specifically two relevant questions:

> *Are children with WS ahead, behind or equal to normally developing children of the same mental age on language measures ?*

and

> *Do children with WS display unique patterns of grammatical morphology in a rich inflected language like Italian?*

Lexical and morphosyntactic abilities in 17 individuals with WS between 4.10 and 15.3 years of age were explored. The mean mental age of these persons with WS was 5.2 years (range 3.8 to 6.8 years), reflecting a mean IQ of 56 (range 38–90). In all of the relevant language measures children with WS were compared with a sample of 116 normally-developing children whose chronological age corresponded to the mental age range of the children with WS. The language measures that were used included both lexical and grammatical measures. Comprehension was evaluated by the Peabody Picture Vocabulary test (PPVT), the Test for Reception of Grammar (TROG). Production was evaluated by the Boston Naming test (BNT), by the Category Test for Semantic Fluency (WF category), by the Phonological Fluency Test (WF phonology), by the Sentence Repetition Test (SRT), and by three Story Description tasks.

Results of the comparison showed that the two groups did not differ on the Peabody test for lexical comprehension, on the Category Test for Semantic Fluency, or on Mean Length of Utterance calculated from the story descriptions. However, individuals with WS did obtain significantly poorer results than normal controls on the TROG test, on the Boston Naming Test, and on the Sentence Repetition Test. In contrast, the individuals with WS performed significantly better than controls on the Phonology fluency test.

Our answer to the first question was that the language produced by persons with WS in this age range was for the most part not ahead of their mental age and that our data offered very little evidence for a dissociation between language and cognition. As to our second question, the language produced by our children with WS was unusual from several points of view. By investigating language development in children with WS exposed to Italian we were able to see some patterns that would be difficult to detect in English. In particular our children with WS produced some grammatical errors that were qualitatively different from anything that has usually been reported for normally developing children acquiring Italian, including errors of gender agreement and verb conjugation, and substitutions of prepositions and function words. We also found word order inversions that have rarely been reported for children acquiring Italian or English.

In order to explore whether these qualitative deviations are determined by a different rate in the language acquisition process, we conducted a detailed longitudinal study of the first stages of cognitive and linguistic development of an Italian girl with WS followed through weekly observations from 18 months to 58 months of age and systematically tested every two months (Capirci, Sabbadini, & Volterra 1996). The results of the study confirmed a delayed and partially atypical profile of language development in children and adolescents with WS.

Despite an initial delay which appeared less marked than is usually reported for children with WS, Elisa's rate and sequence of development seemed to be similar to those observed in control children. However, in contrast to children with typical development, she displayed an uneven pattern of within-domain dissociations. Elisa exhibited fluent vocabulary and proficient use of syntax, at least in some contexts, but failed with simple grammatical agreement: she made several kinds of grammatical errors (gender agreement between article and noun and in pronominalization) that are rarely made by children at the same syntactic level.[1]

In a following paper we have explored the question of variability in performance between individuals within the group with WS. Comparing Italian children and adolescents with WS with a group of younger typically developing children on the same visuo-spatial and linguistic tasks, our results suggested that children with WS do not exhibit a single cognitive profile. Instead, considerable variability across individuals with WS has been found. In the four individual cases we examined in detail, each of the children showed a different pattern of sparing and impairment on the linguistic and visual-spatial tasks. But in all four cases a particular difficulty in visuo-motor construction test (block construction test) was recognized (Pezzini, Vicari, Volterra, Milani, & Ossella 1999).

In another study reporting a case of dizygotic twins, one boy with WS and one typically developing girl, our goal was to verify whether the child with WS displayed a cognitive profile unique to the syndrome (Volterra, Longobardi, Pezzini, Vicari, & Antenore 1999). The special case gave us a unique opportunity to compare in more detail the neuropsychological profile of a child with WS with that of a normal control matched for age and family background. Several tests designed to assess visuo-perceptual, visuo-motor, linguistic and memory abilities were administered to both children when they were 10 years and 9 months of age. Compared to his sister, the boy with WS displayed a developmental delay in many non-verbal and verbal abilities. He achieved a level of performance similar to his sister only in facial recognition, phonological word fluency and memory for phonologically similar words. But, despite the overall delayed performance of the boy with WS, both the twins displayed a cognitive profile characterized by strength in lexical comprehension and relative weakness in visuomotor abilities.

In a more recent study two distinct lines of investigation were presented: the study of linguistic competence in the written language of deaf children and adults, and the study of linguistic development in children and adolescents with WS. Italian deaf people demonstrate selective difficulties with aspects of grammatical morphology playing a syntactic rather than a semantic function. Italian people with WS displayed a particular asymmetric fragmentation within linguistic abilities: a profile of strength in phonological abilities but serious deficits in semantic and morphosyntactic aspects of language. The case of these two very different populations offered us important clues for investigating which aspects of language and specifically of grammar are influenced by modality of perception.

Studies conducted by our laboratory have demonstrated that children with WS present, in the presence of well preserved phonological processes, slightly impaired lexical-semantic and morphosyntactic abilities challenging the popular view that people with WS present a peculiar and remarkable dissociation between relatively preserved linguistic abilities and visuo-spatial deficits. A complex pattern of spared and impaired functions both in the linguistic and visuo-spatial domains is the emerging picture for WS children's mental architecture, replacing the previous interpretation of a dichotomy between language and visuo-spatial abilities (Karmiloff-Smith, Grant, Berthoud, Davies, Howlin, & Udwin 1997). Dissociations within the linguistic domain in WS subjects and, particularly, a better efficiency of phonological than lexical-semantic encoding processes, is also supported by recent studies conducted in both short-term and long-term memory (Vicari, Carlesimo, Brizzolara, & Pezzini 1996; Vicari, Brizzolara, Carlesimo, Pezzini, & Volterra 1996; Vicari, Bellucci, & Carlesimo 2001).

Children with Down syndrome, although there are rare exceptions (Vallar & Papagno 1993; Rondal 1995) usually exhibit impairments in language acquisition. Problems in morphology and syntax are frequently reported (Fowler 1990; Miller 1992; Chapman 1995; Schaner-Wolles 2000).

Fabbretti, Pizzuto, Vicari and Volterra (1997) compared linguistic production on a story description task administered to older children and adolescents with DS (from 6 to 15 years) with that of normally developing subjects matched on mean length of utterance. The results revealed strong individual differences in the sample of individuals with DS. Data analysis focused on a subset of lexical, morphological and syntactic aspects of language use. The results showed that the individuals with DS and their normal matches used a similar lexical repertoire. However, the two groups differed with respect to omissions of free morphemes, and some aspects of syntactic and pragmatic abilities.

In recent years we have focused our attention on early communicative and linguistic development in Italian children with DS.

Two studies investigated the relationship between gestures and words in the early stages (Caselli, Vicari, Longobardi, Lami, Pizzoli, & Stella 1998; Caselli, Longobardi, & Pisaneschi 1997), revealing a more extensive use of communicative gestures by children with DS compared with normally developing children at the same stage of communicative-linguistic development. This "advantage" in the gestural modality can be interpreted as an indirect sign of a verbal ability that is having trouble developing adequately.

Another study (Vicari, Caselli, & Tonucci 2000) explored the acquisition of language in children with DS focusing on the potential dissociation between mental age and specific aspects of language. Particular attention was given to the emergence of morphosyntactic abilities compared with the lexicon. Fifteen children with DS (from 4 to 7 years) and fifteen normal controls matched on mental age participated in the study. For children with DS the results showed a lower performance in language abilities with respect to the normal controls. No dissociation was evident between lexical and cognitive abilities in either group, but specific morphosyntactic difficulties emerged both in comprehension and production for the DS group.

A more recent study by Iverson, Longobardi, and Caselli (2003) has analyzed early word and gesture communicative use in children with DS in spontaneous interaction with their mothers. Ten children from upper-middle class families participated in the study. The five children with DS had an average chronological age of 47.6 months, an average mental age of 22.4 months, and an average language age of 18 months. Each child with DS was matched to a typically developing child on the basis of gender, language age, and observed expressive vocabulary size. Results showed that although children with DS had significantly smaller gestural repertoires than their language age-matched peers, there was no reliable difference between the two groups in the overall use of gesture. In addition, children with DS produced many crossmodal combinations (gesture-word) but they did not use two-word combinations as their typically developing controls.

Children with DS, consistently with their linguistic difficulties, have been shown to be always very poor when they have to encode and elaborate verbal stimuli. Some studies have reported impairments in phonological short-term as well as long-term memory abilities (Vicari & Carlesimo 2002; Carlesimo, Marotta, & Vicari 1997).

From the above review, it is clear that our studies have been conducted separately on people with WS or DS. For example children with WS were compared with normally developing children whose chronological age corresponded to the mental age of children with WS and their linguistic performance was never directly compared to that of children with DS on the same tasks. In the following sections we are going to summarize two recent studies comparing directly Italian-speaking children with WS and Italian-speaking children with DS of comparable global cognitive level (Vicari, Caselli, Gagliardi, Tonucci, & Volterra 2002; Volterra, Caselli, Capirci, Tonucci, & Vicari 2003).

## Study 1

The goal of this study was to gather more detailed data on language acquisition in Italian-speaking children with WS, in children with DS of comparable global cognitive level, i.e. matched for chronological and mental age, and in typically developing (TD) children matched for mental age. Particularly, we wished to investigate whether infants with WS are as proficient in language processing during infancy as they are reported to be in adolescent and adult life. Another aim of the study was to explore whether language development in atypical populations is merely delayed, in comparison with the developmental stages followed by typically developing children, or whether it follows a different developmental trajectory.

**Table 1.** Mean (in months) and SD of chronological and mental age of children with WS, with DS and TD controls

| GROUPS | CHRON. AGE | MENTAL AGE |
|---|---|---|
| WS CHILDREN (M = 7; F = 5) | 58.2 (22.4) | 34 (14.8) |
| DS CHILDREN (M = 6; F = 6) | 67.2 (9.9) | 32.2 (5.4) |
| TD CHILDREN (M = 7; F = 5) | 29.7 (3.5) | 30 (4.9) |

## Participants

The sample consisted of twelve children with WS, matched on the basis of mental age to a group of twelve children with DS and to a group of twelve TD children. In all three groups mental age was assessed using the Brunet-Lezine Scale (1967) or the Leiter Intelligence Performance Scale (1980).

The children with WS and DS came from the *Children's Hospital Bambino Gesù* of Santa Marinella, Rome and from *La Nostra Famiglia Institute* of Bosisio Parini. The children with WS and DS were also matched for chronological age. The sample was further selected on the basis of the following criteria: a positive FISH test for elastin deletion for children with WS, a free trisomy 21 documented by karyotyping for children with DS, the absence of any neurosensory deficits, such as hypoacusia or serious impairment of visus, the absence of epilepsy and psychopathological disorders. The three groups of children were given the same tests. For evaluation purposes, the children with WS and DS were examined in the hospital on two occasions within approximately a one-week period. The TD controls were examined individually at school. All the observations were videotaped and subsequently transcribed and analyzed after informed consent was obtained from the families.

The chronological and mental age in months for all children (including means and standard deviations within each group) are reported in Table 1.

## Vocabulary and grammatical complexity

The questionnaire Primo Vocabolario del Bambino (PVB), the Italian version of the MacArthur Communicative Development Inventory (Caselli & Casadio 1995) was adopted for assessing lexical and grammatical competence. The Words and Sentences Form used for this study consists of a section on vocabulary production (670 words) and a section on grammatical complexity (37 pairs of sentences). The parents of the children included in the sample were asked to fill out the questionnaire and were told the aim was to collect detailed information about their child's language development. Particularly, in the vocabulary list the parents were asked to cross off the words that their child produced in spontaneous conversation. In the section referring to grammatical complexity, the parents were asked, for each pair

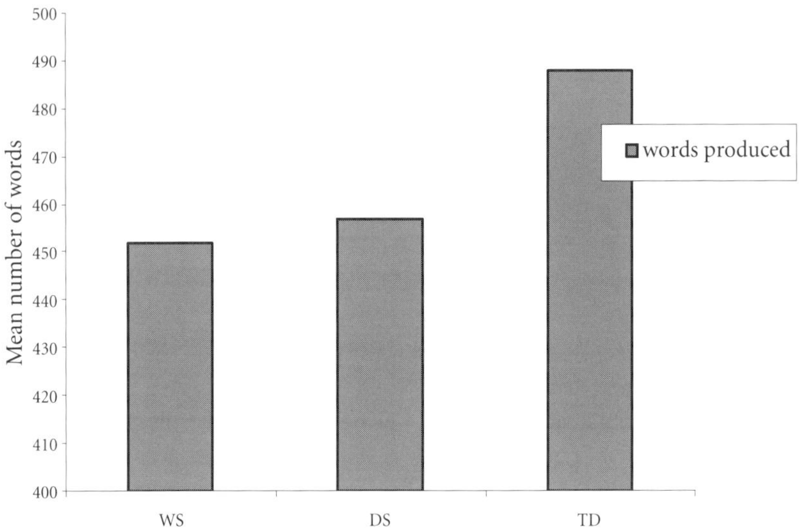


**Figure 1.** Mean number of words produced by children with WS, with DS and TD controls

of phrases, to choose the one closest to the kinds of expressions spontaneously used by their own child. All parents willingly participated in the data collection showing interest in the instrument.

For the purpose of scoring, the total number of words marked by the parents as produced by the child were summed. In addition the types of sentences produced were scored.

The mean number of word types reported by children with WS, DS and TD controls is presented in Figure 1. TD children produced an average of 488 different words (SD = 116.4), while children with WS and DS produced an average of 452 (SD = 157.3) and 457 (SD = 125.4) different words, respectively. An ANOVA was performed treating group as the independent variable and the number of different words produced as the dependent variable. There was no significant difference between the three groups of children [$F(2,33) = 0.25$]. It is worth noting the range of individual variability in the groups: this is typical in the early stages of language development. Therefore, since there were no differences in lexical abilities among children with WS, DS and their TD controls, we have no evidence here for a dissociation between lexical development and non-linguistic cognition.

Differences emerged when the performances of the three groups were considered in the section of the questionnaire referring to grammatical complexity (Figure 2). This section consists of 37 pairs of phrases. Each phrase is presented in two versions: the first without any function words (telegraphic style) and/or lack-

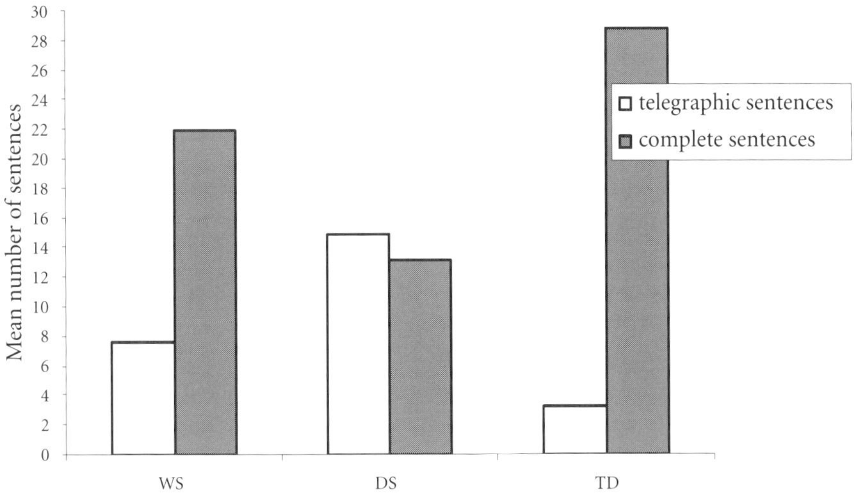


**Figure 2.** Mean number of telegraphic and complete sentences produced by children with WS, with DS and TD controls

ing any predicate and/or necessary argument (incomplete sentence), the second is morphosyntactically complete (for example: (a) *Medicine no*! (b) *I don't want any medicine*).

The three groups of children, with equivalent vocabularies, differed in the type of sentences used. An ANOVA performed with group as the independent variable and the number of simple/telegraphic sentences produced as the dependent variable showed a significant difference between the three groups of children [F (2,31) = 4.7]. Planned comparisons revealed that, on average, children with DS used more simple and telegraphic sentences (M = 14.9, SD = 11.8) than TD controls (M = 3.2, SD = 3.5). Children with WS used a smaller number of telegraphic sentences than children with DS but a higher number than TD controls (M = 7.6, SD = 9.7). Although no statistical difference emerged between WS and TD control groups [F (2,31) = 1.36], a comparison between WS and DS children approached significance [F (2,31) = 3.7, p = .06]. Similar results were obtained by analyzing the number of complete sentences produced by the three groups [F (2,33) = 5.37, p < .05]. TD children produced more complete sentences (M = 28.8, SD = 8.1) than children with WS (M = 21.9, SD = 13.4) and with DS (M = 13.1, SD = 10.4). Once again, the comparison between DS children and TD controls was statistically significant [F (1,30) = 10.6, p < .01], while the DS versus WS comparison only approached significance [F (1,30) = 3.7, p = .06] and the WS versus TD controls' comparison was not significant [F (1,30) = 2.1].

## Sentence comprehension

Comprehension was assessed by the Verbal comprehension test (VCT by Chilosi, Pfanner, & Cipriani 1996). This test explores children's ability to understand increasingly complex phrases. Namely, the child was asked to perform a requested action correctly. The requests included the following: performing motor and verbal routines, pointing to some parts of the body, performing the requested actions by choosing the correct toy lying on the table in front of them.

Children were given one point for each item they answered correctly by performing the requested action.

Each group's performance on this test is shown in Figure 3. They were analysed by an ANOVA in which group was treated as the independent variable and the number of correct responses and actions as the dependent variable [$F(2,33) = 4.14$, $p < .05$].

Children with DS scored lower ($M = 29.9$, $SD = 4.7$) than TD controls ($M = 33.7$, $SD = 1.6$) and children with WS ($M = 31.9$, $SD = 2.4$). Nevertheless, planned comparisons revealed that only the comparison between DS and TD controls groups was significant [$F(1,33) = 8.3$, $p < .01$], while comparisons between DS and WS groups [$F(1,33) = 2.35$] and between WS and TD controls groups [$F(1,33) = 1.8$] failed to reach significance.

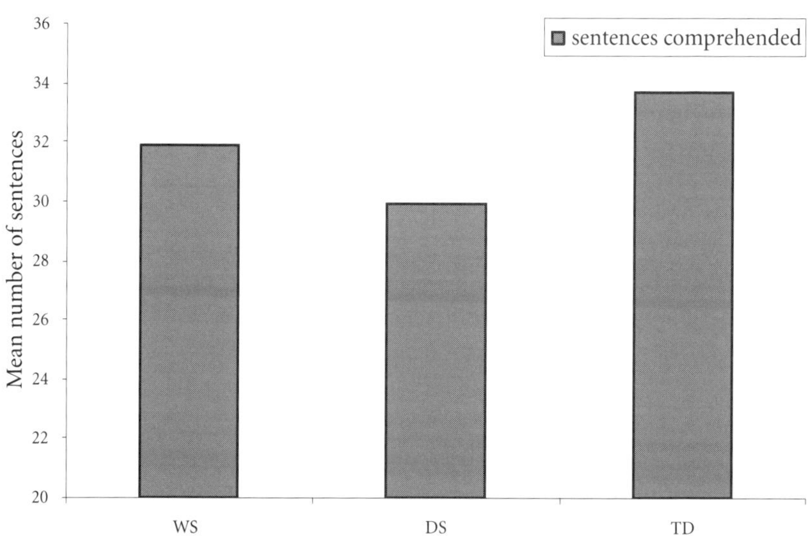


**Figure 3.** Mean number of sentences comprehended by children with WS, with DS and TD controls

## Mean length of utterance in words

Samples of spontaneous production (about twenty minutes per child) were collected and videotaped. In order to compute the mean length of the utterance in words (MLU-w), the spontaneous conversation of each child, corresponding to 50 utterances, was orthographically transcribed. Whenever production was insufficient to provide such a large number of utterances, all of the utterances actually produced were transcribed.

An utterance was defined as a sequence of words preceded or followed by silence (pause) or by a conversational turn. In many studies on children's speech, characterized by poor fluency, a quantitative criterion is also introduced, that is, elements separated by pauses of less than two seconds are considered part of the same utterance.

For each child, all the elements present in the utterances produced were summed and the mean length of the utterances was calculated (that is, the ratio between the sum of all the elements and the number of utterances produced).

Computation of the mean length of utterances in the three groups showed that children with WS have a significantly longer length in their spontaneous production ($M = 3.1$, $SD = 0.8$) than children with DS ($M = 2.4$, $SD = 0.5$) [$F(1,31) = 6.4$, $p < .05$]. TD controls ($M = 2.9$, $SD = 0.7$) did not differ statistically from WS [$F(1,31) = 0.7$] or from DS individuals [$F(1,31) = 2.5$].

These results for MLU are in agreement with results for the grammatical complexity scale on the PVB, relative to the proportion between telegraphic/incomplete and complete sentences.

## Sentence repetition

A phrase repetition test was used (PRT, Devescovi, Caselli, Ossella, & Alviggi 1992 and Devescovi & Caselli 2001) to ascertain children's ability to imitate verbal stimuli: particularly phrases and sentences with different length. The test includes a set of 51 cards plus three training cards. Each card depicts the meaning of each noun and the overall meaning of each utterance. The test was presented to each child individually as a game, introduced as follows: "Now let's play a game together: I will say something and you say the same thing". If the child did not respond to the first presentation of the stimulus phrase, it was repeated a second time, with the figure in view.

The evaluation consisted of the total number of phrases repeated correctly out of the total number of phrases repeated.

In Figure 4 the mean number of correctly repeated sentences expressed as percentage of the total number of repeated sentences by each group is reported. An ANOVA on the phrase repetition results showed a significant difference among

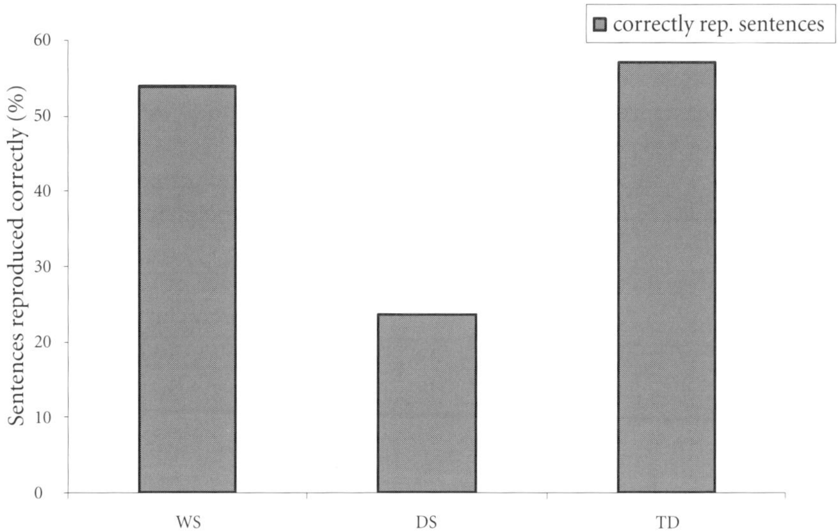


**Figure 4.** Percentage of sentences reproduced correctly by children with WS, with DS and TD controls

groups [F (2,33) = 6.7, p < .01]. Children with DS repeated a smaller number of phrases accurately (M = 23.6, SD = 18.6) than the TD controls group (M = 57.1, SD = 19.9), and a planned comparison revealed this difference to be statistically significant [F (1,33) = 11.05, p < .01]. Also, children with DS repeated a significantly smaller number of phrases than children with WS (M = 54.01, SD = 32.8) [F (1,33) = 9.1, p < .01]. Finally, no significant difference was found when WS and TD controls groups [F (1,33) = 0.9] were compared.

## Relations between grammar and vocabulary size

In this study, children with WS and DS and the TD controls did not differ significantly in lexical measures. However, the three groups have different performance profiles on measures of grammar, with DS children obtaining the lowest scores. The grammar measures that revealed group differences included the following: the Complexity section of the PVB, a measure of mean length of utterance based on laboratory observations, and a measure of correctly repeated sentences on the Repetition test, PRT. These findings suggest there may be a dissociation between lexical and grammatical development in WS and DS populations. On the other hand, several studies of typically developing children showed a strong correlation between grammar and lexical growth. Vicari, Caselli and Tonucci (2000) observed a significant correlation in children with DS between vocabulary size and sentence complexity on the PVB ($r = .75$, $p < .001$), the laboratory measure of mean length of utterance in words ($r = .51$, $p < .05$), and the percentage of correctly repeated sentences on the PRT ($r = .62$, $p < .01$). To verify this result and to extend this observation also to the Italian Williams syndrome population, we performed the same type of analyses. Significant correlations were observed between vocabulary size and sentence complexity on the PVB both in children with DS ($r = .80$, $p < .01$) and with WS ($r = .92$, $p < .001$). Significant correlations were also found between vocabulary size and the laboratory measure of mean length of utterance in words (DS, $r = .49$, $p < .05$; WS, $r = .85$, $p < .001$), and the percentage of correctly repeated sentences on the PRT (DS, $r = .72$, $p < .01$; WS, $r = .84$, $p < .001$).

In other words, grammar and vocabulary are still correlated in the DS and WS populations, even though DS children have a significant disadvantage in grammar compared with WS children and TD controls, matched for mental age. This result suggests that grammar is not independent from lexical development even in populations with atypical development.

## Study 2

In a second study (Volterra et al. 2003) we have concentrated our attention on a qualitative analysis of linguistic repetitions of a small number of young children with WS comparing their performance with that of children with DS and typically developing children. A restricted sample was selected consisting of six children with WS, individually matched on the basis of chronological and mental ages, and productive vocabulary size to six children with DS and six typically developing children matched on the basis of MA and vocabulary size.

The chronological and the mental ages in months, and the vocabulary size for the 18 children examined, (including means and ranges within each group), are reported in Table 2.

As can be seen in the table, chronological age (mean and range) is very similar for the WS and DS children. As expected, the TD children are about 2 years younger than the other two groups, but the mental age (mean and range) for each group is equivalent: 29 months for the WS and for the DS groups and 30 months for the TD group. The means and standard deviations for vocabulary size were very similar in the three groups of children and corresponded to the mean number of words reported for the Italian normative sample on the PVB for 30-months-old toddlers ($M = 446$; $SD = 168$, in Caselli & Casadio 1995). An ANOVA performed with group as the independent variable and number of words produced as the dependent variable showed no significant differences among the three groups.

**Table 2.** Mean (in months) and range of chronological and mental age of children with WS, with DS and TD controls

| Subjects | Children with Williams Syndrome (WSC) | | | Children with Down Syndrome (DSC) | | | Typical Developing Children (TDC) | | |
|---|---|---|---|---|---|---|---|---|---|
| | C.A. | M.A. | W.P. | C.A. | M.A. | W.P. | C.A. | M.A. | W.P. |
| 1 | 44 | 27 | 306 | 64 | 27 | 298 | 31 | 28 | 331 |
| 2 | 58 | 30 | 345 | 48 | 25 | 385 | 29 | 28 | 395 |
| 3 | 41 | 31 | 349 | 61 | 30 | 430 | 31 | 30 | 478 |
| 4 | 62 | 30 | 369 | 58 | 27 | 433 | 30 | 29 | 530 |
| 5 | 56 | 24 | 578 | 64 | 36 | 500 | 31 | 37 | 565 |
| 6 | 55 | 33 | 630 | 51 | 30 | 521 | 28 | 25 | 603 |
| Mean | 52.7 | 29.1 | 429.5 | 57.7 | 29.1 | 427.8 | 30.0 | 29.5 | 484.7 |
| Range | 41–62 | 24–33 | 306–630 | 51–64 | 25–36 | 298–521 | 28–31 | 25–37 | 331–603 |

In order to make sure that the children were matched for vocabulary size not only measured by parents report but also on lexical production directly measured in the laboratory, all children performed a picture naming task. A subscale for lexical production of nouns taken from the First Language Test (TPL by Axia 1995) has been used. The subscale consists of 20 pictures (plus two training pictures) depicting very common items from different lexical categories: vehicles, animals, people and everyday objects. No significant differences were found among the groups. A qualitative analysis of substitutions revealed no differences across the three groups. The majority of substitutions were from the same semantic category and the labels produced by the children were very similar across groups. Children with WS, at this early age did not use rare or strange words compared to the other children. Similar results have been recently replicated with older children with WS performing the Boston Naming Test (for further details see Bello, Capirci, & Volterra 2004).

After we ascertained that the children in the three groups had very similar lexical competence in vocabulary size reported by the parents and in the ability to name pictures evaluated in the laboratory we conducted a more detailed analysis of their performance in the PRT, the phrase repetition test designed to ascertain the children's ability to imitate verbal stimuli and particularly their morphological and syntactic aspects.

The evaluation consisted not only of the total number of phrases repeated correctly out of the total number of phrases repeated, the total number of errors was also computed and the type of error produced (omission, lexical substitution, error of bound morphology, addition of new elements, word order inversions) was also considered.

Table 3 presents for each child the number of repeated sentences and the number of the correct ones, in addition to means and ranges for each group.

**Table 3.** TRF: Repeated and correct sentences

| Subjects | WSC | | DSC | | TDC | |
|---|---|---|---|---|---|---|
| | Repeated | Correct | Repeated | Correct | Repeated | Correct |
| 1 | 49 | 21 | 51 | 10 | 51 | 38 |
| 2 | 51 | 23 | 34 | 4 | 51 | 38 |
| 3 | 50 | 27 | 49 | 0 | 50 | 26 |
| 4 | 35 | 20 | 27 | 4 | 15 | 9 |
| 5 | 49 | 33 | 11 | 7 | 51 | 38 |
| 6 | 51 | 48 | 47 | 35 | 28 | 3 |
| Mean | 47.5 | 28.7 | 36.5 | 10.0 | 41.0 | 25.3 |
| Range | 35–51 | 20–48 | 11–51 | 0–35 | 28–51 | 3–38 |

The children with DS repeated fewer sentences (M = 36,5) than the children with WS and the TD children (M = 47,5 and M = 41 respectively). Nevertheless, an ANOVA analysis did not show any significant difference among the three groups, $F(2,15) = 1.12$.

More evident is the difference in the mean of correct sentences repeated by children with DS (M = 10) and by the other two groups (M = 28,7 for the children with WS and M = 25,3 for the TD children). An ANOVA analysis approaches significance, $F(2,15) = 3.41$, $p = .06$.

Sentences correctly repeated, but in which one or more words were added, were counted as correct sentences. Sentences with additions were produced by the children with WS (M = 7.3), and were very rarely observed in the other two groups (M = 0.6 and M = 0.5 for the children with DS and TD children respectively). Examples of additions produced by children with WS, were: target sentence "Il bimbo va a casa" (The child goes home) was repeated with a local addition as "Il bimbo va a guardare la casa" (The child goes to look the house); target sentence "Il topo" (The mouse) was repeated as "Il topo mangia il formaggio" (The mouse eats the cheese).

The total number of additions for children with WS was 44 (25 final additions and 19 local addition), only 4 and 3 for children with DS and TD children respectively.

Finally, we have considered the total number of errors produced by children, counting: each element omitted (specifying also the number of omissions in obligatory contexts) or substituted (the child repeated the target sentence omitting or substituting one or more elements – article, name, verb, preposition etc. – in the sentence repeated); each morphological modification of a word (the child used in the repeated sentence a different morphological form of the same word – a singular form instead of a plural one, a feminine instead of a masculine form, etc.); each repetition with word order inversion (a different order of one or more elements in the sentence repeated), without taking into account the number of inverted elements.

Table 4 presents for each child the type of errors produced, in addition with means and ranges for each group. The total number of errors is 179 for children with WS, 360 for children with DS and 174 for TD children.

The mean number of errors produced was very similar for children with WS and TD children. The mean number of errors produced by children with DS was almost twice than that produced by children with WS and TD children. Nevertheless, an ANOVA analysis did not show any significant difference among the three groups: $F(2,15) = 3.05$, $p = .07$. Probably, the absence of a significant difference in this analysis was due to the particular performance of the two children with DS (#5 and #6).

In order to analyze in more detail the type of errors produced from a qualitative perspective the proportion of the different types of errors produced by the three groups of children has been considered. Omissions were proportionally the most frequent error produced by all groups of children. In the children with WS, the percentage of omissions was lower (71%) compared to both, children with DS (87%) and typically developing children (87%).

Errors in bound morphology were present in an appreciable proportion in both children with WS and DS (10% and 4% respectively), but they were almost absent in the TD children (0,5%). In this category of errors, only children with WS and DS produced sentences with an incorrect agreement between article and noun, but in the repetitions produced by the children with WS the percentage of this type of errors was markedly higher (44.4%) than in the repetitions produced by children with DS (18.7%). Lexical substitutions were proportionally produced more frequently by children with WS (15%) in respect to children with DS (7%) and to TD children (4%). Lexical substitutions produced by TD children are on nouns while lexical substitutions produced by children with WS and DS, are also on articles, prepositions and verbs.

Finally, word order inversions were produced in a higher proportion by typically developing children (8%), in an appreciable percentage by children with WS (4%) and in a lower proportion by children with DS (2%). All the word order inversions produced were at the sentence-level (not noun-phrase internal), in addition, only children with WS and DS produced sentences in which the order inversion generated semantically and/or grammatically unacceptable sentences.

Some examples of atypical errors and additions produced by children with WS are reported below.

The child #5 repeats the target sentence “I cani” (The dogs) with an incorrect agreement between article and noun: “Le cani” (feminine plural article “le” instead of masculine plural article “i”).

The same child (#5) repeats the target sentence “Il bimbo va a casa” (The child goes home) with an addition in the middle of the phrase: “Il bimbo va a guardare la casa” (The child goes to look the house). Another child (#3) shows a difficulty

Table 4. PRT: Number and type of errors

| Subjects | WSC | | | | DSC | | | | TDC | | | |
|---|---|---|---|---|---|---|---|---|---|---|---|---|
| | Total omissions (*) | Lexical substit. | Bound morphol. | Word order inversion | Total omissions (*) | Lexical substit. | Bound morphol. | Word order inversion | Total omissions (*) | Lexical substit. | Bound morphol. | Word order inversion |
| 1 | 43 (13) | 2 | 2 | 4 | 76 (19) | 4 | 7 | 4 | 13 (11) | 0 | 0 | 0 |
| 2 | 21 (11) | 13 | 6 | 0 | 73 (18) | 3 | 2 | 0 | 23 (9) | 1 | 0 | 0 |
| 3 | 35 (16) | 0 | 4 | 0 | 90 (43) | 7 | 3 | 1 | 43 (10) | 3 | 1 | 7 |
| 4 | 12 (7) | 4 | 5 | 1 | 45 (22) | 6 | 1 | 0 | 14 (3) | 0 | 0 | 3 |
| 5 | 14 (8) | 8 | 0 | 1 | 16 (3) | 0 | 1 | 0 | 18 (5) | 1 | 0 | 1 |
| 6 | 2 (1) | 0 | 1 | 1 | 13 (1) | 5 | 2 | 1 | 41 (28) | 2 | 0 | 3 |
| Mean | 21.2 | 4.5 | 3.0 | 1.2 | 52.2 | 4.2 | 2.7 | 1.0 | 25.3 | 1.2 | 0.2 | 2.3 |
| Range | 2–43 | 0–13 | 0–6 | 0–4 | 13–90 | 0–6 | 1–7 | 0–4 | 13–43 | 1–3 | 0–1 | 1–7 |

(*) Omissions in obligatory contexts are reported in parenthesis

in vocabulary selection also reported in other studies (Capirci et al. 1996). For example given the target sentence "Le volpi" (The foxes), he repeats "Cagnolino...c'é Tom e Jerry...e voppi" (Little dog...here is Tom and Jerry...the foxes). A child (#2) repeats the target sentence "Maria mette la bambola a letto" (Maria puts the doll in the bed) with a word order inversion that generates an unacceptable sentence: "Maria mette il letto a bambola" (Maria puts the bed in the doll). Finally, given the target sentence "La macchina" (the car), the subject #1 produces "Maria dà il gelato" (Maria gives the ice cream), a phrase presented many items before during the same test.

## Discussion

The results of our study can be summarized as follows: the expressive vocabulary size of the three groups, as reported in the PVB, is very similar and corresponds to the mean number of words reported for the Italian normative sample on the PVB for 30-month-old toddlers (Caselli & Casadio 1995). This finding contrasts with a recent report by Mervis and Robinson (2000). These authors used the English version of the CDI Words and Sentences for 24 children with WS and 28 children with DS (mean chronological age of both groups was 30 months). In that study, children with WS exhibited a significantly larger vocabulary than children with DS. The discrepancy between their findings and ours may be explained by differences in the age range examined and in the methodology used for recruitment. Our children were more than two years older than the children examined by Mervis and Robinson. Also, these authors matched their participants only on the basis of chronological age, while ours were matched for both mental and chronological age. This is an important methodological difference. Indeed, looking only at chronological age, IQ differences among individuals can be missed and an advantage in lexical production may simply reflect higher global cognitive capacities.

Considering the mean chronological age of the participants, our results seem more comparable to those reported by Singer-Harris et al. (1997). In their study, no significant differences were found in vocabulary size for children with DS and children with WS, when children who produced more than 600 words (considered the ceiling for the CDI) were excluded.

Data on sentence production from parental reports also revealed interesting findings: children with DS were reported to produce a significantly higher proportion of telegraphic and incomplete sentences than children with typical development. Similar findings were reported in Singer-Harris et al. (1997), and confirmed in a recent Italian study of 15 children with DS using the PVB (Vicari et al. 2000). Children with DS were also reported to produce more telegraphic sentences than individuals with WS, although this comparison only approached significance. In contrast, no difference was found comparing the children with WS and the TD controls.

Similarly, in spontaneous production, children with DS used significantly shorter utterances than children with WS.

Problems in comprehension were also observed at a very early age. In fact, the verbal comprehension test showed that the children with DS had greater problems in understanding simple sentences than the typically developing and WS children. Once again, no difference emerged between WS and TD controls.

Finally, examination of the phrase repetition test as well as mean length of utterance further confirmed the difficulties of children with DS in the morphosyntactic aspects of language. Indeed, data on the phrase repetition test showed that children with DS produced far fewer complete sentences (proportionally) than WS children with the same mental age and vocabulary size. In turn, WS individuals did not differ from typically developing children in the number or proportion of complete repetitions.

Our results may be compatible with the modular account provided by Clahsen and Almazan (1998, 2001), who argued that the computational, rule based system for language is selectively spared in WS while lexical representations and/or their access procedures are impaired. However, Clahsen and Almazan's theoretical interpretation assumes a clear dissociation between lexical and morphosyntactic performance also at an early age.

In order to explore this hypothesis, we investigated whether grammatical development and lexical ability were or were not dissociated in our special populations by examining the correlations among morphosyntactic capacities, sentences and vocabulary size in the DS and WS groups respectively. Consistent with a previous report (Vicari et al. 2000), we found a robust correlation between grammatical and lexical performance in the DS sample. A similar correlation also appeared in the WS group, confirming findings reported by Stojanovik, Perkins and Howard (2001). Although children with intellectual disabilities, especially those with DS, may have a grammatical disadvantage compared with TD children at the same mental age and vocabulary size, we cannot conclude that grammar is dissociated from other aspects of language in these special populations.

## Conclusion

The results of studies reported in the present chapter conducted with younger children confirm and extend previous findings with older children and adolescents with WS. They confirm that language is not ahead of mental age in the Williams population in this early age range, in line with a revised view of Williams Syndrome that has already been suggested by research within the older age range explored in previous studies (Volterra et al. 1996).

Our data further suggest that the apparently spared linguistic abilities of WS children is in part an artifact of comparisons made with children with DS, whose morphosyntactic abilities are more compromised relative to their non verbal mental age and to their lexical repertoire. Children with WS do not speak like normally developing peers at the same chronological age, they have an expressive lexical repertoire and use sentences like younger typically developing children at a comparable level of non-verbal abilities. In addition, they often produce, like children with DS, sentences that are unacceptable semantically, pragmatically and/or very rarely produced by typically developing children (Capirci et al. 1996). Thus, these differences with typically developing children could be related to cognitive impairment and not to a specific syndrome.

Nevertheless, there are intriguing qualitative differences between the groups at a more detailed level, including a tendency for children with WS to produce errors that are rarely observed in children with DS or in typically developing children at any age. In particular, the tendency for children with WS to add material that was not present in the model. In many cases the material added was not consistent with the picture shown at that time but was present in a target sentence presented some items before. In the case of children with WS, their spared ability to hear and store speech sounds may permit them to acquire some aspects of language that are especially difficult for children with DS, but this ability is not enough to guarantee productive control over all grammatical aspects of language.

The theoretical relevance of prospective studies on genetic disorders, tracing language development from its earliest manifestations, may lie in what they reveal about how different cognitive and perceptual capacities affect the process of language development.

Linguistic abilities and the relationships among linguistic sub-domains seem to vary over time as a function of subjects' developmental level, the characteristics of the language they are learning and individual differences in the rate and nature of this learning process. For example, in children with DS the discrepancy between lexical and morphosyntactic abilities, evident in the early stages of development, may gradually decrease with age, leading to a pattern of residual deficits in both domains. Similarly, the linguistic skills of individuals with WS are usually reported to be particularly sophisticated in adolescence, while the linguistic capacities of very young children are described as poor and consistently delayed.

Such findings argue for a dynamic approach to intellectual disorders (Karmiloff-Smith 1998) and for a change in cognitive and linguistic profiles over time: dissociation in linguistic and cognitive functioning in children with intellectual disabilities could be the product of a developmental trajectory.

## Acknowledgements

The financial support of Telethon-Italy (Grant n. E.C. 685) and FIRB is gratefully acknowledged. We especially thank the children who participated in the study and their parents.

## Note

1. We have also conducted a detailed analysis on Elisa's visuo-spatial and drawing abilities but that study is not immediately relevant to the topic of the present chapter (Stiles, Sabbadini, Capirci, & Volterra 2000).

## References

Bello, A., Capirci, O. & Volterra, V. (2004). "Lexical Production in Children with Williams Syndrome: Spontaneous use of gesture in a naming task". *Neuropsychologia, 42*(2), 201–213.

Bellugi, U. & St. George, M. (Eds.). (2001). *Journey From Cognition to Brain to Gene. Perspectives from Williams syndrome.* Cambridge, MA: The MIT Press.

Brunet, O. & Lézine, I. (1967). *Scala di Sviluppo Psicomotorio della Prima Infanzia.* Firenze: Organizzazioni Speciali.

Capirci, O., Sabbadini, L., & Volterra, V. (1996). "Language development in Williams syndrome: A case study". *Cognitive Neuropsychology, 13*(7), 1017–1039.

Carlesimo G. A., Marotta, L., & Vicari S. (1997). "Long-term memory in mental retardation: Evidence for a specific impairment in subjects with Down syndrome". *Neuropsychologia, 35*(1), 71–79.

Caselli, M. C. & Casadio, P. (1995). *Il Primo Vocabolario del Bambino. Guida all'uso del questionario MacArthur per la valutazione della comunicazione e del linguaggio nei primi anni di vita.* Milano: Franco Angeli.

Caselli, M. C., Longobardi, E., & Pisaneschi, R. (1997). "Gesti e parole in bambini con sindrome di Down". *Psicologia Clinica dello Sviluppo, 1*, 45–63.

Caselli, M. C., Vicari, S., Longobardi, E., Lami, L., Pizzoli, C., & Stella, G. (1998). "Gestures and words in early development of children with Down syndrome". *Journal of Speech, Language and Hearing Research, 41*, 1125–1135.

Chapman, R. S. (1995). "Language development in children and adolescents with Down syndrome". In P. Fletcher & B. MacWhinney (Eds.), *The Handbook of Child Language* (pp. 641–663). Oxford: Blackwell.

Chilosi, A., Pfanner, L., & Cipriani, P. (1996). "Dati preliminari di una prova di comprensione grammaticale per bambini tra 15 e 40 mesi". *Workshop di Neuropsicologia dello Sviluppo.* Nuovi strumenti di valutazione, Calambrone, Pisa.

Clahsen, H. & Almazan, M. (1998). "Syntax and morphology in Williams syndrome". *Cognition, 68*, 167–198.

Clahsen, H. & Almazan M. (2001). "Compounding and inflection in language impairment: Evidence from Williams syndrome and SLI". *Lingua, 111*, 729–757.

Devescovi, A., Caselli, M. C., Ossella, T., & Alviggi, F. G. (1992). "Strumenti di indagine sulle prime fasi dello sviluppo linguistico: Risultati di una prova di ripetizione di frasi con bambini fra i due e i tre anni e mezzo". *Rassegna di Psicologia, 2*(9), 29–54.

Devescovi, A. & Caselli, M. C. (2001). "Una prova di ripetizione di frasi per la valutazione del primo sviluppo grammaticale". *Psicologia Clinica dello Sviluppo, 3*, 341–364.

Fabbretti, D., Pizzuto, E., Vicari, S., & Volterra, V. (1997). "A story description task with Down syndrome: Lexical and morphosyntactic abilities". *Journal of Intellectual Disability Research, 41*, 165–179.

Fowler, Anne (1990). "Language abilities of children with Down syndrome: Evidence for a specific syntactic delay". In D. Cicchetti & M. Beeghly (Eds.), *Children with Down Syndrome: A developmental perspective* (pp. 302–328). Cambridge: CUP.

Karmiloff-Smith, A. (1998). "Development itself is the key to understanding developmental disorders". *Trends in Cognitive Sciences, 2*, 289–298.

Karmiloff-Smith, A., Grant, J., Berthoud, I., Davies, M., Howlin, P., & Udwin, O. (1997). "Language and Williams syndrome: How intact is 'intact'?" *Child Development, 68*(2), 246–262.

Iverson, J. M., Longobardi, E., & Caselli, M. C. (2003). "The relationship between gestures and words in children with Down syndrome and typically-developing children in the early stages of communicative development". *International Journal of Language and Communication Disorders, 38*, 179–197.

Leiter, R. G. (1980). *Leiter International Performance Scale.* Illinois, USA: Stoelting Co.

Maratsos, M. & Matheny, L. (1994). Language specificity and elasticity: Brain and clinical syndrome studies. *Annual Review of Psychology, 45*, 487–516.

Mervis, C. B. & Robinson, B. R. (2000). "Expressive vocabulary ability of toddlers with Williams syndrome or Down syndrome: A comparison." *Developmental Neuropsychology, 171*, 111–126.

Miller, J. F. (1992). "Development of speech and language in children with Down syndrome". In J. Y. Lott & E. E. Mc Loy (Eds.), *Clinical care for persons with Down Syndrome* (pp. 39–50). Cambridge, MA: The MIT Press.

Pezzini, G., Vicari, S., Volterra, V., Milani, L., & Ossella, M. T. (1999). "Children with Williams syndrome: Is there a single Neuropsychological profile?" *Developmental Neuropsychology, 15*(1), 141–155.

Pinker, S. (1994). *The Language Instinct: How the mind creates language.* New York, NY: William Morrow.

Pinker, S. (1999). *Words and Rules.* London: Weidenfeld and Nicholson.

Rondal, J.A. (1995). *Exceptional Language Development in Down Syndrome.* Cambridge: CUP.

Schaner-Wolles, C. (2000). "Within-language dissociations in mental retardation: Williams-Beuren and Down syndrome". In S. C. Howell, S. A. Fish, & T. Keith-Lucas (Eds.), *BUCLD 24: Proceedings of the 24th annual Boston University Conference on Language Development* (pp. 633–644). Somerville, MA: Cascadilla Press.

Singer Harris, N., Bellugi, U., Bates, E., Jones, W., & Rossen, M. (1997). "Contrasting profiles of language development in children with Williams and Down syndromes". *Developmental Neuropsychology, 133*, 345–370.

Stiles, J., Sabbadini, L., Capirci, O., & Volterra, V. (2000). "Drawing abilities in Williams syndrome: A case study". *Developmental Neuropsychology, 18*(2), 213–235.

Stojanovik, V., Perkins, M., & Howard S. (2001). "Language and conversational abilities in individuals with Williams syndrome: How good is 'good'?" *International Journal of Language and Communication Disorders, 36*, 234–239.

Vallar, G. & Papagno, C. (1993). "Preserved vocabulary acquisition in Down syndrome children: The role of phonological short-term memory". *Cortex, 29*, 467–483.

Vicari, S., Brizzolara, D., Carlesimo, G. A., Pezzini, G., & Volterra, V. (1996). "Memory abilities in children with Williams syndrome". *Cortex, 32*, 503–514.

Vicari, S., Carlesimo, G., Brizzolara, D., & Pezzini, G. (1996). "Short-term memory in children with Williams syndrome: A reduced contribution of lexical-semantic knowledge to word span". *Neuropsychologia, 34*(9), 919–925.

Vicari, S., Tonucci, F., & Caselli, M. C. (2000). "Asynchrony of lexical and morphosyntactic development in children with Down Syndrome". *Neuropsychologia, 38*, 634–644.

Vicari, S., Bellucci, S., & Carlesimo, G. A. (2001). "Procedural learning deficit in children with Williams syndrome". *Neuropsychologia, 39*, 240–251.

Vicari, S. & Carlesimo, A. (2002). "Children with intellectual disabilities". In A. Baddley & M. Kopelman (Eds.), *Handbook of Memory Disorders* (pp. 501–518). Chichester: Wiley.

Vicari, S., Caselli, M. C., Gagliardi, C., Tonucci, F., & Volterra, V. (2002). "Language acquisition in special populations: A comparison between Down and Williams syndromes". *Neuropsychologia, 40*, 2461–2470.

Volterra, V., Capirci, O., Pezzini, G., Sabbadini, L., & Vicari, S. (1996). "Linguistic abilities in Italian children with Williams syndrome". *Cortex, 32*, 663–677.

Volterra, V., Longobardi, E., Pezzini, G., Vicari, S., & Antenore, C. (1999). "Visuo-spatial and linguistic abilities in a twin with Williams Syndrome". *Journal of Intellectual Disability Research, 43*, 294–305.

Volterra, V., Caselli, M. C., Capirci, O., Tonucci, F., & Vicari, S. (2003). "Early linguistic abilities of Italian children with Williams syndrome". *Developmental Neuropsychology, 23*, 33–58.

# Language in Hungarian children with Williams syndrome

Ágnes Lukács*†, Csaba Pléh*‡, and Mihály Racsmány*#
Research Group on Neuropsychology and Psycholinguistics* / Reseach Institute of Linguistics† / Budapest University of Technology and Economics‡ / University of Szeged#

Four studies of a group of Hungarian individuals with Williams syndrome (WS) are presented tapping controversial aspects of atypical organization in the WS mental lexicon and grammar. Two tasks aimed at clarifying the issue of frequency: a *Semantic Fluency task* and a *Picture Naming Vocabulary Task*. In a *Morphology Task*, we elicited regular and irregular affixation patterns. A *Spatial Postpositions and Suffixes* task tested knowledge of spatial expressions. Overall findings show that WS language lags behind verbal age as measured by receptive vocabulary scores, but no evidence of atypical organization was found. We do not take this as evidence that language in WS is typical: more fine-grained studies of representation, temporal processing, and mechanisms of language acquisition are needed.

## Introduction

In this chapter, we are going to present four studies all of which were designed to tap different aspects of the issue of atypical organization in the WS mental lexicon and grammar. All of the studies form part of a broader project (Hungarian Williams Syndrome Project) in which different aspects of cognitive and linguistic development in Hungarian WS children are investigated. The four studies reported here are summarized in Table 1.

We wanted to clarify the issue of frequency by a *Fluency task* which uses a wider range of categories, because fluency studies in the literature indicate that performance might be influenced by the specific category being tested (Jarrold et al. 2000). Most studies asked children to list as many animals as they can: animals are a category very much in the focus of interest of children, this might be one of the reasons that WS subjects can list more or more peculiar ones than older controls.

Table 1. Summary characterization of the studies reported here

| Task | Behavioral task | Rationale |
|---|---|---|
| Fluency | Verbally list members of a category | Atypical lexical organization |
| Picture vocabulary | Picture naming | Frequency effects |
| Morphology task | Picture based suffix elicitation | Overgeneralizations as a function of stem types |
| Spatial postpositions and suffixes | Elicited suffixes and postpositions | Qualitative nature of spatial language impairments |

To test knowledge in different kinds of categories, we used eight categories, which were hypothesized to be of different familiarity to children. The issue of frequency effects on WS vocabulary was tapped by two other tasks in earlier studies (Lukács et al. 2001; Pléh et al. 2003; Racsmány et al. 2001): a *Picture Naming Vocabulary Task* and a *Morphology Task* for eliciting regular and irregular affixation **patterns** in WS children as a function of frequency and regularity. The fourth was a *Spatial Postpositions and Suffixes* task to test pattern of performance on spatial expressions.

## Frequency and lexical organization in WS

The organization of the lexicon is the aspect of language that is most widely and from the earliest times accepted to be atypical in Williams syndrome: it is both an everyday observation and a result of several studies that WS people tend to use unusual and contextually unexpected words (see Bellugi et al. 2000). The most famous examples come from Ursula Bellugi and her colleagues' description of a WS child saying e.g. 'I have to evacuate the glass' instead of 'I have to empty the glass'. People with WS generally perform at a high level on standardized vocabulary tests, but several tasks show that their semantic organization is different from that of normal controls. It is claimed that WS people tend to list infrequent items in a category fluency task, a frequently cited example of this is a WS list for animals: 'tiger, owl, sea lion, zebra, hippopotamus, turtle, lizard, reptile, frog, beaver, giraffe, chihuahua' (Bellugi et al. 1994).

Different observations also point to the fact that in WS people frequency is not as strong in weighting connections within the lexicon as in normals, and WS people access infrequent words just as easily as frequent ones (see Bellugi et al. 2000). Bellugi and her colleagues (e.g. 1994) noted that WS individuals perform better than controls matched on mental age, almost reaching the performance of controls matched on chronological age regarding the number of items produced in a category. They also observed that WS individuals listed more infrequent words within categories, and that performance on the fluency tasks improved dramatically between the age of 9 and 15 years in WS. Another observation revealing unusual organization of the lexicon and its relation to frequency is that of Vicari et al. (1996a, 1996b): when subjects have to recall words from a word list, normal controls typically recall more high frequency words; in people with WS no bias is shown towards frequent words in recall.

Tapping the nature of semantic organization, Rossen et al. (1996) tested WS subjects on three homonymy task. In a free associations task, where subjects had to say the first word that came into their minds hearing a homonym, WS subjects, just as normal controls, responded mainly with words related to the primary (i.e. more frequent) associate of the homonym. In the similarity judgment task, however, WS people judged words related to the primary and secondary associates to be equally similar to the target homonym, while normal subjects consistently judged words related to the primary associate more similar. In a definition task, WS subjects gave definitions of the secondary associate significantly more frequently than normal controls.

One of the main areas of debate with regard to the frequency issue is performance on fluency tasks. Rossen and colleagues (1996) found controversial results: their findings show that WS and Down Syndrome subjects did not differ in the average number of unusual items they produced, but WS people produced more infrequent category members towards the end of the list.

Volterra and her colleagues (1996) tested 17 individuals with WS between 4;10 and 15;3 years of age, comparing their performances to typically developing children matched on mental age (3;8 to 6;8 years). The two groups were tested on both category and phonological fluency. On the Category Test for Semantic Fluency, the two groups did not display any difference: only two of the 17 subjects performed above their mental age on the number of items, and there was no tendency in the WS group to list particularly unusual category members. In general, the WS group did not perform better than the MA control group on any linguistic measures, while they performed significantly poorer on some (TROG, Boston Naming, and Sentence Repetition tasks). The only task they were significantly better on was the Phonological Fluency test, which is explained by the authors by the fact that WS children have many school experience while controls below 6 years none.

Semantic fluency was also tested by Jarrold and his colleagues (2000) in WS subjects with a mean age of 16;9 in two categories: Animals and Body Parts. Their results showed that subjects with Williams syndrome were comparable to the control group matched on vocabulary level on measures of number, frequency and typicality of items they produced. They found differences between the two groups, however, in the ordering of items during production, which they interpreted as reflecting abnormal underlying semantic organization in WS. As another observation they noted that WS individuals produced more repetitions, which is accounted for by executive dysfunction instead of a purely linguistic deficit.

A recent study aimed at clarifying the issue of frequency and semantic fluency in WS within a wider project of testing lexical skills. Temple and her colleagues (2002) examined different lexical skills in four WS subjects in the age range of 11;2–15;4. Results showed that receptive vocabulary scores were above mental age, but they proved to be anomic on a naming task relative to their vocabulary knowledge, and performed poorer on confrontation naming than mental age (MA) controls. Comprehension was also significantly poorer than for MA controls, when they had to point to pictures on the basis of spoken names in the presence of semantic distractors. Children were also tested on phonological fluency, with the letters F, A and S, and on semantic fluency in two categories, animals and 'things you would find in the house'. Scores on the FAS were above mental age, and were above or at mental age on the semantic categories, with a general tendency of WS children producing more items of low frequency. These results show that WS children are good at lexical tasks that do not require fine semantic distinctions (British Picture Vocabulary Test – BPVT, fluency). Language in WS is said to be atypical, partly because naming errors are atypical, and more low frequency items are listed in the fluency task. The low frequency advantage was found with 'things in the house', but not with animals. Volterra et al. (1996) did not find a low frequency advantage with animals either. Temple et al. argue that the anomia of the children is a semantic one, in which "the representations are either inadequately specified or incompletely activated in both naming and pointing from spoken names" (Temple et al. 2002:487).

In the following studies we tried to obtain additional evidence on the proposed frequency insensitivity and peculiar semantic organization in WS in a different language than that of studies cited earlier.

## Regular and irregular morphology in WS

One approach to WS language integrates lexical peculiarities observed in this population into a model claiming a within-language dissociation of grammatical rules and lexical processes, based on the finding that WS individuals have problems accessing irregularly inflected forms, while they produce regularly inflected forms correctly (Bellugi et al. 1988; Bromberg et al. 1994; Clahsen & Almazan 1998; Zukowski 2001). On this view, WS children have a relatively intact grammar, combined with a much weaker lexical system. As a consequence of this, overregularizations of irregular forms are characteristic of their performance. This conception is based on dual-route models of normal language processing and production (Pinker 1991; Pinker & Prince 1994; and Clahsen 1999). Clahsen's model is more explicit and specific in adopting Minimalist Morphology's approach to inflection and in working with internally structured lexical representations. This hybrid model is also proposed to explain linguistic behavior in WS (Clahsen & Almazan 1998; Clahsen 1999). According to this perspective, there are two distinct systems within the language faculty, a computational symbol-manipulating rule system of grammar and an associative network constituting the mental lexicon. These two distinct systems of language can be selectively impaired, as exemplified by individuals with Williams syndrome having an intact rule system with an atypically operating mental lexicon. Such a dissociation of the grammar and the lexicon is manifested in morphology so that regularly inflected forms (e.g. *talk→talked*; purportedly generated by the rule system) are produced easily and correctly, but the retrieval of irregular forms (e.g. *go→went;* stored as a whole in the mental lexicon) is impaired, often resulting in overgeneralizations.

In Clahsen and Almazan's study (1998) of elicited production of regular and irregular plurals and past tense forms, English-speaking WS children could inflect existing regular stems virtually as well as unimpaired controls (matched on mental age), while their performance on irregulars was poor; they often overgeneralized the regular suffix both to existing irregular forms and to novel words rhyming with existing irregulars, and failed to generalize irregular patterns to novel forms, showing, according to the authors, an impairment in "associating phonological patterns of novel verbs to corresponding strings of existing irregular verbs" (p. 193). This dissociation is also reflected in their performance on inflecting derivational forms: their performance was similar to controls and showed sensitivity to morphological structure in contexts where verbs were presented as denominal derivatives, prohibiting irregular inflection even with verbs that are homophonous with existing irregulars (*He ringed/*rang the city with artillery*, 'formed a ring around'). The results are interpreted as a selective impairment of the lexical module of language, as an inability to retrieve information from subnodes of lexical entries. Krause and Penke (2002) confirmed these findings with data on German participles and plurals from two WS adolescents. WS and control participants did not differ in their overall performance rates on regular and irregular participles, both groups making errors with irregulars, but while control children tended to overregularize rare items, in the WS group, overregularization of frequent verbs was common as well. With irregular plurals, WS subjects' performance was poorer.

There have been several studies on regular and irregular morphology in WS carried out in this vein. Zukowski (2001) tested the selective lexical impairment proposal in a larger sample of 12 WS children (8–16 years) and controls matched on mental age in a different task, in elicited production of synthetic noun-noun compounds. In English, there is a constraint on plurals appearing within compounds that bans regular forms (**rats-eater*), but tolerates irregulars (*mice-eater*). In producing simple plurals, corroborating Clahsen and Almazan's observations, the WS group was much better with regulars, but showed a relatively low rate of overregularization with irregulars and instead produced singulars where they could not retrieve the correct plural form.[1] Their performance on compounds shows that they obey the morphosyntactic constraint disallowing regulars but allowing irregular plurals to appear in compounds. In fact, WS children produced higher rates of irregular plurals in the compound task than in the task where they only had to give the plural form. On the whole, Zukowski summarizes her findings with the following conclusion: "we have replicated the finding that WS children exhibit lexical access problems, and we have seen that in a test of morphosyntactic knowledge that does not require the retrieval of rote-stored lexical information, WS children perform at ceiling" (2001:45).

This interpretation of WS performance is much discussed in the literature, and just as there is much debate over typical production and processing data concerning the dual route model, the above view of WS pattern is also challenged, most importantly by Thomas et al. (2001). They argue that since typically developing children also show poorer performance on irregulars than regulars, poorer performance on irregulars in itself does not suffice for postulating a selective deficit: "Rather, it must be shown that their level of past tense formation is poorer than we would expect *given their level language development* (p. 147). Thomas et al. tested 21 WS individuals (mean age: 22;8, range: 10;11–53;3) and compared them to controls from different age ranges (from 5;5–45;0) on the task used in the Clahsen and Almazan (1998) study, and another also assessing knowledge of past tense forms on a larger set of verbs, making it possible to test effects of frequency and imageability. There was great variability between performance patterns of different WS subjects. Controlling for chronological age they found that the WS group's performance was significantly worse in general, and the difference was greater for irregulars than regulars. Overall performance was similarly poorer in the WS group than in controls when they were controlled for verbal mental age, but the difference in this case was not greater in irregulars than in regulars. Thomas et al. take their results as evidence that the WS group does not have a selective deficit with irregulars, but they show lower rates of generalization to novel strings. The WS group was atypical, though, in displaying frequency effects: for typically developing controls, Thomas et al. found the generally observed pattern of frequency effects observed with irregulars and lack of frequency effects in performance on regulars. In the WS group, frequency did not affect irregulars, but, surprisingly, it had an effect on regulars. These results are interpreted as arguing against the dual route model, and for the hypothesis that language development in WS is not only delayed, but follows atypical constraints, possibly due to atypical phonological representations. More specifically, the WS language system is argued to show a greater than typical reliance on phonology and weaker reliance on semantics. Reduced rates of overgeneralizations are explained as a consequence of deviant phonological representations: "in WS, they might contain too much detail to support robust generalization" (p. 169).

Later studies by Clahsen and colleagues (Clahsen & Temple 2003; Clahsen, Ring, & Temple, this volume) took up some of the criticism by Thomas et al., and enlarged the number of their WS subjects to 8. On the other hand, they made their own criticism of the Thomas et al. study by arguing against lack of proper matching (treating children between 5 to 10 as a single group) between WS and control individuals. Besides extending their studies of past tense forms of existing and nonce verbs and denominal verbs to new WS individuals, Clahsen and his colleagues also tested them on a different task tapping comparative adjective formation. The different classes of stimuli in this task included adjectives that form their comparatives with (a) *-er*, (b) *more*, (c) *either* (d) in an irregular way (e.g. *bad*) and it also included e) nonce adjectives. WS children tended to mark the comparative almost exclusively with *-er* (erring on both suppletives and on *more*-adjectives) while controls used both *-er* and periphrastic *more* in their comparatives. These findings, together with results from studies of lexical skills and complex syntax, are taken by the authors to confirm that the performance pattern observed in WS results from impairment of a subcomponent of the normal language system: what we see in WS is selective lexical deficit, accompanied by an intact computational i.e. rule-based system. In Clahsen's model, the nature of this lexical impairment is conceived in a framework where lexical representations are structured sets of semantic and grammatical features. The difficulty of WS individuals would not be with accessing the basic lexical entry (this is done in regular inflection as well) but with retrieving information from subnodes of entries, as manifested by the inability to access relevant features for morphological exceptionality, or semantic features needed for fine-grained distinctions.

The rich morphology of Hungarian with its different stem classes provides possibilities to test these claims in an agglutinative language. We tested production of regular and irregular forms together with possible frequency effects on inflection in Hungarian WS subjects. Agreeing with Thomas et al.'s claim, we compared performance to verbal controls, but matching was done on an individual basis. As the system of Hungarian differs in important respects from English and German, we give a brief introduction to the relevant grammar in the section below in presenting our study.

## The language of space in WS

There have been several studies of spatial language use in WS, most motivated by finding out the nature of intersection of language and spatial cognition, a peak and a valley in WS cognition. What most studies expected to gain from research on spatial language in WS was an answer to the following question: in the light of the severe impairment in spatial cognition and relatively good language, how do WS people perform when they have to use language to describe spatial relationship, or have to construct spatial relations by comprehending spatial language (see Bellugi et al. 2000)?

As already mentioned, several studies have concluded that there is a selective deficit of spatial terms in language in Williams syndrome. Lichtenberg and Bellugi (1998) tested WS subjects on both comprehension and production of spatial terms, and compared their performance to younger typically developing (TD) controls. In the comprehension task, subjects had to chose from among four pictures the one matching the auditorily presented spatial description. Controls performed at ceiling, the WS group erred on 11.5% of items on average. In the production test, the task was to describe pictures depicting spatial arrangements, and give the position of a target item relative to a referent. Again, WS subjects performed poorly relative to younger TD children, making an average of 30.2% of errors: for example, to describe a scene where an apple is in a bowl, WS subjects gave answers like 'apple without the bowl' and 'the bowl is in the apple' and 'the apple is around the bowl'. They made errors where they reversed figure and ground in the description, while retaining the preposition (e.g. *The bowl is in the apple*), used the opposite preposition (*The apple is around the bowl*) or gave completely inappropriate answers. They also made errors that were atypical, never produced by normally developing children, whose errors were mostly giving a response that was too general. Bellugi et al. (2000:23) conclude that "it appears that WS individuals in particular may be having difficulty in the mapping between spatial representation and language representation". Another possibility is that they do not have any specific difficulty in *mapping* between the two representations; it is the spatial representations that are impaired or underspecified, which, then, even without a problem in mapping, result in an inappropriate linguistic description.

Several studies pointed out that WS children have especially low scores on spatial items on the TROG on the following blocks: K (*longer/bigger/taller*); M (*in/on*) and P (*above* and *below*) (e.g. Clahsen & Almazan 1998; Jarrold et al. 2001; Phillips et al. 2002). Italian children made many preposition errors in a Sentence Repetition test, that in addition were quite unlike anything seen in typically developing children: e.g. *The grandchildren pick up flowers with their grandmother* → *The grandchildren pick up flowers *on top of the grandmother* (Volterra et al. 1996). In the Phillips et al. study, the subjects' task was to understand both spatial and non-spatial comparisons (*above* or *lighter*), presented in the TROG format, but there was a larger sample of both spatial and non-spatial items. WS subjects had lower scores than either TD children, or subjects with mild learning difficulty.

All these results were interpreted as evidence for a specific interaction between cognition and language, and arguing against any strict modularity of language. As the argument above points out, though, we suggest that an overall deficit in spatial terms in the presence of a serious deficit in spatial cognition seems to be trivial and teaches us little about the language-cognition interface. We believe, for reasons specified above, that examining spatial language seems to be crucial for different reasons: fine-grained scrutiny in the study of impaired spatial terms might lead to findings on the more specific organization and the structure of the spatial deficit. The only study of WS language conceived in this spirit that examined spatial language in its more specific organization was Landau and Zukowski (in press) which we discuss in more detail, and although while most studies of spatial language in WS emphasize the reflection of severe spatial deficit in language the authors claim that "non-linguistic spatial deficits shown by children with Williams syndrome have, at most, limited effects on their spatial language" (p. 1), and they have a nontrivial explanation for the pattern of performance on spatial descriptions observed in the WS group.

Landau and Zukowski elicited descriptions of 80 videotaped motion events (40 of which showed a single object moving, the other showed a Figure object moving and a stationary Ground object) from 12 WS children, their mental age matched controls, and adults. They checked representation and linguistic encoding of all components of spatial representation of motion events (Figure and Ground, Manner of Motion and Path, as listed by Talmy 1975), which can all be potentially selectively impaired, since they differ in the spatial elements they describe, and the mode and complexity of the linguistic encoding of that spatial element. Figure objects were encoded at ceiling level by all groups. WS children showed more omission of Ground objects than control children, and, unlike participants in the control groups, they omitted significantly more in describing FROM paths than either TO or VIA paths. The WS group used significantly less specific manner of motion verbs to describe the scene than adults, but the ratio of simple/specific verbs did not reliably differ from that of control children. Path turned out to be the most vulnerable category in WS, with control children producing more correct answers on all path types. All groups followed semantic constraints regarding spatial terms: they used *off* for surfaces and *out* for containers. WS children performed significantly better on bounded TO paths than on FROM and VIA paths (this tendency was also present in controls, but did not reach significance), with more correct answers and less omissions and ambiguous intransitives on the first than on the latter two, a similar pattern as Landau and Zukowski found with Ground object omissions.

WS children could represent Figure and Ground objects, their relative spatial roles, and they could map them onto their appropriate syntactic role of subject/object of preposition. They also correctly encoded, and thus perceived manner of motion. Path seemed to be the most difficult element of the motion event for WS children. But even here, WS children tended to use largely the same set of expressions for all three path types as controls, and they made errors by using an expression from one path type to describe another. In contrast to previous observations, most of their mistakes were not using inappropriate spatial terms, but using either a vague expression (like *over*) or omitting the path expression altogether. This tendency was strong with FROM and VIA paths, but not with TO paths.

The authors take an interesting position in interpreting their data. They explain this selective fragility as the interaction of language with the impaired non-linguistic spatial system. This deficit, as they say, "appears most prominently in tasks requiring the retention of visual-spatial information over time, for example, the representation of spatial relationships which then must be reconstructed in an adjacent but separate space". They link it to the findings of Vicari et al. (1996b) that there is normal recency effect but no primacy effect in recall in WS. With FROM and VIA paths, the Figure's final resting place does not coincide with the ground. If the child cannot retain the representation of Ground object or Path over time, he will not be able to talk about them. Although Landau and Zukowski take this fragility to be residing in spatial cognition, they do not link it to findings that point exactly to the special difficulty of WS individuals with retaining spatial representations in memory: one of the most established findings in WS is the dissociation between different components of working memory, with individuals showing relatively preserved capacity in verbal short-term memory and serious limitations in spatial span (Wang & Bellugi 1994; Jarrold et al. 1999; Vicari et al. 1996a; Racsmány 2002; Racsmány et al. 2001). We will return to this issue in more detail in our discussion of our results from the study of spatial language in Hungarian WS individuals.

## Study 1: Semantic fluency

### Participants

12 individuals with Williams syndrome and 12 control subjects completed this task. The mean age of the WS group was 13,5 years (range: 7–19 years; SD 4.4). WS subjects were recruited through the Hungarian Williams Syndrome Association. The control group consisted of children matched on receptive vocabulary as measured by the Peabody Picture Vocabulary Test (Peabody scores: WS group: 99,3 (SD: 28,5), verbal control (VC) group: 101,3 (SD: 26,5)). The mean chronological age of the control group was 7,5 years (range: 6–9 years; SD 1,3). Verbal age was used for matching on similar basis as in Jarrold and his colleagues' study: we were particularly interested in the possible differences in the organizational *patterns* of the lexicon, and such differences are expected to manifest themselves when performance of groups with the same vocabulary *size* is compared.

## Procedure

All participants were tested individually in a quiet room, either in our laboratory, or in their respective schools. In addition to the PPVT, they were given a semantic fluency task with 8 categories, in which we asked them to list as many members for the given category as they could within 1 minute. Eight categories were used: Food, Animals, Drinks, Musical Instruments, Occupations, Things to read, Furniture and Clothes. Responses were audiotaped and then transcribed for further analysis. Frequency data for assessing the answers were taken from Kónya and Pintér (1986), a semantic fluency study conducted for these eight categories with 366 secondary school students. Although the procedure in the Kónya and Pintér study was different from ours in that ours required participants to list as many items as they could orally and within 1 minute, while they asked them to do it in writing and within 30 seconds, we consider the Kónya and Pintér (1986) measures appropriate and certainly the best available for Hungarian. We do not have real methodological worries about using these measures, and we again refer to the Jarrold et al. (2000)'s arguments: we are not assessing a group by these norms, but comparing the performance of two groups with each other, using the same measures for each. We applied two measures of the three proposed by Kónya and Pintér. The first was the *Frequency* of a given item: the number of times it was mentioned within a given category in the sample, and *Rank*, showing the average position of an item on the participants' lists. If there was an item mentioned by participants in the current study that did not appear in the Kónya and Pintér sample, we decided to give it a score of 0 on both measures.

## Results

We tested several measures for the fluency task: for each category we counted (a) the number of correct answers, (b) the number of non-category answers, (c) the number of repetitions, (d) the frequency and (e) rank of items, and the (f) number of items with zero frequency mentioned by the participant. A two way ANOVA on the number of items produced with the two-level factor GROUP (WS, VC) and the eight-level factor CATEGORY did not show any main effect for GROUP ($F(1,176) = 2{,}44$; n.s.). The main effect of CATEGORY was significant ($F(7,176) = 11{,}09$; $p < 0{,}001$). The interaction between the two factors was not significant (GROUP × CATEGORY: $F(7,176) = 1{,}5$; $p = 0{,}17$). The factor CATEGORY had a significant main effect on each type of dependent variable we tested; for clarity of exposition, we will only consider the effect of group here in detail, and reflect on some of the specific comparisons later. GROUP had a significant effect on the number of non-category answers the individuals produced, with the WS group producing significantly more ($F(1,176) = 5{,}5$; $p < 0{,}05$). The GROUP effect was

**Table 2.** Examples of answers on the fluency task from a WS child and his VC pair

| Animals | | Furniture | |
|---|---|---|---|
| WS | VC | WS | VC |
| horse | squirrel | table | chair |
| goat | butterfly | chair | bed |
| deer | deer | bed | bench |
| moufflon | reindeer | rocking chair | desktable |
| squirrel | crocodile | | wardrobe |
| lion | swine | | armchair |
| frog | guinea-pig | | shelf |
| hen | mouse | | |
| rooster | wolf | | |
| goose | cat | | |
| duck | fox | | |
| dinosaur | rabbit | | |
| mammoth | bird | | |
| monkey | turtle | | |
| gazella | fish | | |
| ostrich | frog | | |
| snake | owl | | |
| owl | thrush | | |
| mouse | | | |
| cat | | | |
| dog | | | |

also significant in the number of repetitions, the WS group producing more (F (1,176) = 15,43; p < 0,001). There was no effect of GROUP on the frequency (F (1,165) = 0,62; n.s.) or the rank (F (1,165) = 0,45; n.s.) of the items as measured by Kónya and Pintér (1986). The main effect of GROUP was significant, though, on the number of answers listed by the two groups that received a zero score for not appearing in the Kónya and Pintér corpus (F (1,176) = 8,08; p < 0,01): the WS group produced more of those.

The effect of CATEGORY was significant on all variables, showing that familiarity and size of a category do have an effect on the responses, but in this study it is of concern only where the performance of the two groups differ. Table 2 gives examples for two categories, one with many and one with few members, from a WS boy, aged 14 and his VC control, aged 9.

Figure 1 shows the number of answers by group and by category: the WS group produced significantly more answers only in the 'DRINKS' category, marked in capitals. The answers are listed by categories in decreasing order for the WS group: the ranking of the categories would be slightly different for the control group, with CLOTHES, FURNITURE and JOBS taking over MUSICAL INSTRUMENTS, a cat-

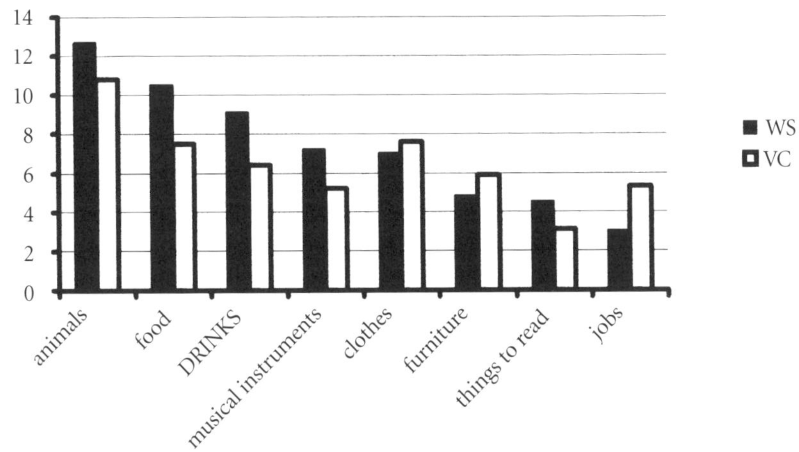


**Figure 1.** Mean number of answers by WS subjects and by controls matched on verbal age on the Fluency task

egory that is probably more familiar and richer for the WS group because of the musical therapy many of them engage in. The WS group produced significantly more answers that were not acceptable members of the given category: the mean number of non-category answers for the eight categories together for the WS group was 3,8 (SD = 3,6), for the VC group it was 1,8 (SD = 2,2). The WS made most mistakes in the OCCUPATIONS category, for the VC group THINGS TO READ proved to be the most difficult category. The WS group tended to repeat more items in all categories, the difference between the two groups being largest in the CLOTHES category.

Regarding the issue of frequency, we obtained the following results. There were no differences between the two groups in the average frequency and rank of the items they produced. There were differences, though, in the number of items with zero frequency, with WS subjects producing more in general. As can be seen on Figure 2, the two groups displayed the largest differences in the following 3 categories: ANIMALS, FOOD and DRINKS, probably the categories the WS subjects are most familiar with and/or interested in. Even in these categories, though, the items with zero frequency produced by the WS subjects are often not unusual or rare, but rather pet names for food or animals, examples of which are not found in the control sample, in which children are past the age at which typically developing children use such names. Both groups had items listed that scored zero frequency on the Kónya and Pintér scales that did not appear in the older sample because of the time lapse between the two studies. New brandnames, kinds of food and drinks appeared on the market in Hungary since then: *pizza*, *hamburger*, *Fanta*, are men-

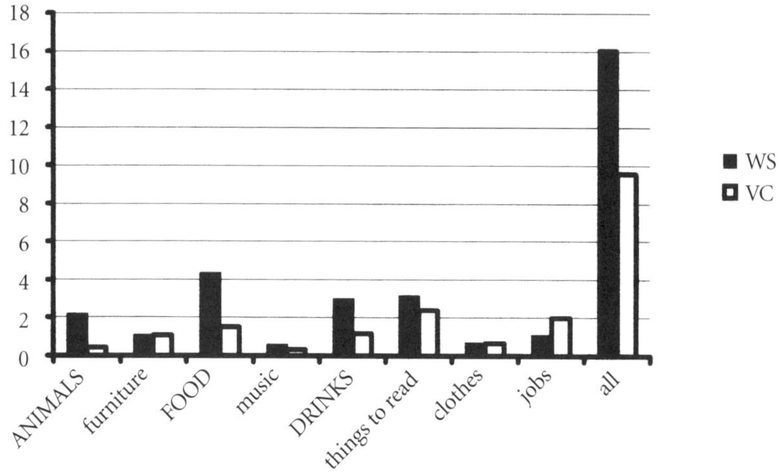


**Figure 2.** Number of answers with zero frequency on the Fluency task

tioned by individuals in both groups, and get a zero score for frequency and rank, although they are mentioned by almost every individual in our sample.

## Discussion

We can summarize the results of the Fluency task in the following way:

There was no significant difference between the WS and the VC group in:

- the number of items they produced
- the frequency and rank of items

There were, however, differences between the two groups in:

- the number of non-category members they listed, with WS subjects producing more
- the number of repetitions, with WS subjects producing more
- the number of answers with zero frequency, with WS subjects producing significantly more in 3 categories: animals, food and drinks

The results of the Fluency task suggest that WS individuals are not more fluent than typically developing children matched on receptive vocabulary, and they do not differ in the frequency effects governing retrieval and production of lexical items belonging to a semantic category. There were two significant differences. WS subjects tended to produce more repetitions, a difference reflecting problems with executive function, rather than language. They also produced more answers that fell outside the category they were listed in: most errors appeared in categories that were not too familiar for the WS subjects (furniture and jobs). We will discuss these findings together with results of the Picture Naming Vocabulary Task.

## Study 2: Picture Naming Vocabulary Task

### Participants

15 WS subjects, children and young adults (ranging from 7,2 to 19 years) participated in the Picture Naming Vocabulary Task, matched by two control groups: one matched on chronological age (AC), another matched on verbal age (VC) based on Peabody scores. WS subjects were mostly assessed in a summer holiday camp for WS children and their families. Control children were assessed individually in their school or kindergarten. Table 3 summarizes data of the participants.

### Materials

Pictures to be named were selected according to word class and Hungarian word frequency. To obtain a good and reliable sample, different sources of picture pools were used. Pictures in the naming task were black and white line drawings (Székely & Bates 2000; Bates et al. 2000; Druks & Masterson 2001; Masterson & Druks 1998), printed on cardboard paper.[2] Stimuli came in three categories: the *NOUNS* group had 30 line drawings of objects or animals and plants, the *VERBS* group consisted of 30 pictures displaying actions, and the *COMPOUNDS* group consisting of 20 items showing objects and creatures again, with the condition that their names were compound nouns. Half of the names of the items in each category were frequent words, half were rare, according to norms in the frequency dictionary of Hungarian (Füredi & Kelemen 1989). Examples are given in Table 4.

**Table 3.** Participants in the Picture Naming Vocabulary Task

| | AC | VC | WMS |
|---|---|---|---|
| Age (years) | 13,4 (SD = 4,3) | 7,1 (SD = 0,9) | 13,4 (SD = 4,38) |
| Peabody scores | 140,9 (SD =7,8) | 100 (SD = 22,1) | 98 (SD = 28,6) |
| Male | 7 | 7 | 7 |
| Female | 8 | 8 | 8 |

**Table 4.** Examples of stimuli from the vocabulary task

| | NOUNS | VERBS | COMPOUNDS |
|---|---|---|---|
| Frequent | *macska* 'cat' | *táncol* 'dance' | *babakocsi* 'pram' |
| Rare | *piramis* 'pyramid' | *térdepel* 'kneel' | *karmester* 'conductor' |

## Procedure

Participants were tested individually. They were given the pictures one by one by the experimenter, and were asked to name it with questions like '*What is it*?' in the case of NOUNS and COMPOUNDS, and '*What is he/she/it doing*?' in the case of VERBS. Responses were tape-recorded for later assessment; there was no time limit on the response of the subject. The independent variables were the category and the frequency of the word, the dependent variable was the correctness of the response. A response was coded correct if it corresponded to the dominant response of normal subjects to the picture (established by Székely & Bates 2000; Bates et al. 2000; Druks & Masterson 2001) or were synonymous with it in the NOUNS and VERBS group; in the case of compounds, only responses that were compounds were accepted.

## Results

A mixed 3-way (GROUP × WORD CLASS × FREQUENCY) ANOVA comparing the WS and the AC groups showed main effects of GROUP ($F = 16{,}44$; $p < 0{,}001$), WORD CLASS ($F = 4{,}8$; $p < 0{,}02$), and FREQUENCY ($F = 46{,}3$; $p < 0.001$) The interaction between the GROUP × FREQUENCY factors was also significant ($F = 23{,}1$; $p < 0.001$), but the interaction between GROUP and WORD CLASS did not reach significance ($F = 2{,}5$; $p > 0.1$). To summarize, the WS group obtained significantly poorer scores on the naming task than their age matched controls, but there was no difference in the pattern of performance of the two groups concerning the distribution of scores according to word class. The frequency effect, was stronger in the WS group (although the lack of frequency effects in the AC group does not mean that this group is insensitive to frequency: it is explained in their case by near ceiling performance).

The same comparison of the WS and the VC groups showed significant main effects for all three factors. (GROUP: $F = 5{,}4$; $p < 0{,}03$; WORD CLASS: $F = 18{,}6$; $p < 0{,}001$; and FREQUENCY: $F = 87{,}03$; $p < 0{,}001$). Here neither the GROUP × WORD CLASS ($F = 1{,}8$; $p > 0.1$) nor the GROUP × FREQUENCY ($F = 2{,}9$; $p > 0.09$) interaction was significant. Thus, the group matched on receptive vocabulary performed significantly better on the productive task, but the effects of syntactic

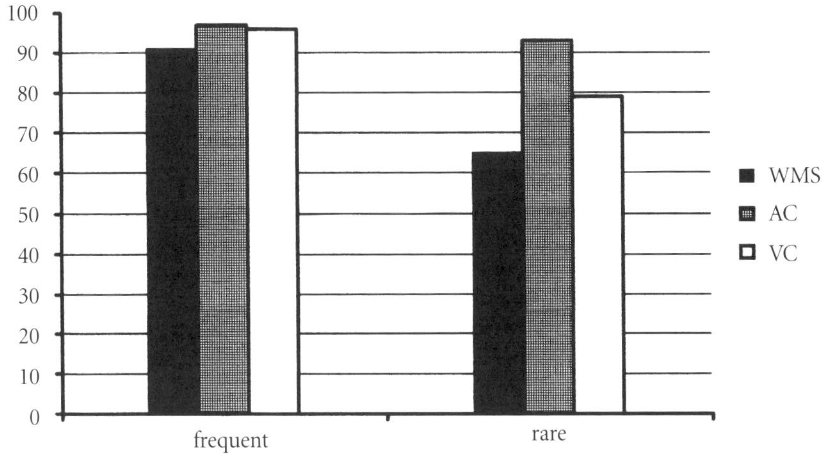


**Figure 3.** Percentage of correct answers on the vocabulary task by frequency and group

category and frequency were not different in the two groups. Performance of the three groups averaged over word classes is shown on Figure 3.

## Discussion

To summarize results of the naming task, our findings were the following. Both the chronological age and the verbal controls performed significantly better on this task than WS individuals. Naming performance lags behind receptive vocabulary level, in line with findings of Temple and her colleagues (2002), who found that receptive vocabulary scores were above mental age in the four WS individuals they tested, but they proved to be anomic on a naming task relative to their vocabulary knowledge, and performed poorer on confrontation naming than MA controls. A relative naming difficulty in WS is also in accord with results of Volterra et al. (1996) who found that the 17 WS individuals they tested was at an equal level to mental age matched typically developing controls, on PPVT scores, a receptive vocabulary test, while they were poorer on the Boston naming test. In our study, frequency effects in the WS group were stronger than in the AC group (although this difference might be due to a ceiling effect in the latter group) and are the same as frequency effects for the VC group, both groups performing better with frequent than with rare items. Results of this study, together with findings from the Fluency task show that frequency effects operate in the normal way in WS. This of course does not rule out the possibility that as a consequence of mental retardation, more input might be needed in stabilizing items in the WS lexical system. This result is in line with conclusions of previous studies (Johnson & Carey 1998; Jarrold et al.

2000; Temple et al. 2002), that instead of the lack of frequency effects, it is atypical organization or underspecification of conceptual knowledge that could explain the phenomena characteristic of lexical organization in Williams syndrome. Further research needs to be conducted in this direction.

## Study 3: Morphology task

### The system of Hungarian noun allomorphs

Hungarian, as an agglutinating language, has a very rich suffix-system. Suffixes play an important role and encode much more grammatical information than in a configurational language like English. In our view, testing regular and irregular morphology with Hungarian WS individuals does not simply extend studies to another language, because the Hungarian system of allomorphs, as will be clear from the presentation below, is different from the English system in several relevant respects. In Hungarian, irregular forms seem to be less frequent, and, accordingly, these are not the first ones that the child learns in typical acquisition. As for the type frequency of regular forms, our language is rather like English (and not like German: see Marcus et al. 1995): the great majority of stems belong to productive regular classes, and the minority of irregulars form closed classes. The basic structure of the noun is Noun-Number-Case, singular number and nominative case are unmarked. The accusative suffix is the same for singular and plural forms (e.g. *szoba* 'room', *szobát* 'room acc.', *szobák* 'rooms', *szobákat* 'rooms acc.').

Most importantly, Hungarian is different from both English and German in that the suffix is invariable and identifiable with all stem types, regular and irregular: for example, the plural form of every noun ends in *-k*; it is either the stem that alternates, or the quality of the linking vowel or allomorphy in general that changes in irregular forms (for previous research on Hungarian see Lukács & Pléh 1999).

On the basis of their morphophonological behavior, noun stems are classified into different stem types. Potential stem alternations are not elicited by all nominal suffixes: they appear with the plural, accusative, superessive, possessed and comitative forms of nouns, i.e. with bound suffixes that attach to the stem with a linking vowel.[3] We tested plural and accusative forms and we present different stem classes through these forms based on Kiefer (1998), Nádasdy and Siptár (1994) and Törkenczy (1994). We do not present accounts of particular stem classes in full detail; we only provide the information relevant to understanding the behavior of plural and accusative forms under study.

*Non-productive stem classes*[4]

1. *Epenthetic stems.* These stems have two forms. The free form of the stem ends in a -VCVC (*bokor* 'bush', *terem* 'hall') sequence, in which the final vowel alternates with Ø, so some bound forms of stems (accusative and plural, among others) are closed by a -VCC- sequence (*bokr*ot 'bush, acc.', *term*et 'hall, acc.'). Other suffixes take the free form of the stem: *bokorban* 'bush, iness.' and *teremben* 'hall, iness'.
2. *Lowering stems.* Stems in this class do not themselves alternate, but instead of the typically middle linking vowel, the linking vowel of the suffix is low: the resulting vowel follows the rules of vowel harmony and is *a* after a back vowel in the stem (e.g. *ház* 'house" ~ *házak* 'houses' as opposed to the productive *gáz* 'gas' ~ *gázok* 'gases'), and after front vowels (even after round *ö*, *ü*) the linking vowel is *e* (e.g. *hölgy* 'lady' ~ *hölgyek* 'ladies' as opposed to the productive form *rög* 'clod' ~ *rögök* 'clods').
3. *Shortening stems.* The vowel of the last syllable, which in free forms of these stems is long, shortens when one of the suffixes listed above is attached to the stem. (e.g. *egér* 'mouse' ~ *egerek* 'mice'; *bogár* 'beetle' ~ *bogarak* 'beetles'. Other suffixes take the free form: *egérben* 'mouse, iness.' and *bogárban* 'beetle iness.'). Shortening stems, like lowering stems, require a low vowel as a linking vowel.
4. *v-inserting stems.* This class contains one-syllable stems ending in a long vowel. In bound forms of stems, a /v/ is inserted between the stem final and the linking vowels, and at the same time, the stem final vowel shortens. (*tő* 'stem' ~ *tövek* 'stems' vs. *tőben* 'stem, iness.', *ló* 'horse' ~ *lovak* 'horses' vs. *lóban* 'horse, iness.'). These stems are at the same time lowering stems.

*Productive stem classes*

Stems in these classes appear in the same form with all suffixes.

5. *Stems ending in a low vowel.* Low vowels (*a*, *e*) lengthen (to *á* and *é*, respectively) when a suffix is attached to the stem (*kamra* 'chamber' ~ *kamrák* 'chambers'; *csésze* 'cup' ~ *csészék* 'cups').
6. *Stems ending in a consonant.* The vowel of suffixes with a linking vowel always shows up after these stems (like the plural suffix which can be represented as -*Vk*; e.g. *mester* 'master' ~ *mesterek* 'masters'; *alap* 'basis' ~ *alapok* 'bases'). The behavior of the accusative -*t* is more complicated; with some consonants, it forms a cluster (with coronal nasals, with liquids, and with sibilant fricatives e.g. *mester* 'master' ~ *mestert* 'master, acc.'), with the rest, it requires a linking vowel (e.g. *alap* 'basis' ~ *alapok* 'basis, acc.')
7. *Stems ending in a nonlow vowel.* With these stems, the linking vowel of suffixes is dropped, and the stem-final vowel does not change (*hajó* 'ship' ~ *hajók* 'ships'; *buli* 'party' ~ *bulik* 'parties').

## Morphology task

Participants in this study were the same as in the Picture naming vocabulary task with the exclusion of 1 WS participant and his matched controls.

### Materials

28 picture pairs were used in this experiment, those from the NOUN ALLOMORPHS subtest of a screening method developed earlier for language impaired children by Pléh, Palotás and Lőrik (2002). These stimuli were complemented by new picture pairs to adjust for frequency, as our questions also concerned effects of frequency on regular and irregular suffixation. The first picture of each pair shows an object, the second one is supposed to elicit either its accusative or plural form. The test had 4 items in each of the 3 regular and 4 irregular stem classes in Hungarian, 2 frequent and 2 rare, based on Füredi and Kelemen (1989). Table 5 gives some examples.

### Procedure

Participants were given the pictures one by one by the experimenter, the one depicting an individual object shown first from each pair. After providing the name for the object, they were shown the second picture from the pair, and were asked questions prompting either a plural ('What are these?') or an accusative (e.g. 'What

**Table 5.** Examples of stimuli used in the morphology task

| Stem class | Example | |
|---|---|---|
| | Frequent | Rare |
| 1. Epenthetic | *majom-majmok*<br>'monkey-monkey acc.' | *bagoly-baglyot*<br>'owl-owl acc.' |
| 2. Lowering | *hal-halak*<br>'fish-fish pl.' | *sál-sálak*<br>'scarf-scarf pl.' |
| 3. Shortening | *kenyér-kenyerek*<br>'bread-bread pl.' | *bogár-bogarak*<br>'beetle-beetle pl.' |
| 4. v-insertion | *kő-követ*<br>'stone-stone acc.' | *távcső-távcsövet*<br>'telescope-telescope acc.' |
| 4. 'Low V'-final | *kutya-kutyát*<br>'dog-dog acc.' | *teve-tevék*<br>'camel-camel pl.' |
| 5. C-final | *asztal-asztalok*<br>'table-table pl.' | *pingvin-pingvinek*<br>'penguin-penguin pl.' |
| 6. 'Nonlow V'-final | *cipő-cipőt*<br>'shoe-shoe acc.' | *hattyú-hattyút*<br>'swan-swan acc.' |

is the boy eating?') forms. Responses were tape-recorded; there was no time limit on the response of the subject. Independent variables were stem type and frequency of the word, the dependent variable was the correctness of the response. A response was coded as correct if it was properly inflected; it was considered incorrect if it was overregularized or unmarked.

## Results

Controls matched on chronological age produced a ceiling effect with zero errors, so their results are again not included in the analysis below. Results of the WS and VC groups are shown in Figure 4. A 2 × 2 × 2 ANOVA with the factors GROUP, and REGULARITY and FREQUENCY revealed a significant main effect for all factors: GROUP ($F\ (1,28) = 4{,}96$; $p < 0{,}05$) REGULARITY ($F\ (1,28) = 66{,}2$); $p < 0{,}001$) and FREQUENCY ($F\ (1,28) = 16{,}9$; $p < 0{,}001$). The interaction of GROUP with REGULARITY and with FREQUENCY was not significant ($F\ (1,28) = 0{,}52$; n.s. and $F\ (1,28) = 2{,}8$; n.s., respectively), but the interaction of REGULARITY × FREQUENCY ($F\ (1,28) = 18{,}05$; $p < 0{,}001$) and of the three factors was ($F\ (1,28) = 9{,}5$; $p < 0{,}05$). The VC group performed significantly better on both frequent ($t = -2{,}84$; $p < 0{,}05$) and infrequent regulars ($t = -3{,}27$; $p < 0{,}05$), and on frequent irregulars ($t = -2{,}86$; $p < 0{,}05$), but not on infrequent irregulars ($t = 0{,}89$; n.s.). Pairwise comparisons of different morphological types in the two groups show that both groups score significantly higher on regulars than on irregulars (VC: $t = -14{,}22$; $p < 0{,}001$; WS: $t = -4{,}06$; $p < 0{,}01$), this effect was found analyzing both frequent and infrequent words by regularity. The effect of frequency was different in the two groups, though: Verbal Controls performed significantly better on frequent irregulars than on infrequent ones ($t = 8{,}56$; $p < 001$), but their scores were just as high on infrequent regulars as on frequent ones ($t = 0{,}34$; n.s.). In the WS group, there is no effect of frequency in either regulars or irregulars (frequent regulars-infrequent regulars: $t = 1{,}15$; n.s.; frequent irregulars-infrequent irregulars: $t = 1{,}13$; n.s.). Figure 4 shows results for the two groups.

## Error types

We classified errors to look for possible differences in error patterns, since this issue also seemed relevant concerning contrasting findings and debates on overregularization (see above). The control group did not make enough errors to allow proper comparison, so we analyzed performance and error types of 30 control children between 3;8–6;3 years on the same morphology task. Taking errors of both groups, five types of errors were distinguished. An error was considered OVERGENERALIZATION if the plural or accusative form of the noun was regularized, i.e. a noun

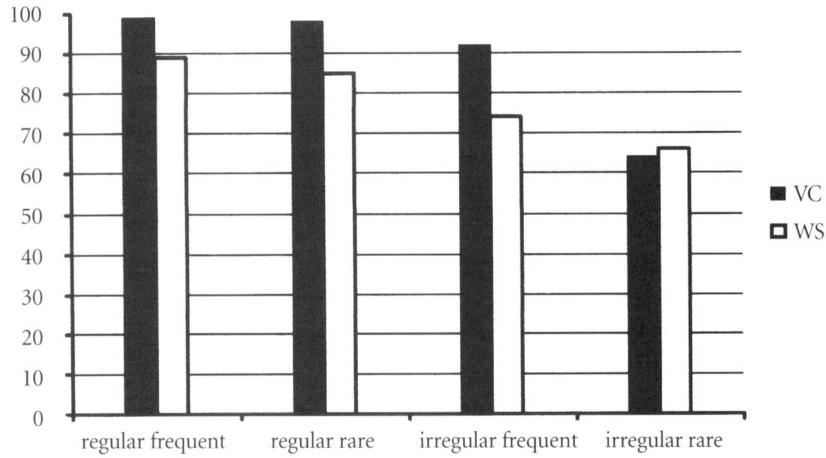


**Figure 4.** Percentage of correct answers in the morphology task

belonging to a specific pattern was inflected according to the general one (*kő* 'stone' ~ *kőt instead of correct *követ* 'stone, acc.'). An answer was coded UNMARKED when the participant answered with the unmarked nominative form of the noun (*kő* ~ **kő* instead of *követ*). Perhaps surprisingly for the reader, overgeneralization errors occurred with regulars as well, because stem alternations characterize regular stems as well. There were two kinds of overgeneralization errors in regulars: lack of lengthening of the stem-final low-vowel (e.g. *teve* ~ **tevek* instead of *tevék* 'camel ~ camels') or inserting a linking vowel between the accusative and a consonant with which it forms a cluster (e.g. *pingvin* ~ *pingvinet* instead of *pingvint* 'penguin ~ penguin, acc.'). The category DOESN'T KNOW included cases when the participant did not answer or said s/he didn't know the answer. Another type of error category included AVOIDING ANSWERS: these were answers where the participant, not knowing the correct answer, answered with a properly inflected form of a noun similar in meaning or in form to the target noun (*ló* 'horse' ~ *pacit* 'gee-gee, acc.' instead of *lovat* 'horse, acc.'). The OTHER category included errors that did not fit any of the four categories listed above. Rates of different error types in the two groups are given in Table 6 below. Percentages for single error types are calculated as error rates of all errors for the given morphological type.

There are a couple of differences between the two groups that are worthy of consideration. The DOESN'T KNOW answer type did not occur in the WS group, but it was as common in the TD group as unmarked answers. In contrast, avoiding answers were more common in the WS group. This might reflect the pursuit of the WS group to the answer by any means, thus a social compliance tendency in WS on the one hand and better understanding of the task by TD children on the other.

**Table 6.** Percentages of different types of errors in the WS and TD groups

| | WS Irregular | Regular | All | TD Irregular | Regular | All |
|---|---|---|---|---|---|---|
| Overgeneralization | 60,7 | 8,3 | 45 | 83,6 | 28 | 74,5 |
| Unmarked | 32,14 | 66,6 | 42,5 | 8,6 | 36 | 13,07 |
| Doesn't know | 0 | 0 | 0 | 7,03 | 36 | 11,76 |
| Avoiding answer | 3,5 | 16,66 | 7,5 | 0,78 | 0 | 0,6 |
| Other | 3,5 | 8,3 | 5 | 0 | 0 | 0 |
| All | 70 | 30 | 100 | 83,6 | 16,4 | 100 |

**Table 7.** Number of overgeneralization and other errors in the two groups

| | WS Irregular | Regular | All | TD Irregular | Regular | All |
|---|---|---|---|---|---|---|
| Overgeneralization | 34 | 2 | 36 | 107 | 7 | 114 |
| Other | 22 | 22 | 44 | 21 | 18 | 39 |

Overgeneralizations were more common in the group of typically developing children than in the WS group, and this was true for both irregulars and regulars: in the TD group, they made up two-thirds of all errors, whereas in the WS group, overregularizations constituted less than half of the errors. Table 7 shows number of overgeneralization errors and all other errors (sum of unmarked, avoiding, doesn't know, and other answers) in the two groups. Comparing rates of overgeneralization answers to all other answers, we find that in irregulars, this rate is significantly higher in the control group: irregulars: $\chi^2 = 11{,}4$; $p < 0{,}001$; regulars: $\chi^2 = 3{,}16$; n.s.). Rates of overgeneralization errors for irregulars and regulars did not differ between the two groups ($\chi^2 = 0{,}02$; n.s.), neither did rates of all other answers for irregulars and regulars ($\chi^2 = 0{,}12$; n.s.).

Rates of unmarked answers were much higher in the WS than in the TD group, for both irregulars and regulars. One possible explanation, following Zukowski (2001), is that WS individuals were much older and also had higher verbal mental ages than the control group used for comparing error patterns. WS individuals might have had some knowledge of the irregularity of irregulars, that is why they did not inflect them like regulars, but they were unable to access the correct form, leading to an unmarked answer. The account that unmarked answers reflect sensitivity to irregularity is contradicted by rates of unmarked answers for regulars, which are high even if we take into account that these are relative rates of the much smaller proportion of errors on regulars (in fact, as rates of all errors, percentages of unmarked answers for regular and irregulars are very similar: 22,5% percent of all errors were unmarked irregulars and 20% of all errors were unmarked regulars).

Although the WS group shows lower rates of overregularization and higher rates of unmarked answers than controls, both groups gave more OVERGENERALIZATION than UNMARKED answers. As we have seen above, relative rates of overgeneralizations differed across previous studies as well: Clahsen and Almazan (1998) found robust overgeneralization, while in Zukowski (2001)'s plural prompt task singular answers were the most common error. As referred to above in Note 1, Zukowski puts this down to either individual differences in strategies to solve the task, or methodological differences between studies. Individual differences can be a real reason, and further investigation is needed to uncover whether there is some underlying factor behind choice of one strategy over the other (it can be a function of chronological or verbal age). Constraining our discussion to irregulars, the type of error, we would add, can also be item-specific. Most errors with the nouns *kerék* ('wheel') or *majom* ('monkey') included unmarked answers (**kerék* instead of *kerekek* 'wheels'[5] and **majom* instead of *majmok* 'monkeys'), while for *kenyér* ('bread') and *távcső* ('telescope') most frequent errors were overgeneralizations (*kenyért* (bread-ACC) instead of *kenyeret* and *távcsők* ('telescopes') instead of *távcsövek*). This dissociation was observed within individuals as well.

## Discussion

Results of the morphology task reveal the superiority of performance on regulars over irregulars in WS, observed by others (Clahsen & Almazan 1998; Clahsen, Ring, & Temple, this volume; Zukowski 2001). However, the same pattern was found in the control group matched on receptive vocabulary obtaining significantly higher scores than the WS group in all morphological types except for rare irregulars, where performance of the two groups did not differ. We agree with the conclusion of Thomas et al. (2001) that we do not find a selective deficit for irregulars, and although we are also convinced by arguments for the general theoretical position that we cannot take developmental deficits to be cases of residual normality, our own data do not argue for atypical processes in acquisition of inflectional morphology.

Frequency in our study seemed to play a different role in the two groups: in line with predictions of the dual route model (Pinker 1991), it affects performance on irregulars but not regulars in typically developing children. In the WS group, though, performance on frequent and infrequent items did not differ in regulars and in irregulars either. Although Thomas et al. (2001) also found atypical frequency effects in the WS group (frequency affected regulars and not irregulars), our finding of a lack of frequency effect in the WS group on the morphology task is hard to explain and interpret as arguing for atypical processes underlying WS language development, especially in the light of the results of lexical skill studies presented above, where the WS showed similar effects of frequency as typically developing children. This finding probably reflects the wide age range of the WS group: older children might perform better on rare items than younger typically developing children, while they still make occasional errors with frequent items.

Clahsen, as a reviewer of this chapter, pointed out that "WS children were *not* matched with mental age controls, but rather on the basis of receptive vocabulary scores, and that this is problematic because children with WS have receptive vocabulary scores above the level of their mental ages (see e.g. Bellugi et al. 1990; Tyler et al. 1997; Temple et al. 2002). Consequently, by matching the WS group to the controls based on an elevated skill (i.e. receptive vocabulary), we end up with a control group that disadvantages the WS group." As he argues, this critically affects the results and interpretation of the present data set, e.g. the claim that the controls are significantly better in regular inflection than the WS children. We find the problem of matching crucially important in interpreting results. We decided against matching on mental scores because we find that as a composite measure, (1) it might mask differences between individuals having similar scores, (2) it is not clear that all nonlinguistic abilities required for language are bundled up in this measure, and (3) it is also not obvious how these abilities relate to language either in typically developing or impaired children. In our view, matching on verbal age is important if we want to establish differences in patterns of linguistic abilities between groups. Besides, data in the error analysis also shows that with a younger group probably closer in mental age to our WS group, we find larger rates of errors (and more specifically) overregularization on irregulars in the group of typically developing children than in the WS group. This is strong support against selective difficulty of Hungarian WS children with irregulars.

To summarize, results from an agglutinative language argue against a selective deficit of the lexicon in Williams syndrome, and show that rule application posits similar difficulties. We matched our WS participants to a group of verbal controls individually, looking for differences in the pattern of performances in the two groups. The pattern of errors could be explained by a general retardation, as suggested by Thomas et al. (2001) but is not conclusive for the debate concerning the dual route model: our data are reconcilable both with single route models of language and proposals of two distinct mechanisms for the lexicon and grammar, with a general deficit equally affecting both systems of language. The data presented here do not argue for the dual route model, although findings do not strictly argue against it either: the above results are compatible with an explanation working with two systems of a lexicon and a computational system of rules within language, supplemented with a claim that none of them are intact in WS. For this reason, our data from Williams syndrome do not present a case which supports the validity of the model by displaying selective impairment to one of its components.

## Study 4: Spatial postpositions and suffixes

### The language of space in Hungarian

As all languages, Hungarian has several means of encoding spatial relations: suffixes, postpositions, verbal prefixes and adverbs. We focus on suffixes and postpositions, because our studies revolve around these two types of spatial expressions, which are used together with noun phrases in descriptions making reference to the reference object as well. Suffixes encode simpler relations (IN, ON) and obey the rules of vowel harmony. The system of postpositions is used to encode cognitively more complex relations (BEHIND, UNDER) and is structurally more systematic than suffixes, as can be seen from Table 8 and Table 9. Each kind of spatial relation can be encoded in three forms according to the dynamic aspect of coding the location and the path. For each spatial relation, Hungarian has a STATIC LOCATIVE term, and two dynamic forms, one encoding the GOAL or end of the path, the other the SOURCE or starting point of the path. Hungarian is very systematic in encoding all three directions with terms of the same formal complexity (and differs in respect from English, for example, which in some cases uses expressions of different complexity: *above the picture* vs. *from above the picture*. Thus for our studies of these spatial terms in WS, we can cite MacWhinney (1976), taken as a starting point for previous research on spatial terms in Hungarian (Pléh, Vinkler, & Kálmán 1997): "Hungarian inflections differ little in terms of formal complexity. Thus, differences in their emergence can be attributed to semantic pragmatic factors" (MacWhinney 1976:409). Similarly, specific pattern possibly emerging in WS usage will reflect the influence of such factors instead of the effect of linguistic complexity.

Table 8. Postpositions used in the study

| spatial relation | Static | Goal | Source |
|---|---|---|---|
| BEHIND | *mögött* | *mögé* | *mögül* |
| IN FRONT OF | *előt* | *elé* | *elől* |
| UNDER | *alatt* | *alá* | *alól* |
| NEXT TO | *mellett* | *mellé* | *mellől* |
| BETWEEN | *között* | *közé* | *közül* |

Table 9. Suffixes used in the study

| spatial relation | Static | Goal | Source |
|---|---|---|---|
| ON | *-on/en/ön* | *-ra/re* | *-ról/ről* |
| IN | *-ban/ben* | *-ba/be* | *-ból/ből* |

## Participants

Participants in this study were the same as participants in the previous two studies, with the exception of two WS individuals and their controls. For studying performance on spatial expressions, we also included a control group matched on spatial performance as measured by the Block Design test of the WISC-R. This group consisted of 13 children, with a mean age of 4,6 (SD = 0,9), almost ten years less than mean age of the WS group.

## Procedure

For testing production of spatial terms, we used a SPATIAL POSTPOSITIONS AND SUFFIXES subtest of Pléh et al. (2002). Spatial postpositions were elicited with two toy wardrobes as reference objects, and small, coloured token circles, triangles and squares as target objects. Spatial suffixes were tested with the same target objects and two glasses as reference objects. The experimenter put the target objects to different positions, and asked 3 kinds of questions, which code the directionality aspect of the answer. Examples of questions are 'Where is the blue circle?' (STATIC), 'Where did I put the blue circle?' (GOAL) and 'Where did I take the blue circle from?' (SOURCE). Knowledge of 15 postpositions, SOURCE, STATIC and GOAL forms of the Hungarian words for *in front of, behind, below, between*, and *next to*, and 6 suffixes (SOURCE, STATIC and GOAL forms of the Hungarian equivalents of *in* and *on*) was tested.

## Results

The group matched on chronological age produced a ceiling effect with zero errors, so their results are again not included in the analysis below. Results for the Williams syndrome (WS) group, for controls matched on verbal age (VC) and controls matched for spatial performance (SC) are presented in Figure 5, contrasted to their performance in Study 3, i.e. on plurals and accusatives.

The WS group obtained significantly lower scores than the VC group on both spatial postpositions ($F(1,26) = 37,8$; $p < 0,001$) and spatial suffixes ($F(1,26) = 25,7$; $p < 0,001$). Spatial controls also performed significantly better than the WS group on suffixes ($F(1,26) = 3,8$; $p < 0,05$) but not on postpositions ($F(1,26) = 0,64$; p < n.s.). Analyzing results on postpositions by directionality (results are shown on Figure 6 below) revealed that both the main effect of GROUP ($F(2,39) = 15,25$; $p < 0,001$), and the main effect of DIRECTIONALITY ($F(2,78) = 13,15$; $p < 0,001$) is significant, with a significant interaction ($F(2,78) = 3,94$; $p < 0,01$). Posthoc Sheffé-tests showed that the difference between the WS and the verbal control and the spatial and the verbal control group was significant, but the WS and

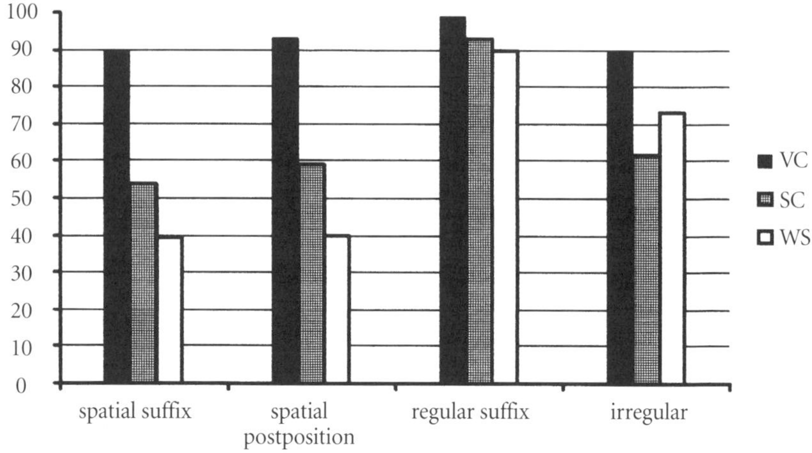


**Figure 5.** Performance of the three groups on the spatial and non-spatial task

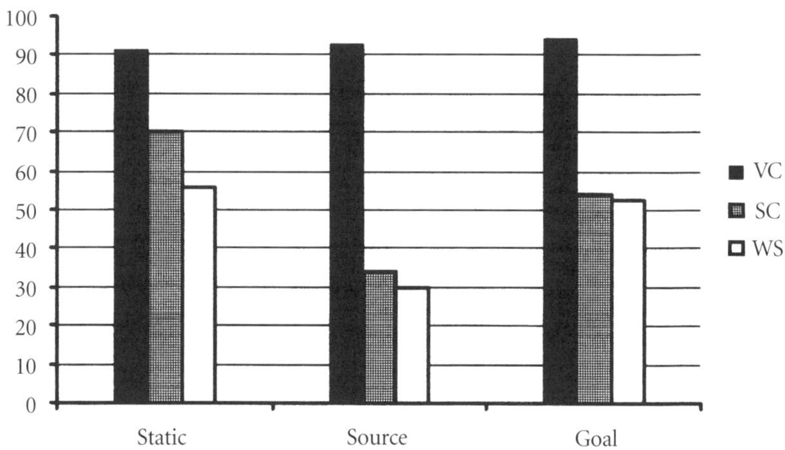


**Figure 6.** Performance of subjects with Williams syndrome (WS) and two control groups (verbal control (VC), spatial control (SC)) on the spatial expressions task by directionality

the spatial control group performed at the same level (WS-VC: $F(1,26) = 22{,}52$; $p < 0{,}001$; SC-VC: $F(1,26) = 36{,}75$; $p < 0{,}001$; WS-SC: $F(1,26) = 0{,}53$; n.s.). Pairwise comparisons showed that there were no significant differences between the WS and the spatial control group on any directions. Comparison with the VC group reveals worse performance in the WS group for all directions (STATIC: $t(26) =$

3,06; $p < 0{,}01$; SOURCE: $t(26) = 5{,}95$; $p < 0{,}001$; GOAL: $t(26) = 3{,}6$; $p < 0{,}01$). Figure 6 shows performance of the three groups by directionality.

On nonspatial morphology, we have already seen that the VC group performs better than the WS group. When comparing WS subjects with spatial controls, we find that they do not differ in producing regular inflection correctly, ($F(1{,}26) = 0{,}4$; $p > 0{,}1$), but on irregulars, WS subjects actually outperform spatial controls ($F(1{,}26) = 4{,}5$; $p < 0{,}05$), who perform at the level corresponding to their chronological age (mean: 4,6 years).

## Discussion

As previous research has already demonstrated, spatial language is impaired in WS. They performed significantly worse than verbal controls groups, and their performance matched that of spatial controls. Comparison with the group matched on spatial cognition, though, suggests that linguistic performance on spatial expressions reflects degree of deficit in spatial cognition, and not a manifestation of a real interaction between language and spatial cognition. This is also confirmed by patterns of relative difficulty of postpositions by directionality. Our results concerning directionality were in line with previous developmental data (Pléh et al. 1997, 2002; Király et al. 2001). Source proved to be most difficult for all three groups. The VC controls, as predicted by previous results, showed a goal-preference and performed almost as well on static as goal expressions. Performance of the WS group was very similar, and although the performance of the SC group shows higher scores for static expressions, the difference between static and goal expressions did not reach significance. Although the WS group is delayed on spatial expressions relative to their verbal age, they perform at the level of spatial controls, and they show the same pattern of performance as controls, suggesting a similar organization and no sign of atypical mapping to language.

## Conclusions

Our Hungarian data imply that the use of unusual and partially inappropriate words in WS is not due to insensitivity to frequency. In the Fluency task, there were no systematic differences between the frequency of items produced by the WS and the VC groups. The WS group produced the same frequency effects as verbal controls on the picture naming task. WS subjects' problems with integrating semantic representations into context might be one of the reasons for the slight differences in lexical organization, and underspecified semantic representations can also explain the data, but the nature of underspecification awaits further study.

As for morphological overgeneralizations, Hungarian data imply a strong tendency to overgeneralize in WS. There was no selective deficit in irregulars as suggested by Clahsen and Almazan (1998): WS children's performance was worse on both irregulars and regulars. The pattern of errors could be explained by a general retardation, as suggested by Thomas et al. (2001) but is not conclusive for the debate concerning the dual route model: our data are reconcilable both with single route models of language and proposals of two distinct mechanisms for the lexicon and grammar, with a general deficit equally affecting both systems of language.

Results concerning elicited production of spatial terms show that WS children are delayed relative to their verbal age, but their performance matches their degree level of sophistication of spatial cognition. Taken together, our findings on spatial language provide strong support for Landau and Zukowski's hypothesis that the difficulty with retaining spatial information in memory can account for special difficulty with SOURCE paths. Our results pointed out the relative difficulty of SOURCE, and confirmed that scenes that do not charge spatial memory (STATIC and GOAL) are easier to describe. This finding is exactly what we would expect based on Landau and Zukowski's hypothesis, that SOURCE paths are difficult because they have a memory component missing from GOAL and STATIC scenes.

We would like to take Landau and Zukowski's argument one step further, though. They backed up their argument by findings from Vicari et al. (1996b) that in list learning, WS children show normal recency effect, but no primacy effect, pointing to problems in retention, and they allow for the possibility that effects observed in spatial descriptions are due to overall problems of retention, which might be a general consequence of mental retardation. A more natural possible explanation is the selective impairment of the spatial component of working memory. Besides results in the literature arguing for a dissociation of verbal and spatial short term memory, previous results from our research group (Racsmány et al. 2001; Racsmány 2002) have shown that Corsi span (taken to be a measure of spatial working memory capacity) is just a strong factor in predicting performance of WS children on spatial postpositions as digit span (measuring verbal working memory capacity).

Results from the four studies we presented show that WS language lags behind verbal age as measured by receptive vocabulary scores in several respects, but no evidence of atypical organization was found. This of course, does not mean that language in WS is typical (as many previous studies have shown it is not), but more fine-grained studies of representation, temporal processing aspects, and detailed studies of mechanisms of acquisition are needed to uncover those structures and processes that are different from typical. Also, more studies analyzing complex individual profiles would be needed in interpreting the group differences.

## Acknowledgements

The research reported here owes much to the help and support of the Hungarian Williams Syndrome Association and the devoted help and attention of its scholarly leaders, Gábor Pogány and Dóra Scheiber. We thank the assistance and enthusiastic help of all the parents and the children participating in the study. Financial support for the research was provided by OTKA (Hungarian National Science Foundation) T 029514 provided to Csaba Pléh, by an NSF Grant Award No. BCS-0126151 to Ilona Kovács and Csaba Pléh as principal investigators, and a NKFP Hungarian National Research Grant for the project 'Cognitive and Neural Plasticity', No. 02151079. Mihály Racsmány was supported by the Jánas Bolyai scholarchip.

## Notes

1. Zukowski hypothesizes that differences between rates of overregularization in her study and Clahsen and Almazan might reflect individual differences in strategies to solve the task where they do not have the correct answer. We will return to this in discussing error patterns in our study.

2. Interestingly, in Hungarian, even irregular inflected forms are disallowed in compounds. In contrast, many derivations (including noun-verb ones) contain the irregular allomorph: *kanál* 'spoon, n' ~ *kanalaz* 'spoon, v', *halom* 'pile, n' ~ *halmoz* 'pile, v', kő 'stone, n' ~ *kövez* 'stone, v'). In contrast, Ackermann (2002) cites two languages, Finnish and Sepečides-Romani, where regularly inflected forms *can* occur as nonheads in compounds.

3. The reason for designing our own vocabulary test instead of using a standardized one was that there were no tests in Hungary that would have fit our specific questions concerning frequency and categories.

4. Morphemes belong to this suffix type that do not form a syllable on their own, their linking vowel is dropped if they attach to a stem ending in a vowel, and attach to the bound form of the stem (Kiefer 1998).

5. This was also observed by MacWhinney (1976), as being related to the final *-k* as a pseudo-plural.

## References

Ackermann, F. (2002). "Pausing to consider: A lexicalist appraisal of dual mechanism models and Williams syndrome research in morphology". *Paper presented at the Williams syndrome and the issue of Neurogenetic Developmental Disorders, Budapest, Hungary, May* 1–5.

Bates, E., Andonova, E., D'Amico, S., Jacobsen, T., Kohnert, K., Lu, C-C., Székely, A., Wicha, N., Federmeier, K., Herron, D., Iyer, G., Pechmann, T., Devescovi, A., Orozco-Figueroa, A., Gutierrez, G., Hung, D., Hsu, J., Tzeng, O., Gerdjikova, G., Mehotcheva, T., & Pléh, C. (2000). "Introducing the CRL International Picture-Naming Project (CRL-IPNP)". *Center for Research in Language Newsletter, 12*(1). La Jolla: University of California, San Diego.

Bellugi, U., Bihrle, A., Jernigan, T., & Doherty, S. (1990). "Neuropsychological, neurological and neuroanatomical profile of Williams syndrome". *American Journal of Medical Genetics, 6*, 115–125.

Bellugi, U., Lichtenberger, L., Jones, W., & Lai, Z. (2000). "The neurocognitive profile of Williams syndrome: a complex pattern of strengths and weaknesses". *Journal of Cognitive Neuroscience, 12*, 17–29.

Bellugi, U., Marks, S., Bihrle, A., & Sabo, H. (1988). "Dissociation between language and cognitive functions in Williams syndrome". In D. Bishop & K. Mogford (Eds.), *Language Development in Exceptional Circumstances* (pp. 177–190). Hillsdale, NJ: LEA.

Bellugi, U., Wang, P. P., & Jernigan, T. L. (1994). "Williams syndrome: An unusual neuropsychological profile". In S. Broman & J. Grafman (Eds.), *Atypical Cognitive Deficits in Developmental Disorders: Implications for brain function* (pp. 23–56). Hillsdale, NJ: LEA.

Bromberg, H. S., Ullman, M., Marcus, G. Kelly, K. B., & Levine, K. (1994). "The dissociation between lexical memory and grammar in Williams syndrome: Evidence from inflectional morphology". *Paper presented at the Williams Syndrome Professional Conference, San Diego, July.*

Clahsen, H. & Almazan, M. (1998). "Syntax and morphology in Williams syndrome". *Cognition, 68*, 167–198.

Clahsen, H. (1999). "Lexical entries and rules of language: A multidisciplinary study of German inflection". *Behavioral and Brain Sciences, 22*, 991–1060.

Clahsen, H. & Temple, C. (2003). "Words and rules in children with Williams syndrome". In Y. Levy & J. Schaeffer (Eds.), *Language Competence across Populations* (pp. 323–352). Mahwah, NJ: LEA.

Druks, J. & Masterson, J. (2001). *An Object and Action Naming Battery*. London: Psychology Press.

Füredi, M. & Kelemen, J. (Eds.). (1989). *A mai magyar nyelv szépprózai gyakorisági szótára* 1965–1977. Budapest: Akadémiai.

Jarrold, C., Baddeley, A. D., & Hewes, A. K. (1999). "Genetically dissociated components of working memory: evidence from Down's and Williams syndrome". *Neuropsychologia, 37*, 637–651.

Jarrold, C., Hartley, S., Phillips, C., & Baddeley, A. D. (2000). "Word fluency in Williams syndrome: Evidence for unusual semantic organisation"? *Cognitive Neuropsychiatry, 5*, 293–319.

Jarrold, C., Phillips, C., & Baddeley, A. (2001). "Comprehension of spatial and nonspatial language in Williams syndrome". Poster presented at the SRCD Biennial meeting, Minneapolis, April 2001.

Johnson, S. C. & Carey, S. (1998). "Knowledge enrichment and conceptual change in folkbiology: Evidence from Williams Syndrome". *Cognitive Psychology, 37*, 156–200.

Kiefer, F. (1998). "Alaktan". In K. É. Kiss, F. Kiefer, & P. Siptár (Eds.), *Új magyar nyelvtan* (pp. 187–293). Budapest: Osiris.

Király, I., Pléh, Cs., & Racsmány, M. (2001). "The language of space in Hungarian". In E. Németh T. (Ed.), *Cognition in Language Use: Selected papers from the 7th International Pragmatics Conference* (pp. 181–192). Antwerp: IprA.

Kónya, A. & Pintér, G. (1986). "Kategórai norma a verbális emlékezet vizsgálatához". (Category norms for testing verbal memory.) *Magyar Pszichológiai Szemle, XX*, 93–111.

Krause, M. & Penke, M. (2002). "Inflectional morphology in German Williams syndrome". *Brain and Cognition, 48*, 253–631.

Landau, B. & Zukowski, A. (2001). "Objects, motions and paths: Spatial language in children with Williams syndrome". In C. Mervis (Ed.), *Developmental Neuropsychology: Special Issue on Williams Syndrome.*

Lichtenberger, L. & Bellugi, U. (1998). "Intersection of spatial cognition and language in Williams syndrome". *Journal of cognitive neuroscience, SS*, 80.

Lukács, Á. & Pléh, Cs. (1999). "Hungarian cross-modal priming and treatment of nonsense words supports the dual process hypothesis". Commentary on Harald Clahsen's Rules of Language. *Behavioral and Brain Sciences, 22*(6), 1030–1031.

Lukács, Á., Racsmány, M., & Pléh, Cs. (2001). "Vocabulary and morphological patterns in Hungarian children with Williams syndrome: A preliminary report". *Acta Linguistica, 48*, 243–269.

MacWhinney, B. (1976). "Hungarian research on the acquisition of morphology and syntax". *Journal of Child Language, 3*, 397–410.

Marcus, G. F., Brinkmann, U., Clahsen, H., Wiese, R., & Pinker, S. (1995). "German Inflection: The exception that proves the rule". *Cognitive Psychology, 29*, 189–256.

Masterson, J. & Druks, J. (1998). "Description of a set of 164 nouns and 102 verbs matched for printed word frequency, familiarity and age-of-acquisition". *Journal of Neurolinguistics, 11*, 331–354.

Nádasdy, Á. & Siptár, P. (1994). "A magánhangzók". In F. Kiefer (Ed.), *Strukturális magyar nyelvtan. 2. kötet: Fonológia* (pp. 42–181). Budapest: Akadémiai Kiadó.

Phillips, C. E., Jarrold, C., Baddeley, A. D., Grant, J., & Karmiloff-Smith, A. "Spatial language difficulties in Williams syndrome". Manuscript.

Pinker, S. (1991). "Rules of language". *Science, 253*, 530–535.

Pinker, S. & Prince, A. (1994). "Regular and irregular morphology and the psychological status of rules of grammar". In S. D. Lima, R. L. Corrigan, & G. K. Iverson (Eds.), *The Reality of Linguistic Rules* (pp. 321–350). Amsterdam: John Benjamins.

Pléh, Cs., Lukács, Á., & Racsmány, M. (2003). "Morphological patterns in Hungarian children with Williams syndrome and the rule debates". In press *Brain and Language.*

Pléh, Cs., Palotás, G., & Lõrik, J. (2002). *A New Screaning Method for Hungarian Language Impaired Children.* Budapest: Akadémiai. (in Hungarian)

Pléh, Cs., Vinkler, Zs., & Kálmán, L. (1997). "Early morphology of spatial expressions in Hungarian children: A CHILDES study". *Acta Linguistica Hungarica, 44*(1–2), 249–260.

Racsmány, M. (2002). "A munkamemória alrendszereinek szerepe a megismerésben". (The role of subcomponents of working memory in cognition.) Unpublished Ph.D. dissertation.

Racsmány, M., Lukács, Á., Pléh, Cs., & Király, I. (2001). "Some cognitive tools for word learning: The role of working memory and goal preference". *Behavioral and Brain Sciences, 24*(6), 1115–1117.

Rossen, M. L., Klima, E. S., Bellugi, U., Bihrle, A., & Jones, W. (1996). "Interaction between language and cognition: Evidence from Williams syndrome". In J. H. Beitchman, N. Cohen, M. Konstantareas, & R. Tannock (Eds.), *Language, Learning and Behavior Disorders: Developmental, biological and clinical perspectives* (pp. 367–392). New York, NY: CUP.

Székely, A. & Bates, E. (2000). "Objective visual complexity as a variable in studies of picture naming". *Center for Research in Language Newsletter, 12*(2). La Jolla: University of California, San Diego.

Talmy, L. (1975). "Semantics and syntax of motion". In H. Kimball (Ed.), *Syntax and semantics*, Volume 4. New York, NY: Academic Press.

Temple, C., Almazan, M., & Sherwood, S. (2002). "Lexical skills in Williams Syndrome: A cognitive neuropsychological analysis". *Journal of Neurolinguistics, 15*, 463–495.

Thomas, M,. Grant, J., Barnham, Z., Gsödl, M., Laing, E., Lakusta, L., Tyler, L. L, Grice, S., Patterson, S., & Karmiloff-Smith, A. (2001). "Past tense formation in Williams syndrome". *Language and Cognitive Processes, 16*, 143–176.

Törkenczy, M. (1994). "A szótag". In F. Kiefer (Ed.), *Strukturális magyar nyelvtan. 2. kötet: Fonológia* (pp. 273–393). Budapest: Akadémiai.

Tyler, L. K., Karmiloff-Smith, A., Voice, J. K., Stevens, T., Grant, J., Udwin, O., Davies, M., & Howlin, P. (1997). "Do individuals with Williams syndrome have bizarre semantics? Evidence for lexical organization using an on-line task". *Cortex, 33*, 515–527.

Vicari S., Brizzolara, D., Carlesimo, G. A., Pezzini, G., & Volterra, V. (1996a). "Memory abilities in children with Williams syndrome". *Cortex, 32*, 503–514.

Vicari, S., Carlesimo, G., Brizzolara, D., & Pezzini, G. (1996b). "Short-term memory in children with Williams syndrome: A reduced contribution of lexical-semantic knowledge to word span". *Neuropsychologia, 34*(9), 919–925.

Volterra, V., Capirci, O., Pezzini, G., Sabbadini, L., & Vicari, S. (1996). "Linguistic Abilities in Italian Children with Williams Syndrome". *Cortex, 32*, 663–677.

Wang, P. P. & Bellugi, U. (1994). "Evidence from two genetic syndromes for a dissociation between verbal and visual-spatial short-term memory". *Journal of Clinical and Experimental Neuropsychology, 16*, 317–322.

Zukowski, A. (2001). "Uncovering grammatical competence in children with Williams syndrome". Ph.D. dissertation, Boston University.

# Lexical and morphological skills in English-speaking children with Williams syndrome

Harald Clahsen, Melanie Ring, and Christine Temple
University of Essex

In previous work, we have argued that Williams syndrome (WS) presents us with a dissociation of the two core modules of language in which the computational (rule-based) system for language is selectively spared, while lexical representations and/or their access procedures are impaired. However, this account of WS has been challenged, and an alternative non-modular connectionist model has been proposed which is claimed to simulate the actual performance of WS subjects more accurately.

Against this background, the present study reports results from new cases of WS and groups of normal children closely matched to the WS participants examining morphological skills, particularly past-tense formation and comparative adjective formation, as well as lexical skills, specifically receptive vocabulary and naming. The results, we will argue, provide further support for a modular account and for a selective lexical deficit in WS.

## 1. Introduction

In a series of previous studies, we have investigated a group of four English-speaking children with Williams-syndrome (WS) with respect to a range of linguistic phenomena and skills, among them the comprehension of passives and anaphoric pronouns (Clahsen & Almazan 1998), past-tense inflection (Clahsen & Almazan 1998), noun plurals and compounding (Clahsen & Almazan 2001), comparative adjective formation (Clahsen & Temple 2003), receptive vocabulary skills and naming (Temple et al. 2002), and reading (Temple 2003). The findings from these studies were interpreted within modular theories of linguistic representation and processing. Within such theories, language performance should reflect normal linguistic function minus impaired function, such that exhibited skills are indicative of intact normal skills and part of a normal linguistic functional architecture.

This has been termed subtractivity (Saffran 1982) or transparency (Caramazza 1984) or residual normality (Thomas & Karmiloff-Smith 2003). Evidence against subtractivity in linguistic domains would come from cases in which the underlying functional architecture of the language system itself had changed in ways that do not exist in the normal mind/brain. However, there is no such empirical evidence in relation to language development in either adults or children.

We have argued that WS represents a dissociation within the language system itself. Adopting the view that the knowledge of language consists of two separate components, a lexicon of stored entries and a computational system of combinatorial operations to form larger linguistic expressions (e.g. Chomsky 1995; Pinker 1999), we proposed that these two core modules of language are dissociated in WS such that the computational (rule-based) system for language is selectively spared, while lexical representations and/or their access procedures are impaired (Clahsen & Almazan 1998; Clahsen & Temple 2003). This account of the linguistic difficulties of children with WS has recently been challenged by Thomas, Karmiloff-Smith and their collaborators, on the basis of empirical data and simulations (Thomas et al. 2001; Thomas & Karmiloff-Smith 2003). Investigating a group of 18 cases with WS, Thomas et al. (2001) did not find evidence for a selective deficit in their cases of WS with irregular past-tense formation, in contrast to what Clahsen and Almazan (1998) found. Moreover, Thomas et al. (2001) claimed that the results from their studies are more persuasive than our findings, since theirs are based on a larger sample of WS subjects, while ours due to the smaller sample size are potentially misleading.

The contrasting view to subtractivity is that the performance of those with developmental language disorders does not bear any relationship to normality but reflects the abnormal developmental form of the entire system as a consequence of the abnormality which created the disorder. Thomas and Karmiloff-Smith (2003) argue for just such a qualitatively abnormal end-state in children with WS that has "a different functional structure in children". On this basis language disorders provide no insight into normal development. Thus, one of the contemporary debates in the study of children with WS has implications for the question of whether or not developmental disorders have any relevance for understanding normal function. The specific issue is whether children with developmental disorders have modular impairments with residual intact skills or whether they have generalised disorders that affect components throughout the system.

One example of relevant data addressing the general issue comes from research into specific language impairment (SLI). Detailed longitudinal studies on groups of English (Rice 1999) and German SLI children (Rothweiler & Clahsen 1994) demonstrate (i) a selective delayed onset of finiteness marking, (ii) the same developmental trajectory as in normal children, and (iii) a persistent selective delay in the area of finiteness marking into late childhood. Thus, the case of SLI shows that impairments in the onset will not necessarily lead to atypical developmental trajectories nor generalised abnormality throughout the system.

The present study reports further new data relevant to this debate. We present results from new cases of WS and groups of normal children closely matched to the WS participants. We examine morphological skills, particularly past-tense formation and comparative adjective formation, as well as lexical skills, specifically receptive vocabulary and naming. The results, we will argue, provide further support for a modular account and for a selective lexical deficit in WS.

## 2. Previous studies on morphological and lexical skills in WS

### 2.1 Morphological skills

Most previous studies of morphological skills in English-speaking subjects with WS have focused on two phenomena, the past tense and noun plurals (Bromberg et al. 1994; Clahsen & Almazan 1998, 2001; Thomas et al. 2001; Zukowski 2001). Clahsen and Almazan (1998, 2001) found that subjects with WS performed excellently on regular past tense and regular plural inflection. On the other hand, their scores on irregular past tense and irregular plural forms were lower than those of unimpaired mental age controls, and the subjects with WS used regular rules of inflection excessively, even in circumstances in which unimpaired children (and adults) would not use them. Similar results were obtained by Bromberg et al. (1994), an unpublished study with 6 WS participants (speaking American English) which reported spared production of regular past tense formation, but impaired production of irregulars, with overregularizations largely produced instead. Moreover, Zukowski (2001) investigated 12 children with WS with respect to English noun plural formation and found that the children with WS apply the regular plural affix to existing nouns and to nonce nouns at near-ceiling rates, just like control children, but that they performed worse than the unimpaired children on irregulars. Another piece of evidence for the dissociation between lexical storage and rules of grammar in WS comes from Clahsen and Temple's (2003) study of *-er* comparative adjective formation (*cool* → *cooler*). It was found that children with WS heavily overapply *-er* affixation and that they seem to ignore the constraints and lexical exceptions that hold for *-er* affixation in English producing forms such as **expensiver*, **dangerouser, etc.*

Different results for past-tense formation in English-speaking children and adults with WS were obtained by Thomas et al. (2001). Results from two elicited production experiments displayed no selective deficit in irregular past tense performance. Instead, 'the WS group showed the same relation between performance on regular and irregular verbs as the typically developing group' (Thomas et al.

2001: 166f.). However, as pointed out by Clahsen and Temple (2003), Thomas et al. did not properly match their cases of WS to normal controls of comparable age levels. Instead, they discuss average scores collapsed across 18 cases of WS with ages ranging from 11 to 53 years and mental ages ranging from 5 to 16 years and compare them to normal children from 5 to 10 years treating them as if they were a single group. Data presented in their figure 3 also implied matching of verbal mental ages but the actual descriptions of the controls' ages of those tested and the case-by-case verbal mental ages indicate that such precise matches are not possible from their data. In a reanalysis of Thomas et al.'s data, Clahsen and Temple (2003) showed that if the WS data are properly matched with those of the normal controls for mental age, Thomas et al.'s data do indeed confirm that the participants with WS perform worse on irregulars than unimpaired children and produce significantly fewer overapplications of irregular inflection than mental age controls.

## 2.2 Lexical skills

Within the spontaneous speech of those with WS, the use of relatively low frequency lexical items has been noted (Bellugi et al. 1992; Bradley & Udwin 1989). The production of unusual low frequency category members has been reported as increased, relative to controls, on semantic fluency tasks, e.g. *salamander* and *ibex* in the category of animals (Bellugi et al. 1992; Rossen et al. 1996; Temple et al. 2002) though not in all studies (Johnson & Carey 1998; Mervis et al. 1999; Volterra et al. 1996). Several studies have also found an increased number of responses on oral fluency tasks, which require the generation of words to specific phonemic or semantic cues (e.g. Bellugi et al. 1994; Temple et al. 2002; Volterra et al. 1996) though not all (Rossen et al. 1996). In the study of young children with WS, increased responses in phonological fluency was the only task on which they were found to be better than mental age controls (Volterra et al. 1996).

This production of low frequency vocabulary items in spontaneous speech and oral fluency and generation of increased numbers of responses on oral fluency could reflect more extensive stores of lexical items. Consistent with such a view, the expressive language of children with WS is reported to contain a larger number of different lexical items than that of children with Down syndrome both during the period of first word combinations (Singer Harris et al. 1997) and as toddlers (Mervis & Robinson 2000), though results from toddlers are conflicting (Singer Harris et al. 1997). Performance on traditional receptive vocabulary tasks in WS would be consistent with such a theory of enlarged lexical stores. Performance on the Peabody Picture Vocabulary Test [PPVT] (Dunn & Dunn 1981) has been found to be better than expected relative to mental age controls in some studies (Bellugi et al. 1990) and to be at normal chronological age level in other studies (Mervis et al. 1999). Performance on the British Picture Vocabulary Scale [BPVS] (Dunn et al. 1997) has also been reported as above mental age level (Tyler et al. 1997; Temple et al. 2002). Furthermore knowledge of semantic concepts as measured by the similarities subtest of the Wechsler Intelligence Scale for Children [WISC-III] (Wechsler 1992) is also above mental age level (Temple et al. 2002).

However, not all lexical tasks are performed well. Bellugi et al. (1990) report scores as weak as for controls with Down syndrome in defining words in the vocabulary subtest of the WISC-R (Wechsler 1976), though they attribute this to the cognitive demands of the task rather than knowledge of the lexical items themselves. Bromberg et al. (1994) report an impairment in naming, although since the difficulty was in accessing irregularly inflected forms, the underlying basis of the difficulty might be associated with the morphological problems discussed above rather than any naming difficulty per se. However, Temple et al. (2002) also report naming ages well below receptive vocabulary levels and in most cases also below mental age levels arguing that the discrepancy between receptive vocabulary and naming constituted an anomia. This anomia was evident in the simple retrieval of base lexical forms in confrontation naming tasks. As this study was based on data from just four children there is a need to attempt to replicate this new finding with more cases of WS.

Temple et al. (2002) also explored receptive vocabulary in more detail, using the traditional paradigm of matching a spoken word to a picture from an array. Their arrays contained 23 semantically related distracters, and therefore required fine grain semantic knowledge. In this context, the performance of children with WS was significantly impaired in comparison to mental age controls. On the basis of these naming and receptive vocabulary results they argued that either semantic representations are impoverished or access to these representations is impoverished and "sloppy". Previous reports of good performance on semantic fluency and in judging semantic concepts may argue for the latter. In two children they also describe lexical access which is significantly faster than mental age controls and is therefore both fast and sloppy. However, an alternative interpretation is that the receptive vocabulary weakness identified by Temple et al. (2002) is unconnected with semantic representations for lexical items and has a perceptual basis linked to impaired perception when there are multiple, simultaneous distracters.

It is evident from the above summary of previous studies that more research is needed to resolve the controversial issues surrounding the linguistic strengths and weaknesses of children with WS. On the one hand, as pointed out by Thomas et al. (2001), those studies supporting a lexical deficit in WS are based on relatively small sample sizes. On the other hand, Thomas et al.'s larger studies fall short of matching the WS participants to normal controls of a comparable age level. Hence, what is needed are studies with a less small sample size which also have control matching encompassing a relatively narrow mental age span. The present study employs double the number of children we have previously described and incorporates close mental age matches and relatively narrow mental age and chronological age spans.

## 3. Participants

The results of the present study of past tense formation and comparative adjective formation come from nine cases of WS, five of whom are new cases and four are the same as those examined in previous studies from our group. The results from the present study of receptive vocabulary and naming come from seven new cases of WS. In this case, it was not possible to combine the data with the earlier cases studied as the experiments reported are new in design. Mental ages were derived from scores on the WISC-III$^{UK}$ (Wechsler 1992). The children had chronological ages ranging from 10;3 to 16;2 and mental ages ranging from 5;3 to 7;9. The chronological and mental ages of the participants with WS are summarised in Table 1. All of the participants with WS live with a parent or parents and attend a special school, or units within mainstream schools where they interact with other children with learning disabilities.

The data from the WS subjects will be compared to control groups of monolingual English-speaking younger children of normal intelligence whose chronological ages match the mental ages of the children with WS. The control children live in native homes and were randomly selected by date of birth from state schools in Essex and Suffolk, England. Details concerning the size and the age ranges of the control groups will be presented below, separately for each experiment. Subjects who had any known neurological abnormality, learning difficulties or a history of special needs were excluded.

**Table 1a.** Mental and chronological ages of the WS participants employed in the studies of past tense formation and comparative adjective formation

| | Chronological Age | Mental Age |
|---|---|---|
| Olivia | 13;3 | 5;3 |
| Emily | 13;1 | 5;4 |
| Jane | 11;2 | 5;7 |
| David | 10;3 | 5;7 |
| Florence | 12;7 | 7;5 |
| Susan | 12;2 | 7;6 |
| Martin | 15;4 | 7;6 |
| Helena | 13;2 | 7;9 |
| Jackie | 16;2 | 7;9 |

**Table 1b.** Mental and chronological ages of the WS participants employed in the studies of receptive vocabulary and naming

| | Chronological Age | Mental Age |
|---|---|---|
| Olivia | 13;3 | 5;3 |
| David | 10;3 | 5;7 |
| Nathan | 13;2 | 6;3 |
| Megan | 16;0 | 6;6 |
| Susan | 12;2 | 7;6 |
| Helena | 13;2 | 7;9 |
| Jackie | 16;2 | 7;9 |

## 4. Past-tense formation

Two elicited production experiments were performed, the first one eliciting past tense forms of existing and nonce verbs, and the second one eliciting past-tense forms of denominal verbs. We present the results of these experiments separately.

### 4.1 Experiment I: Existing and nonce verbs

The experimental procedure and materials were adopted from Ullman (1993). The test items included 14 existing irregular verbs (*swim, dig, swing, wring, bend, bite, feed, make, give, think, stand, keep, drive, send*); 14 novel irregular verbs with stems which rhymed with existing irregulars (*strink, frink, strise, crive, shrell, vurn, steeze, shrim, cleed, sheel, blide, prend, shreep, drite*); 16 existing regular verbs (*scowl, tug, flush, mar, chop, flap, stalk, scour, slam, cross, rush, rob, drop, look, stir, soar*); and 12 novel verbs with stems which do not rhyme with any existing irregular verb (*spuff, dotch, stoff, cug, trab, crog, vask, brop, satch, grush, plam, scur*).[1] Each verb was presented in the context of two sentences which were spoken by the experimenter. After hearing the first sentence, e.g. *Everyday I play football*, the child was asked to repeat the whole sentence. This was followed by the test sentence, e.g. *Just like everyday, yesterday I _____ football*. The child was asked to repeat the test sentence from *yesterday* and to fill in the missing word. All responses were recorded on tape and coded as *regular* (correct *-ed* application), *overregularized* (incorrect *-ed* application), *irregular* (correct irregular form), *overirregularized* (irregular form used on regular verbs) or *unmarked* (bare stem form).

The task was administered to the nine participants with WS detailed in Table 1a and two groups of unimpaired control children who had similar chronological ages to the mental ages of our WS subjects. There were 18 five-year old controls (age range: 4;10 to 5;10) and 21 seven-year old controls (age range: 7;1 to 7;11).

## Results

The results for the four kinds of verbs tested separately for the four groups of participants are presented in Tables 2 and 3. In the analysis, we only included responses that incorporated the target stem, i.e. either one of the past-tense forms or a bare stem form of the target verb. The mean scores and standard deviations present a breakdown of the relative percentages of these responses. Responses in which the children produced (unintelligible) mispronunciations or in which they substituted the target verb with some other lexeme were not included in the analysis; such responses made up 5.2% of the total responses of the 5-year-old controls, 3.2% for the 7-year-old controls, and 13.3% of the total responses in the WS data.

Analyses were carried out in a two-step manner. In Table 2, the number of *-ed* and irregular past tense markings were combined and compared to the percentage of forms which remained unmarked. In Table 3, we compared the types of past-tense marking (regular vs. irregular). The purpose of this two-step analysis is to clearly tease apart proper morphological errors from other kinds of error. For responses in which the children produced a past-tense marked verb form (irrespective of whether it is regular or irregular), it is possible to determine whether or not this form is morphologically correct. Responses, however, in which the child simply repeated the unmarked stem form in this task, producing e.g. *play* for a test item such as *Everyday I play football. Just like everyday, yesterday I *play football*, allow for different interpretations. One possibility would be that the child misunderstood the task thinking that she had to repeat the verb form given, rather than to form its past tense. Another possibility is that a form such as *play* in the above example is a non-finite verb, i.e. a form that is underspecified for tense and/or agreement features. Several studies of early English child language have found that unaffected children produce such forms, even in contexts in which the adult language requires finite verb forms, and it has been argued that such errors are syntactic in nature (see e.g. Wexler 1994). A third possibility would be that *play* in the above example is a present-tense form used in a past-tense context, but again the form would be morphologically correct. For these reasons, it is difficult to decide what such responses might mean. In any case, the two-step analysis employed here allows us to clearly distinguish these kinds of responses from proper morphological errors, e.g. cases of *-ed* overregularizations on irregular verbs.

With respect to the marking and non-marking of verbs (Table 2), combining age groups such that all WS are compared to all controls, the WS subjects did not produce significantly higher levels of unmarked responses than the normal controls. However, in the existing irregular condition, the WS-5 subjects used significantly more unmarked forms than the 5-year-old controls (CTR-5 vs. WS-5: $z = 2.114$, $p = 0.03$); the corresponding difference in this condition for the WS subjects taken as one group and compared to all controls came out marginally significant

**Table 2.** Elicited production of past-tense forms: marked and unmarked responses

| | | WS | | CTR | |
|---|---|---|---|---|---|
| | | 5 | 7 | 5 | 7 |
| Existing Regulars | marked | 70.3 | 92.5 | 85.2 (11.1) | 91.1 (14.0) |
| | bare stem | 29.7 | 7.5 | 14.8 | 8.9 |
| Existing Irregulars | marked | 47.1 | 75.3 | 81.9 (13.7) | 87.4 (13.7) |
| | bare stem | 52.9 | 24.7 | 18.1 | 12.6 |
| Novel Regulars | marked | 91.7 | 96.7 | 84.5 (17.7) | 87.0 (17.3) |
| | bare stem | 8.3 | 3.3 | 15.5 | 13.0 |
| Novel Irregulars | marked | 56.8 | 65.2 | 77.3 (21.0) | 78.7 (24.8) |
| | bare stem | 43.2 | 34.8 | 22.7 | 21.3 |

Responses given in % (s.d. in parentheses)

**Table 3.** Elicited production of past-tense forms: breakdown of marked responses

| | | WS | | CTR | |
|---|---|---|---|---|---|
| | | 5[2] | 7 | 5 | 7 |
| Existing Regulars | *-ed* | 100.0 | 100.0 | 100.0 (0.0) | 100.0 (0.0) |
| | irregular | 0.0 | 0.0 | 0.0 | 0.0 |
| Existing Irregulars | *-ed*[3] | 73.6 | 39.1 | 23.0 (22.5) | 19.8 (28.9) |
| | *overreg.* | *73.6* | *34.1* | *15.9 (13.6)* | *13.2 (21.5)* |
| | irregular | 26.4 | 60.9 | 77.0 (22.5) | 80.2 (28.9) |
| Novel Regulars | *-ed* | 100.0 | 100.0 | 100.0 (0.0) | 100.0 (0.0) |
| | irregular | 0.0 | 0.0 | 0.0 | 0.0 |
| Novel Irregulars | *-ed* | 96.7 | 82.9 | 50.4 (35.7) | 57.0 (39.3) |
| | irregular | 3.3 | 17.1 | 49.7 | 42.9 |

Responses given in % (s.d. in parentheses)

(Existing Irregular: CTR vs. WS: $z = 1.749$, $p = 0.08$). The combined WS group also used more unmarked forms in the novel irregular condition than the unimpaired controls (Novel Irregular: CTR vs. WS: $z = 1.964$, $p = 0.05$). For the other conditions, there were no statistically significant differences in the percentages of marked/unmarked responses given by the WS and normal control groups shown in Table 2. On an individual level, there was one child with WS (Olivia) who never marked the verbs for past tense, producing only stem forms and forms classified as 'other', which were excluded from the analyses. It is possible that this child misunderstood the task. Moreover, one WS-5 subject (Emily) and two WS-7 subjects (Susan and Jackie) produced significantly more unmarked forms in the existing irregular condition than their age-matched controls.

With respect to the type of marking on existing verbs, the data in Table 3 clearly show that the WS subjects achieved high *-ed* marking rates for regulars, the same as the unimpaired controls, whereas on irregulars they performed significantly worse than the control subjects (CTR vs. WS: z = 2.881, $p$ = 0.004). Both the 5-year old controls and the 7-year-old controls achieved significantly higher 'irregular marking' rates on existing irregular verbs than the two corresponding groups of children with WS (CTR-5 vs. WS-5: z = 2.266, $p$ = 0.02; CTR-7 vs. WS-7: z = 1.951, $p$ = 0.05).

Concerning overregularizations, it is important to note that for these counts we only included those *-ed* forms produced for existing irregular verbs that are clearly ungrammatical and not permitted as past tense forms in the spoken language of the region where the children were living; see '*overreg.*' in Table 3. The figures in Table 3 show that the children with WS frequently overgeneralized *-ed* to existing irregular verbs. By contrast, unimpaired children preferred irregular past tense forms and rarely used regular *-ed* forms which are not permitted regional variations. Overall, the children with WS had significantly higher overgeneralization rates than the control children on existing irregular verbs (CTR vs. WS: z = 3.398, $p$ = 0.001). Furthermore, the two groups of children with WS produced significantly more *-ed* overapplications than the corresponding control groups (CTR-5 vs. WS-5: z = 2.470, $p$ = 0.01; CTR-7 vs. WS-7: z = 2.329, $p$ = 0.02).

With respect to novel verbs, Table 3 shows the children with WS applied *-ed* to novel regular verbs, as did the unimpaired children. Irregular past-tense patterns, however, were significantly less often applied to novel irregular verbs by the children with WS than by the unimpaired controls (CTR vs. WS: z = 2.132, $p$ = 0.03). Table 3 shows that this is particularly clear for the WS-5 group (compared to the corresponding control group), but that the WS-7 group also produced less than half as many irregular past-tense forms for novel verbs as the normal controls.

These findings replicate those of Clahsen and Almazan (1998) and Bromberg et al. (1994) and confirm a marked dissociation between regular and irregular past-tense formation in the WS subjects. The *-ed* affixation rule is applied under appropriate conditions, i.e. to existing regular verbs and to non-rhyming novel verbs, whereas for irregular inflection, the WS subjects achieve low scores on existing verbs and do not extend irregular patterns to (rhyming) nonce verbs. Spared regular inflection paired with difficulties in irregular inflection leads to relatively high overregularization rates in the WS subjects.

### 4.2 Experiment II: Denominal verbs

In English, verbs derived from nouns are regularly inflected with the past tense *-ed*, irrespective of the word's phonological properties, e.g. *He ringed/*rang the city with artillery* meaning that he formed a ring around the city. In morphological terms, words derived from other categories are unusual in that they do not have canonical lexical entries (as verbs). When such derived words are inflected for the past tense, access to lexical entries of verbs is blocked, even though they may sound similar to existing verbs as in the case of *ring*, hence the ungrammaticality of the irregular past tense form **rang* for a denominal verb. Affixation of *-ed*, however, can be applied to any element of a given category, hence the grammaticality of regular past tense forms of denominals.

The experimental procedure and materials were adopted from Kim et al. (1994) and consisted of 9 existing irregular verbs (*see, buy, meet, drink, fly, stick, write, leave, ring*) which were presented to the subjects in their base forms in two different context conditions, once as a verb root with the verb's usual meaning (1a), and once as a denominal verb with the meaning of the corresponding homophonous noun (1b). Children were prompted to produce past tense forms of these verbs. All the denominal verbs used in the experiment were made homophonous with existing irregular verbs in order to control for similarity-based generalizations.

(1) a. Verb root condition: *This airplane is going to fly. This airplane is about to fly through the air.* (Experimenter lets airplane fly.) *The airplane just ____.*

b. Denominal condition: *This is a fly. I'm going to fly this board* (Experimenter puts flies on a board.) *I just ____ (the board).*

Participants were presented with 18 test sentences in random order, and responses were tape-recorded. The task was administered to the 9 participants with WS detailed in Table 1a and two groups of unimpaired control children who had similar chronological ages to the mental ages of our WS subjects. There were 6 five-year olds (age range: 4;10 to 5;10) and 5 seven-year olds (age range: 7;1 to 7;5).

## Results

The results for the two conditions are presented in Tables 4 and 5. In the analysis, we only included responses that incorporated the target stem, i.e. either one of the past-tense forms or a bare stem form of the target verb. The mean scores and standard deviations present a breakdown of the relative percentages of these responses. Responses in which the children produced (unintelligible) mispronunciations or in which they substituted the target verb with some other lexeme were not included in the analysis; such responses made up 5% of the total responses of the 5-year-old controls, 10% for the 7-year-old controls, and 12% of the total responses in the WS data.

As in experiment I, analyses were carried out in a two-step manner in order to tease apart proper morphological errors from other kinds of error. In Table 4, the number of *-ed* and irregular past tense markings were combined and compared to

**Table 4.** Elicited production of past-tense forms: marked and unmarked responses

| | | WS | | CTR | |
|---|---|---|---|---|---|
| | | 5 | 7 | 5 | 7 |
| Denominal | marked | 58.3 | 79.2 | 67.6 (22.1) | 87.5 (17.7) |
| | bare stem | 41.7 | 20.8 | 32.4 | 12.5 |
| Verb Root | marked | 68.4 | 95.6 | 97.9 (5.1) | 100 (0.0) |
| | bare stem | 31.6 | 4.4 | 2.1 | 0 |

Responses given in % (s.d. in parentheses)

**Table 5.** Elicited production of past-tense forms: breakdown of marked responses

| | | WS | | CTR | |
|---|---|---|---|---|---|
| | | 5[4] | 7 | 5 | 7 |
| Denominal | *-ed* | 95.2 | 84.4 | 83.3 (18.3) | 84.4 (20.6) |
| | irregular | 4.8 | 15.6 | 16.7 | 15.6 |
| Verb Root | *-ed*[5] | 57.1 | 26.5 | 30.0 (15.2) | 26.8 (20.7) |
| | *overreg.* | *31.3* | *19.8* | *22.8 (6.1)* | *18.9 (12.5)* |
| | irregular | 42.9 | 73.5 | 70.0 (15.2) | 73.2 (20.7) |

Responses given in % (s.d. in parentheses)

the percentage of forms which remained unmarked. In Table 5, we compared the type of past-tense marking used by the groups.

With respect to the data in Table 4, the WS-5 group used significantly more stem forms in the verb root condition than the 5-year-old control group (CTR-5 vs. WS-5: z = 2.042, $p$ = 0.04). Otherwise, there were no significant differences between the WS subjects and the controls in the percentages of marked and unmarked responses. As in experiment I, the WS child Olivia never marked the verbs for past tense and produced only stem forms and forms classified as 'other', which were excluded from the analyses, indicating that she misunderstood the task in both experiments.

The data in Table 5 show that for *denominal* verbs the WS subjects clearly preferred regular past tense forms with scores similar to those of the unimpaired children; indeed with respect to the regular past-tense marking rates in the denominal condition, there are no significant differences between the children with WS and the normal controls for any of the age groups (CTR vs. WS: z = 0.474, $p$ = 0.63; CTR-5 vs. WS-5: z = 1.374, $p$ = 0.17; CTR-7 vs. WS-7: z = 0.430, $p$ = 0.66). In contrast to the denominal condition, both the children with WS and the normal controls gave significantly fewer regular past-tense responses in the verb root condition. The difference between the scores for *-ed* responses in the two experimental conditions (denominal vs. verb root) is significant for the participant groups when combined across ages, and for three (of the four) individual participant groups (CTR: $z = 2.934$, $p = 0.003$; CTR-5: $z = 2.201$, $p = 0.02$; CTR-7: $z = 2.023$, $p = 0.04$; WS: $z = 2.521$, $p = 0.01$; WS-7: $z = 2.023$, $p = 0.04$). The observation that there is lower *-ed* use in the verb root condition than in the denominal condition is also true at an individual subject level for the three WS-5 children included in this part of the analysis and for all five WS-7 children. This shows that there is a strong effect of grammatical structure, indicating that children with WS are sensitive to the derived morphological structure of denominal verbs.

With respect to the verb root condition, the data in Tables 4 and 5 show that the WS-7 group performed similarly to the unimpaired controls on all measures. By contrast, the WS-5 group produced significantly more bare stems than the controls as well more *-ed* overregularizations[6] yielding a marginally significant difference in the overregularization rates of the WS-5 subjects and the corresponding control group (CTR-5 vs. WS-5: $z = 1.765$, $p = 0.07$).

Summarizing, the two past-tense production experiments show that the past-tense system is selectively impaired in WS. While regular *-ed* affixation functions normally and applies under appropriate circumstances, the children with WS performed below their mental age in irregular past tense formation.

## 5. Comparative adjective formation

Gradable adjectives in English can form comparatives by *-er* suffixation (*big – bigger*) and/or by a periphrastic form with *more* (*unusual – more unusual*). In addition, a small number of highly frequent adjectives have suppletive comparative forms (*good – better, bad – worse*). For most adjectives, the suffixed and the periphrastic comparative are in complementary distribution, while for some adjectives, both options exist (see Barber 1964; Aronoff 1976; Frank 1972). The use of *-er* suffixation is to a certain extent constrained by syllable structure, in addition to other factors: monosyllabic adjectives typically form *-er* comparatives, likewise disyllabic adjectives ending in *-y* (e.g. *happy*), while the comparative of most other adjectives with more than one syllable is formed periphrastically (e.g. *more modern*). This distribution, however, is not without exceptions.

The procedures for this experiment were adopted from Dalalakis' (1994) elicited production task in which two items were depicted that differed in terms of a gradable attribute, e.g. size. The pictures were accompanied by two sentences, which were read aloud to the children. For example: *This circle is big. This circle is even _____?* The children were prompted to complete the sentence with a comparative form. Five kinds of target adjectives were used as shown in (2):

| (2) | *ER adjectives* | *MORE adject.* | *EITHER* | *IRREGULARS* | *NONCE* |
|---|---|---|---|---|---|
| | big | dangerous | round | good | weff |
| | funny | expensive | straight | bad | kell |
| | sad | modern | tasty | | bimmy |
| | young | unusual | bitter | | toshal |
| | little | open | | | |

The adjectives in the first column require *-er* comparative forms in adult English, those in the second column have periphrastic comparatives, while those in the third column may take either form. The adjectives *good* and *bad* have irregular (suppletive) comparatives. The first three nonce adjectives were expected to elicit *-er* comparatives, *weff* and *kell* because they are monosyllabic and *bimmy* because of the *-y* ending, while *toshal* should be more likely to yield a periphrastic comparative.

The stimulus materials were presented to each child individually. The children's responses were written down and tape-recorded for verification. The task was administered to the 9 participants with WS detailed in Table 1a and two groups of unimpaired control children who had similar chronological ages to the mental ages of our participants with WS. There were 18 five-year olds (age range: 4;11 to 5;10) and 19 seven-year olds (age range: 7;0 to 7;10).

## Results

The results for the five kinds of adjectives tested are shown in Tables 6 and 7 for each of the four groups of participants. In the analysis, we only included responses that incorporated the target stem, i.e. either one of the comparative forms or a bare stem form of the target adjectives. The mean scores and standard deviations present a breakdown of the relative percentages of these responses. Responses in which the children produced (unintelligible) mispronunciations or in which they substituted the target adjective with some other lexeme were not included in the analysis; such responses made up 9% of the total responses of the 5-year-old controls, 12% for the 7-year-old controls, and 13% of the total responses in the WS data. In addition, there were two double markings each from the 5-year-old and 7-year-old controls, and one from the WS subjects.

Analyses were carried out in a two-step manner. For the data in Table 6, the number of *-er*, suppletives, and *more* marked adjectives were combined and compared to the percentage of forms which remained unmarked. For the data in Table 7, we compared the type of comparative marking used by the groups.

As regards the unimpaired children, the data in Table 7 show that the 5-year olds and the 7-year-olds produced *-er* comparatives as well as periphrastic forms with *more*, even though in both groups of children the suffixed forms were used

Table 6. Elicited production of comparative adjectives: marked and unmarked responses

| | | WS | | CTR | |
|---|---|---|---|---|---|
| | | 5 | 7 | 5 | 7 |
| ER ADJ. | marked | 91.7 | 100 | 95.0 (12.9) | 89.7 (22.6) |
| | bare stem | 8.3 | 0 | 5.0 | 10.3 |
| MORE ADJ. | marked | 58.8 | 86.9 | 51.6 (37.0) | 68.3 (37.5) |
| | bare stem | 41.3 | 13.3 | 48.4 | 31.7 |
| EITHER ADJ. | marked | 62.5 | 90.0 | 76.4 (32.6) | 77.6 (31.1) |
| | bare stem | 37.5 | 10.0 | 23.6 | 22.4 |
| IRREG ADJ. | marked | 100 | 100 | 86.1 (33.5) | 78.9 (38.4) |
| | bare stem | 0 | 0 | 13.9 | 21.1 |
| NOVEL ADJ. | marked | 50.0 | 80.0 | 72.7 (36.9) | 79.2 (31.2) |
| | bare stem | 50.0 | 20.0 | 27.3 | 20.8 |

Responses given in % (s.d. in parentheses)

Table 7. Elicited production of comparative adjectives: breakdown of marked responses

| | | WS | | CTR | |
|---|---|---|---|---|---|
| | | 5 | 7 | 5 | 7 |
| ER ADJ. | *-er* | 100 | 100 | 100 (0.0) | 96.5 (15.3) |
| | more | 0.0 | 0.0 | 0.0 | 3.5 |
| MORE ADJ. | *-er* | 100 | 96.0 | 69.6 (38.7) | 78.2 (39.4) |
| | more | 0.0 | 4.0 | 30.4 | 21.8 |
| EITHER ADJ. | *-er* | 100 | 100 | 90.1 (26.0) | 89.5 (31.5) |
| | more | 0.0 | 0.0 | 9.9 | 10.5 |
| IRREG ADJ. | *-er* | 100 | 80.0 | 81.3 (30.9) | 68.8 (35.9) |
| | more | 0.0 | 0.0 | 3.1 (12.5) | 15.6 (35.2) |
| | suppletive | 0.0 | 20.0 | 15.6 (30.1) | 15.6 (23.9) |
| NOVEL ADJ. | *-er* | 100 | 100 | 92.2 (18.5) | 92.6 (24.6) |
| | more | 0.0 | 0.0 | 7.8 | 7.4 |

Responses given in % (s.d. in parentheses)

more frequently than the periphrastic construction. Table 7 also shows that the comparatives of ER adjectives are most often correctly formed by both groups of unimpaired children, while for MORE adjectives they are less successful. Likewise, as can be seen from Table 6, they produce considerably more unmarked bare stem responses for MORE adjectives than for any other condition. These results from the control children are in line with those of previous studies of unimpaired children's comparative formations (Gathercole 1985; Graziano-King 1999).

The children with WS produced marked and unmarked responses with similar proportions to those of the unimpaired children; see Table 6. There are indeed no statistically significant differences in the percentages of marked/unmarked responses given by the WS and normal control groups shown in Table 6. However, Table 7 shows that the type of comparative responses given by the children with WS is different from the comparative forms produced by the controls. While the controls produced *-er* and suppletive comparative forms as well as periphrastic comparative forms with *more*, the children with WS's comparative form is almost exclusively *-er*. The children with WS only produced one *more* response and two suppletive comparative forms between them. All other comparative responses are with the *-er* suffix.

Summarizing, the data from the children with WS show that they have just one way of forming comparatives, and this is *-er* affixation, which they apply freely to any adjective. This holds for both groups of children with WS studied here. In contrast to that, the unimpaired children produce not only *-er* comparatives, but also periphrastic comparative constructions, and suppletive comparatives. The data also show that the use of *-er* is less constrained in the participants with WS than in the unimpaired children.

## 6. Lexical skills: Naming

Psychometric measures of receptive vocabulary and naming were employed. The BPVSII (Dunn et al. 1997) assessed the ability to match a spoken name to a target presented with three distracters loosely related to the target. The Renfrew Naming Test (Renfrew 1977) assessed lexical access in confrontation naming. Druks and Masterson's (2000) Object and Action Naming Battery [OANB] was also employed. For the BPVS and the Renfrew age equivalents were derived. For the OANB task scores reflected number of items correct.

The tasks were administered to the 7 participants with WS detailed in Table 1b who had a mean age of 6;8 months and a group of unimpaired control children who had similar chronological ages to the mental ages of our WS subjects. There were 16 control children with a mean age of 6;5 (age range: 5;6 to 7;4).

The results from the psychometric tasks of receptive vocabulary and naming are given in Table 8. The results were analyzed using one-way ANOVAs. Since enhancement of receptive vocabulary was predicted as well as impairment of naming, one-tailed tests were used in these comparisons. There was no significant difference between the groups in mental age ($F(1,21) = 0.73$, $p = 0.40$). However, the children with WS were found to have significantly higher receptive vocabulary ages on the BPVSII than controls ($F(1,21) = 3.86$, $p < 0.03$). In contrast, naming age on the

Table 8. Psychometric scores of receptive vocabulary and naming

| | WS | CTR |
|---|---|---|
| BPVS Age Equivalent | 102.29 (sd = 29.11) | 85.81 (sd = 11.84) |
| Renfrew Naming Age | 68.71 (sd = 12.62) | 74.81 (sd = 6.93) |
| DandM Objects Score | 62.86 (sd = 12.14) | 68.88 (sd = 3.07) |
| DandM Action Score | 36.57 (sd = 9.34) | 39.75 (sd = 3.47) |

Renfrew was lower in the children with WS than in controls, though the result was of marginal significance (F (1,21) = 2.27, $p < 0.07$). For the object targets of OANB, the participants with WS were significantly poorer than controls (F (1,21) = 3.61, $p < 0.035$). The impairment was less evident when naming actions (F (1,21) = 1.47, $p < 0.12$). These results confirm, with a new sample, elevation of receptive vocabulary in WS when assessed by a formal psychometric task in which there are three varied distracters. They also confirm with a new sample that the children with WS are anomic.

## 7. Lexical skills: Receptive vocabulary

Our previous study had demonstrated an unexpected contrast (Temple et al. 2002). There was strong receptive vocabulary on the BPVS (Dunn et al. 1997) in which the target picture corresponding to the spoken word had to be selected from an array with only three distracter pictures. Performance on the BPVS was at a higher level than that expected on the basis of mental age and this result has been replicated above. In contrast, our previous study found that there was weak receptive vocabulary on newly constructed tasks in which the target picture corresponding to a spoken word has to be selected from an array also containing 23 distracter pictures which were closely related semantically to the target. Performance on these new tasks was significantly poorer than controls matched for mental age (Temple et al. 2002). Our interpretation of these results was that it was the close semantic relationship of the new items that was significant in creating the impairment for the children with WS. However the new tasks both presented more closely related semantic distracters and presented a larger number of distracters so that two stimulus dimensions varied simultaneously. It has been suggested that perceptual difficulties of children with WS might lead them to have greater difficulty with multi-item arrays and that the deficit we detected was in fact attributable to the size of the forced choice selection rather than to any aspect associated with semantic relationships.

The objective of the new study was therefore to vary the number of distracter items and the semantic similarity of the distracters to the target independently. Two new types of response grids were therefore constructed. The first type consisted of pictures taken from the BPVS. The target was the correct target picture that matched the stimulus label from the BPVS when administered in its standard psychometric form. The distracters were other picture items selected from the stimulus booklet. The semantic relationship between the distracter items and the target was either loose or nil. Three sets of response grids using BPVS pictures were constructed depicting arrays of 8, 12 or 24 pictures. The second type of response grid employed pictures taken from the items of Snodgrass and van der Wart (1980). The target was the picture that matched the stimulus label selected from the Snodgrass and van der Wart (1980) pictures. The distracters were other picture items selected from the same semantic class illustrated in Snodgrass and van der Wart (1980). The semantic relationship between the distracter items and the target was close as all the distracters came from the same semantic class. There were four semantic classes employed: animals, indoor objects, food and clothes. For each semantic class three sets of response grids using BPVS pictures were constructed, depicting arrays of 8, 12 or 24 pictures. For each trial, the name of the stimulus item was spoken aloud and the child had to point to the corresponding target in the grid.

The task was administered to the 7 participants with WS detailed in Table 1b and groups of unimpaired control children who had similar chronological ages to the mental ages of our WS subjects. There were 12 control children (age range: 5;6 to 7;4).

## Results

The results from the contrasting grids are given in Table 9. The results were analyzed using one-way ANOVAs. Given our prediction that BPVS performance would be good and performance with the close semantic distracters would be poor, one-tailed tests were employed. For the 12-item grids, employing BPVS items, the participants with WS were significantly better than controls ($F = 7.29$, $p < 0.016$). For the 24-item grids, employing BPVS items, the participants with WS were also significantly better than controls ($F = 5.34$, $p < 0.034$). These results confirm the advantage demonstrated above in the BPVS when administered as a psychometric instrument. When children with WS have to perform a receptive vocabulary task where approximate semantic knowledge is enough to complete the task as the distracters are not very closely related to the target, they are significantly better than

**Table 9.** Pointing to spoken names on the new grids

| | WS | CTR |
|---|---|---|
| BPVS grid size 12 | 69.22<br>(sd = 10.22) | 59.79<br>(sd = 4.85) |
| BPVS grid size 24 | 60.60<br>(sd = 14.71) | 49.55<br>(sd = 6.18) |
| SandW grid size 12 | 87.30<br>(sd = 11.43) | 96.12<br>(sd = 3.22) |
| SandW grid size 24 | 80.84<br>(sd = 13.37) | 91.61<br>(sd = 5.71) |

control children of the same mental age. Moreover it demonstrates that this advantage holds even when the number of distracters is increased from 3 to 11 and even to 23. Strength on this task remains significant with multiple item arrays.

In contrast to these results for the 12-item grids, employing Snodgrass and van der Wart (1980) items, the participants with WS were significantly poorer than controls (F = 6.51, $p < 0.021$). For the 24-item grids, employing Snodgrass and van der Wart (1980) items, the participants with WS were also significantly poorer than controls (F = 6.08, $p < 0.025$). These results confirm the impairment demonstrated previously in selecting items from among semantically related distracters. When children with WS have to perform a receptive vocabulary task where fine grain semantic knowledge is required to complete the task, in a forced choice paradigm with distracters which are from the same semantic class, then they are significantly poorer than control children of the same mental age. The current experiment in combination with the earlier results demonstrates that this effect cannot be attributed to the number of the distracters but is a consequence of the nature of the items themselves.

## 8. A selective lexical impairment in WS

The present set of findings on lexical and morphological skills in English-speaking children with WS replicate and extend our earlier results with further cases of WS. Concerning morphological skills, we confirmed that productive regular morphology, such as the past-tense *-ed* in English, is functioning normally in children with WS. They were, however, found to perform significantly worse than unimpaired controls on non-productive or semi-productive morphology, such as the irregular past tense and lexical exceptions to *-er* comparative formation in English. For uninflected lexical items, performance in children with WS was found to be effective and intact in tasks in which the target had to be selected from a set of *semanti-*

*cally distinct* candidate items; this was also the case in multiple-items arrays with 23 distracter items. However, when the target had to be selected from a set of *semantically similar* candidate items the children with WS performed significantly worse than unimpaired controls even in arrays with a relatively small number of 11 (semantically related) distracter items.

We suggest that the observed profile of morphological and lexical skills in WS can be derived from a common source, a selective impairment in retrieving information from the lexicon. By contrast, the computational (rule-based) system of language appears to be unimpaired as evidenced by intact regular inflection and complex syntax (see Clahsen & Almazan 1998). We assume that irregularly inflected forms and lexical exceptions such as *drove* or *mice* are stored in long-term memory, as subnodes to the corresponding basic lexical entries, e.g. *drive* and *mouse* respectively, and that children with WS find it difficult to access morphological feature information represented in these subnodes. In contexts in which an exceptional form is required and the WS child does not retrieve the relevant features, the basic lexical entry is still retrieved and an inflected form is generated by applying a general rule (e.g. '*Add -ed*', '*Add -s*'), yielding overregularization errors. The account proposed here also extends to the retrieval of semantic features from lexical entries. We assume that lexical items can be broken down into sets of semantic features, such as [± COUNT], [± ANIMATE], [± HUMAN] which define an item's meaning, and enter into semantic relations, such as entailment and hyponymy, with other lexical items, and in this way yield hierarchical semantic networks. Children with WS, we suggest, have difficulty accessing fine-grain semantic features of lexical items. Hence, when subtle semantic distinctions are required, for example in a task in which a target item needs to be distinguished from a set of semantically similar distracters, performance in children with WS is poorer than in controls. However, when more general semantic features are sufficient, as in the case when target items and distracters come from different semantic fields, their performance is not impaired. Thus, we do not claim a broad lexical deficit in children with WS, but instead a selective deficit in getting access to fine-grain morphological and semantic feature specifications of lexical items.

More generally, there is no evidence from the lexical and morphological skills we have studied that the linguistic system of children with WS has a functional structure different from normal or that it reflects atypical developmental forms (contra Thomas & Karmiloff-Smith 2003). Instead, the results obtained and the interpretation we suggested support the view that the linguistic performance of subjects with WS reflects the architecture of the normal system but with selective components of this system under-developed.

## Acknowledgements

Supported by an Economic and Social Research Council grant jointly awarded to HC and CT (ESRC grant no. R000223511). We are grateful to Andrea Zukowski and Csaba Pléh for detailed and helpful comments on an earlier version of this chapter.

## Notes

1. These items were included to determine the kinds of past-tense forms children use when they cannot form an analogy to any existing irregular.

2. Recall that Olivia did not produce any past-tense form in this task and is therefore not included in this table.

3. The italicized figures in the existing irregulars condition are the overgeneralizations. The top figures ('*-ed*') represent the total proportion of *-ed* forms in this condition, and the bottom figure ('*overreg.*') subtracts from these figures cases in which *-ed* forms are permitted as past-tense forms in the local dialect, e.g. *wringed, digged, keeped*. Thus, the bottom figure represents a more conservative estimate of productive overregularizations.

4. Olivia produced only stem forms in this task, and her data are therefore not included in this table.

5. The top figures ('*-ed*') represent the total proportion of *-ed* forms in this condition, and the bottom figures ('*overreg.*') subtract from these cases in which *-ed* forms are permitted as past-tense forms in the local dialect.

6. Note that as in Experiment I, we counted as 'overregularizations' only those *-ed* forms produced for existing irregular verbs that are clearly ungrammatical and not permitted as past-tense forms in the spoken language of the region where the children were living; see '*overreg.*' in Table 5.

## References

Aronoff, M. (1976). *Word Formation in Generative Grammar*. Cambridge, MA: The MIT Press.

Barber, C. (1964). *Linguistic Change in Present-day English*. Tuscaloosa, AL: University of Alabama Press.

Bellugi, U., Wang, P., & Jernigan, T. (1994). "Williams syndrome: An unusual neuropsychological profile". In S. Broman & J. Grafman (Eds.), *Atypical Cognitive Deficits in Developmental Disorders: Implications for brain function* (pp. 23–56). Hillsdale, NJ: LEA.

Bellugi, U., Bihrle, A., Jernigan, T., Trauner, D., & Doherty, S. (1990). "Neuropsychological, neurological and neuroanatomical profile of Williams syndrome". *American Journal of Medical Genetics, 6,* 115–125.

Bellugi, U., Bihrle, A., Neville, H., Jernigan, T., & Doherty, S. (1992). "Language, cognition and brain organisation in a neurodevelopmental disorder". In M. Gunnar & C. Nelson (Eds.), *Developmental Behavioural Neuroscience: The Minnesota symposium on child psychology* (pp. 201–232). Hillsdale, NJ: LEA.

Bradley, E. & Udwin, O. (1989). "Williams syndrome in adulthood: A case study focusing on psychological and psychiatric aspects". *Journal of Mental Deficiency, 33,* 175–184.

Bromberg, H., Ullman, M., Marcus, G., Kelly, K., & Coppola, M. (1994). "A dissociation of memory and grammar: Evidence from Williams syndrome". Paper presented at the Eighteenth Annual Boston University Conference on Language Development.

Caramazza, A. (1984). "The logic of neuropsychological research and the problem of patient classification in aphasia". *Brain and Language, 21,* 9–20.

Chomsky, N. (1995). *The Minimalist Program.* Cambridge, MA: The MIT Press.

Clahsen, H. & Almazan, M. (1998). "Syntax and morphology in children with Williams syndrome". *Cognition, 68,* 167–198.

Clahsen, H. & Almazan, M. (2001). "Compounding and inflection in language impairment: Evidence from Williams syndrome and SLI". *Lingua, 111,* 729–757.

Clahsen, H. & Temple, C. (2003). Words and rules in children with Williams syndrome. In Y. Levy & J. Schaeffer (Eds.), *Language Competence across Populations* (pp. 323–352). Mahwah, NJ: LEA.

Dalalakis, J. (1994). "English adjectival comparatives and familial language impairment". In J. Matthews (Ed.), *Linguistic Aspects of Familial language Impairment* (pp. 50–66). Montreal: McGill University.

Druks, J. & Masterson, J. (2000). *An Object and Action Naming Battery.* Hove: Psychology Press.

Dunn, L. & Dunn, L. (1981). *Peabody Picture Vocabulary Test – Revised Manual.* Circle Pines, MN: American Guidance Service.

Dunn, L., Dunn, L., Whetton, C., & Pintilie, D. (1997). *The British Picture Vocabulary Scale.* Windsor Berks.: NFER-Nelson.

Frank, M. (1972). *Modern English: A practical reference guide.* Englewood Cliffs: Prentice-Hall.

Gathercole, V. (1985). "More and more and more about more". *Journal of Experimental Child Psychology, 40,* 73–104.

Graziano-King, J. (1999). Acquisition of Comparative Forms in English. Ph.D. dissertation. New York: CUNY Graduate Center.

Johnson, S. & Carey, S. (1998). "Knowledge enrichment and conceptual change in folk biology: Evidence from Williams syndrome". *Cognitive Psychology, 37,* 156–184.

Kim, J., Marcus, G., Pinker, S., Hollander, M., & Coppola, M. (1994). "Sensitivity of children's inflection to morphological structure". *Journal of Child Language, 21,* 173–209.

Mervis C. & Robinson, B. (2000). "Early expressive vocabularies of children with Williams syndrome or Down syndrome: A comparison". *Developmental Neuropsychology, 17,* 111–126.

Mervis, C., Morris, C., Bertrand, J., & Robinson, B. (1999). "Williams syndrome: Findings from an integrated program of research". In H. Tager-Flusberg (Ed.), *Neurodevelopmental Disorders* (pp. 65–110). Cambridge, MA: The MIT Press.

Pinker, S. (1999). *Words and Rules*. London: Weidenfeld and Nicolson.

Renfrew C. (1977). *Word Finding Vocabulary Scale*. Bicester: Speechmark Publishing.

Rice, M. (1999). "Specific grammatical limitations in children with Specific Language Impairment". In H. Tager-Flusberg (Ed.), *Neurodevelopmental Disorders* (pp. 331–360). Cambridge, MA: The MIT Press.

Rossen, M., Klima, E., Bellugi, U., Birhle, A., & Jones, W. (1996). "Interaction between language and cognition: Evidence from Williams syndrome". In J. Beitchman, N. Cohen, M. Konstantareas, & R. Tannock (Eds.), *Language Learning and Behaviour* (pp. 367–392). New York, NY: CUP.

Rothweiler, M. & Clahsen, H. (1994). "Dissociations in SLI children's inflectional systems: A study of participle inflection and subject-verb agreement". *Journal of Logopedics and Phoniatrics, 18*, 169–179.

Saffran, E. (1982). "Neuropsychological approaches to the study of language". *British Journal of Psychology, 73*, 317–337.

Singer Harris, N., Bellugi, U., Bates, L., Jones, W., & M. Rossen (1997). "Contrasting profiles of language development in children with Williams and Down syndromes". *Developmental Neuropsychology, 13*, 345–370.

Snodgrass, J. G. & van der Wart, M. (1980). "A standardized set of 260 pictures: Norms for name agreement, image agreement, familiarity and visual complexity". *Journal of Experimental Psychology: Human Learning and Memory, 6*, 174–215.

Temple, C. (2003). "Deep dyslexia in Williams syndrome". *Journal of Neurolinguistics, 16*, 457–488.

Temple, C., Almazan, M., & Sherwood, S. (2002). "Lexical skills in Williams syndrome: A cognitive neuropsychological analysis". *Journal of Neurolinguistics, 15*, 463–495.

Thomas, M. & Karmiloff-Smith, A. (2003). "Are developmental disorders like cases of adult brain damage? Implications from connectionist modeling". *Behavioral and Brain Sciences*. In press.

Thomas, M., Grant, J., Barham, Z., Gsödl, M., Laing, E., Lakusta, L. Tyler, L., Grice, S., Paterson, S., & Karmiloff-Smith, A. (2001). "Past tense formation in Williams syndrome". *Language and Cognitive Processes, 16*, 143–176.

Tyler, L., Karmiloff-Smith, A., Voice, J., Stevens, T., Grant, J., Udwin, O., Davies, M., & Howlin, P. (1997). "Do individuals with Williams syndrome have bizarre semantics? Evidence for lexical organisation using an on-line task". *Cortex, 33*, 515–527.

Ullman, M. (1993). The computation of inflectional morphology. Unpublished Ph.D. dissertation, Cambridge, MA, MIT.

Volterra, V., Capirci, O., Pezzini, G., Sabbadini, L., & Vicari, S. (1996). "Linguistic abilities in Italian children with Williams syndrome". *Cortex, 32*, 663–677.

Wechsler D. (1976). *Wechsler Intelligence Scale for Children – Revised*. New York: The Psychological Corporation.

Wechsler, D. (1992). *Wechsler Intelligence Scale for Children- Third Edition UK*. Sidcup, Kent: The Psychological Corporation, Harcourt Brace and Co.

Wexler, K. (1994). "Optional infinitives, head movement and the economy of derivations in child grammar". In D. Lightfoot & N. Hornstein (Eds.), *Verb Movement* (pp. 305–350). Cambridge: CUP.

Zukowski, A. (2001). Uncovering grammatical competence in children with Williams syndrome. Ph.D. dissertation, Boston University.

# Regular and irregular inflectional morphology in German Williams syndrome

Martina Penke and Marion Krause
Heinrich-Heine-Universitaet Duesseldorf

A central issue in the investigation of language capacities in Williams syndrome (WS) is whether the inflectional system is affected by a selective deficit with irregular inflected forms as Clahsen and Almazan (1998, 2001) have reported for English WS, or whether the observed problems are an artifact caused by a delay in language development (Thomas et al. 2001). To contribute to this controversy, we present data on German participle and noun plural inflection that come from five German WS subjects. Like Clahsen and Almazan, we find that regular inflection is intact in our WS subjects, whereas the production of irregular forms is impaired. We will argue that our data cannot be accounted for by assuming a developmental delay. Moreover, we will show that there is an additional deficit affecting morphophonological capacities as well.

## 1. Introduction

One of the central controversies in the investigation of Williams syndrome (WS) concerns whether or not there is a dissociation between language and other cognitive skills in individuals with WS. Bellugi and colleagues (Bellugi et al. 1988, 1994; Wang & Bellugi 1994) reported that language skills, including morphosyntactic capacities and the production of passive clauses and multiple embeddings, are relatively spared in WS, whereas other cognitive capacities are severely impaired. In contrast to these studies, other authors (e.g. Volterra et al. 1996; Capirci et al. 1996; Karmiloff-Smith et al. 1997) have argued that performance of subjects with WS is not ahead of their mental-age matched controls in standardized language tasks and is thus not completely spared.

During the last few years, this debate has focussed on the inflectional capacities of WS subjects. In two studies on English participle and noun plural inflection, Clahsen and Almazan (1998, 2001) reported a marked dissociation between regular and irregular inflectional morphology in English WS children. While regular past tense and plural inflection were intact, performance with irregular verbs and nouns was significantly worse compared to unimpaired children. Clahsen and Almazan suggest an explanation that draws upon a dualistic distinction between rule-based regular and stored irregular inflection. They propose that computational operations are unimpaired in WS, whereas the access to stored irregular forms in the mental lexicon is impaired.

This proposal has recently been criticized by Thomas et al. (2001). Based on a cross-sectional study on past tense inflection in English WS subjects, they claim that the selective deficit with irregular verbs disappears when verbal mental age is controlled for. According to Thomas et al., the WS subjects then show the same difference in performance between regular and irregular verbs as the control subjects. Therefore, they argue that a deficit with irregular verbs in WS is only apparent and simply the consequence of a delay in language development. They assume this delay to be due to an atypical developmental trajectory followed by the WS subjects which leads to phonological representations of lexical entries that are overly specific. Thomas et al. refer to a connectionist network simulation to support their claim that this overspecificity of lexical representations causes a delay in the inflectional system which is apparently worse for irregular forms, and to a reduced generalization of regular patterns to novel verbs. In a reaction to the work of Thomas et al., Clahsen and Temple (2003) have presented data on compound formation and on comparative inflection in English in order to prove that the error patterns observed in their WS subjects are deviant from any of the reactions normal children show.

The aim of this paper is to contribute to this controversy whether or not WS is characterized by a selective deficit with irregular inflected forms. We will present data on three experiments on German participle and noun plural inflection that were administered with five German WS subjects.[1]

Similar to English, German draws a distinction between regular and irregular inflected forms in participle and plural formation. There are, however, much less regularly inflected forms in German than in English. According to Marcus et al. (1995), 95% of the English verbs, but only 78% of the German verbs are weak, regular verbs. For noun plurals this difference is even stronger as 98% of the nouns in English, but only 7% of the German nouns are inflected with the regular default affix, which is *-s* in both languages (Marcus et al. 1995; Clahsen 1999). Another difference between English and German concerns the shape of irregular inflected forms. In English, regular forms are built by affixation whereas irregular past tense and plural forms are characterized by a change of the stem vowel. In German, however, regular and irregular participles and noun plurals have endings that are separable from the word's stem. Moreover, there is more than one irregular ending in German plural inflection. These differences in the inflectional systems of

English and German make it possible to disentangle effects in the performance of WS subjects that are caused by the regularity or irregularity of a form from effects that might be caused by the frequency distribution or the shape of these forms. The investigation of regular and irregular inflectional capacities in German WS subjects thus offers the opportunity to examine whether the findings reported for English WS subjects carry over to the different inflectional systems of German. Moreover, a comparison of intact and impaired capacities across different languages is necessary to establish a characteristic and cross-linguistically valid profile of Williams syndrome.

## 2. Subjects

### 2.1 General subject information

We tested five German subjects who were diagnosed with WS. The subjects' chronological age varied between 15 and 18 years. Medical and (neuro)psychological testing was performed by a team of pediatricians and psychologists in a specialized children's hospital and revealed typical physical and cognitive characteristics of WS for all subjects (for more details see Gosch & Pankau 1996).[2] At the time of our testing, all subjects lived in monolingual families of low (K.) or middle socio-economic class and attended a special school for children with (learning) disabilities. Intellectual level was determined from the Hamburg-Wechsler Intelligence Scale for children (HAWIK-R). Intelligence testing gave a mean full scale IQ value of 51 (range: 44–58). To take the dissociation between relatively spared language skills and more impaired non-verbal skills into account (e.g. Bellugi et al. 1988, 1999) and to address the issues raised by Thomas et al. (2001), we determined mental age on the basis of the verbal IQ scores from the HAWIK-R.

Data of the WS subjects were compared to data from a group of 15 normally developing children matching in mental age with the WS subjects (five children with a mean age of 6;5 years = group I, five children with a mean age of 8;1 = group II, and five children with a mean age of 9;6 = group III). In addition, we tested a group of six control subjects matching in chronological age with the WS subjects (mean age 15.9). All control subjects were monolingual German speakers of middle class socio-economic background. The subjects of the mental-age matched control group attended a regular elementary school. The subjects of the chronological-age matched control group were either high school students or still attended a comprehensive school. None of the control subjects had any known cognitive, psychic or physic impairments. Table 1 presents an overview on some relevant subject data.

**Table 1.** Williams syndrome and control subjects

| WS subjects | Chronological age | HAWIK-R IQ verbal/performance/ full-scale | Mental age determined from verbal part | Controls ∅ age (range) | No. |
|---|---|---|---|---|---|
| C | 15;1 | 48/44/<44 | 6;5 | 6;5 (6;1–6;11) | 5 |
| D | 16;5 | verbal:60 | 6;7 | | |
| M | 18;10 | 62/55/53 | 8;3 | 8;1 (7;9–8;3) | 5 |
| K | 17;6 | verbal:60 | 7;5 | | |
| E | 17;9 | 70/55/58 | 9;7 | 9;6 (8;8–10;3) | 5 |
| | | | | 15;9 (14;11–18;9) | 6 |

**Table 2.** Expressive language capacities of WS and control subjects

| | WS | | Mental-age matched controls | |
|---|---|---|---|---|
| | ∅ | (range) | ∅ | (range) |
| MLU $_{\text{word based}}$ | 6.0 | (5.3–6.7) | 7.4 | (5.6–9.9) |
| No. of utterances | 164 | (72–289) | 93 | (40–164) |
| % multi-constit. utterances* | 93.4 | (85–100) | 99.6 | (98–100) |
| % of subordinate clauses** | 8.2 | (0–12.1) | 8 | (1.5–22.5) |
| % of *wh*-clauses** | 5 | (0–6.9) | 1.1 | (0–4.9) |
| Determiner omissions in % | 2.2 | (0–3.9) | 0.2 | (0–2.8%) |
| correct S-V-agreement in % | 97.6 | (94.1–100) | 98.8 | (97–100) |
| V2 in main clauses in % | 99 | (96.1–100) | 99.8 | (97.9–100) |
| $V_{final}$ in subord. clauses in % | 100 | | 100 | |

* Percentages were calculated in relation to the total number of utterances.
** Percentages were calculated in relation to the number of multi-constituent utterances.

## 2.2 Short overview on expressive language abilities

To determine the expressive grammatical abilities of the tested WS subjects and the mental-age matched controls, we elicited speech production data by asking them to describe short picture stories and to tell the "frog story" (Mayer 1969). Descriptions were tape recorded, transcribed and entered into a database. The data were then analyzed with respect to quantitative and morphosyntactic features. Table 2 presents some quantitative and morphosyntactic measures for the utterances produced by the WS subjects and by the mental-age matched control children.

Table 2 shows that the mean length of utterance (MLU) for the WS subjects is between 5 and 7 words. This is within the range of the mean utterance length for normally developing controls that ranges from 5 to 10 words. For both groups of subjects, utterance length increases with age. This increase, however, is somewhat stronger for the controls than for the WS subjects. Like the controls' utterances, most of the WS subjects' utterances are multi-constituent utterances that consist at least of two phrasal constituents. The proportion of subordinate clauses and *wh*-questions contained in these multi-constituent utterances is comparable for WS subjects and controls: 8.2% of the WS subjects' and 8% of the controls' multi-constituent utterances are subordinate clauses. The respective percentages for *wh*-questions are 5% for the WS subjects and 1.1% for the control subjects.

Determiners are almost never omitted in obligatory contexts – neither by the WS subjects (omission rate 2.2%) nor by the control subjects (omission rate 0.2%). Nearly identical and almost error-free performance of the two subject groups can also be seen for subject-verb agreement inflection. Here the mean correctness scores are 97.6% for the WS subjects and 98.8% for the controls.

Concerning word order, the data presented in Table 2 show that the WS subjects do not have problems with verb placement. German is an asymmetric V2 language. The finite verb is in the second structural position in main clauses (V2), but it appears in clause-final position in subordinate clauses that are introduced by a complementizer. This placement pattern is almost flawlessly applied by the WS subjects. In main clauses, 99% of the produced finite verbs are correctly placed in V2 position, whereas in subordinate clauses all finite verbs appear in sentence-final position. These figures are virtually identical to the figures of the mental-age matched control children.

In sum, the data show that the WS subjects' utterances contain complex syntactic structures and are generally grammatically complete and correct. Certainly, these data do not provide an extensive and detailed overview on the expressive morphosyntactic capacities of the WS subjects examined in this study. Nevertheless, the data demonstrate that morphosyntactic capacities in core areas of the language system are at appropriate levels for their mental age. This observation corresponds to previous findings on the morphosyntactic capacities of WS subjects displayed in speech production (Bellugi et al. 1988; Clahsen & Almazan 1998; Rice et al. 1999). It indicates that the WS subjects studied here are in important respects comparable to the WS subjects described in the literature.

## 3. Regular and irregular inflection in German participles

German participles consist of a prosodically determined prefix *ge-*, a verb stem and the endings *-t* or *-n*. Regular verbs do not show stem changes in the preterite or participle form and are suffixed with *-t* (1a, b). In contrast, irregular verbs show a modification of the stem vowel (Ablaut, at least in the preterite) and have the participle ending *-n* (1c, d). Neither the stem vowel, nor the phonological shape of the verb stem are sufficient to indicate whether a verb is regular or irregular. Thus for example, *trinken* in (1d) is an irregular verb, its participle being *getrunken*. The verb *blinken* (1b), in contrast, is a regular verb, the participle form is *geblinkt*.

| (1) | Infinitive | Preterite | Participle | |
|---|---|---|---|---|
| a. | *tanz-en* | *tanz-te* | *ge-tanz-t* | 'dance' |
| b. | *blink-en* | *blink-te* | *ge-blink-t* | 'flash' |
| c. | *les-en* | *las* | *ge-les-en* | 'read' |
| d. | *trink-en* | *trank* | *ge-trunk-en* | 'drink' |

A theoretical account of this inflectional system is given by Wunderlich (1996). Due to the unpredictability of whether a verb is regular or irregular and due to the largely unpredictable stem changes irregular verbs undergo, irregular inflected participle forms have to be stored as fully inflected forms in the mental lexicon. According to Wunderlich's account, irregular participles such as (*ge*)*trunken* are stored in structured lexical entries that spread from an unmarked base node (see (2a)). These entries are schemes that restrict possible irregularities. In contrast, entries for regular verbs only consist of the base node (2b) and participles are built by regular affixation of the affix -*t* to the base.

(2) a. [tʀɪŋk]$_{+verb}$ ('drink')

    [tʀaŋk]$_{+preterite}$ [tʀʊŋkn̩]$_{+participle}$

    [tʀæŋkə]$_{+subjunctive}$

b. [tants]$_{+verb}$ ('dance')

Wunderlich's account draws a qualitative distinction between irregular and regular inflected participles: whereas irregular participles are stored as fully inflected forms in the mental lexicon, regular participles are built by affixation of the suffix -*t* to the verb stem (see Clahsen 1999 for a similar view). This qualitative distinction between stored irregular and affix-based regular forms has meanwhile been confirmed by an impressive number of psycho- and neurolinguistic studies (see Clahsen 1999; Penke 2002 for an overview and discussion).

## 3.1 Elicitation of regular and irregular participles

### 3.1.1 *Method*

Procedure and material of the first experiment were adopted from Penke et al. (1999). Subjects had to complete a sentence by transforming a given 1st person singular present tense form into a participle. The sentences were presented visually on cards (cf. (3)) and were read out aloud to the subjects. The task was administered with the five WS subjects, the 15 mental-age matched controls and the six chronologically matched controls. Although the reading abilities of the youngest control

Table 3. Frequency information on the tested participles

| Participles | | No. | ∅ frequency of participle form |
|---|---|---|---|
| Regular | infrequent | 14 | 10,1 |
| | frequent | 9 | 250 |
| Irregular | infrequent | 12 | 10,2 |
| | frequent | 14 | 342,6 |

Frequency information based on the CELEX-database (Baayen et al. 1993).

children were still quite limited neither the control children nor the WS subjects experienced any problems with this task. Each subject was tested individually. With the exception of WS subject E., all subjects were tested at their homes.

(3)

| | |
|---|---|
| Ich schreibe. | ('I am writing') |
| Ich habe _______ . | ('I have _______ .') |

To shorten the experiment – which was only one in a series of tests addressing different language capacities – we selected a subgroup of the items presented in the original experiment of Penke et al. We chose items that made it possible to look for influences of participle frequency, stem vowel, and ablaut pattern. In total, we elicited 23 regular and 26 irregular participles. Table 3 gives information on the frequency distribution of the test items. A list of the tested verbs can be found in the Appendix.

In addition to these test items, we elicited 100 regular and irregular noun plurals that served as fillers for this study (see Section 4 for the results on noun plurals). The test and filler items were presented in four blocks separated by short pauses and each starting with a short practice phase. To ensure that the items of each stimulus type were evenly distributed across blocks, test and filler items were assigned in a pseudo-random order to the four blocks. Reactions were audio-taped, transcribed and checked twice. Forms that were not overtly marked as participles, i.e. forms which were neither marked with *ge-*, nor with the suffixes *-t* or *-n*, nor with an ablauting stem, were not analyzed. Furthermore, we excluded all those cases from analysis where subjects produced participle forms for other than the presented verbs. An inflectional error was counted if a wrong participle ending was used.

For ease of presentation, the data will henceforth be collapsed into three age groups for the WS subjects (group I: subjects C. and D.; group II: subjects M. and K.; group III: subject E.) and into four groups for the control subjects: three groups of mental-age matched controls and one group of chronological-age matched controls. Where individual variation occurs in the data, this is indicated in the result tables and discussed in the text.

### 3.1.2 *Results*

Table 4 gives the error rates for regular and irregular participles in relation to the number of analyzable regular and irregular participles for each of the WS subject groups and the four control groups.

For regular participles, the correctness scores are above 95% for each individual WS subject. A comparison between the WS subjects and the control children shows that the correctness scores for the WS subjects (mean 98.3%) are virtually identical to the correctness scores of the mental-age (mean 98.2%) and the chronological-age matched control subjects (99.3%). These figures indicate that for the tested WS subjects regular participle formation is not only at an appropriate level for their mental age but completely intact.

In contrast to regular participle formation, the WS subjects' mean correctness score for irregular participles is only 73.1%. For all WS subjects, correctness scores for irregular participles are considerably lower than the correctness scores for regular participles ($\chi^2$, $p < .05$ for each subject group).[3] This finding, however, also holds for the mental-age matched control children. Compared to their performance on regular participles, their correctness scores on irregular participles are much lower ($\chi^2$, $p < .05$ for each control group) and virtually identical to the WS subjects' scores. Only the chronological-age matched controls achieve correctness scores of over 90% for irregular participles.

A clear difference between WS and mental-age matched control children, however, emerges when we consider frequent and infrequent irregular participles separately (see Table 5). Studies on language acquisition have shown that unimpaired children overregularize the regular participle affix *-t* to those irregular verbs for which they have not yet acquired the respective participle form. These overregularizations especially affect infrequent irregular verbs, as infrequent participle forms occur only rarely in children's input and therefore take some time to be learned (e.g. Weyerts 1997). In fact, error analysis for the mental-age matched control children reveals that 85.6% of their errors with irregular participles affect infrequent participles and lead to overregularizations in participle formation (cf. (4)). More-

**Table 4.** Percentages of correctly inflected participles

| % correct | | WS subjects | Mental-age matched controls | Chronological-age matched controls |
|---|---|---|---|---|
| Regular participles | group I | 97.8 | 95.5 | 99.3 |
| | group II | 97.8 | 99.1 | |
| | group III | 100 | 100 | |
| Irregular participles | group I | 69.2 | 67.2 | 95.5 |
| | group II | 75 | 69 | |
| | group III | 76.9 | 82.3 | |

Table 5. Frequency distribution of inflectional errors with irregular participles

| | % errors affecting infrequent irregular participles | | % errors affecting frequent irregular participles | |
|---|---|---|---|---|
| | WS subjects | Mental-age matched controls | WS subjects | Mental-age matched controls |
| Group I | 68.8 | 80.5 | 31.2 | 19.5 |
| Group II | 69.2 | 87.5 | 30.8 | 12.5 |
| Group III | 66.7 | 91.3 | 33.3 | 8.7 |

over, the controls' data exhibit a clear age trend. As age increases, the percentage of errors with irregular participles affecting frequent forms decreases from 19.5% for group I to 8.7% for group III ($r(13) = -.547$, $p = .035$). This age trend reflects the fact that irregular participle forms are learned over time.

(4) a. **geflechtet* instead of *geflochten* ('plait') (N., control group I)
b. **gelügt* instead of *gelogen* ('lie') (C., control group II)
c. **geschwört* instead of *geschworen* ('swear') (I., control group III)

Compared to the mental-age matched controls, the data for the WS subjects reveal a marked difference in the frequency distribution of errors made with irregular participles ($\chi^2$, $p < .05$). A total of 31.4% of the WS subjects' errors with irregular participles result in overregularizations of frequent verbs. In addition, the percentages for errors with irregular participles that affect frequent forms do not decrease with age ($r(3) = 0.287$, $p = .639$), but remain stable at about 30% for all three groups of WS subjects.

### 3.1.3 *Discussion*

For the German WS subjects tested here, regular participle formation is completely intact whereas irregular participles are impaired. This dissociation between intact regular and impaired irregular participle formation is in line with the results on English past tense formation in WS subjects reported by Clahsen and Almazan (1998) and Thomas et al. (2001). Whereas Clahsen and Almazan interpret this dissociation as evidence for a selective impairment of the lexical access to stored irregular inflected forms, Thomas et al. argue that the performance of their WS subjects indicates a mere delay in the system of past tense formation while there is no evidence for a selective impairment of irregular past tense forms in English WS. As evidence for this assumption, Thomas et al. refer to the finding that a dissociation between intact regular and impaired irregular past tense forms also holds for the mental-age matched control children in their study. Reduced correctness scores for irregular participles can also be seen in the mental-age matched control groups of our study. A closer investigation of the error patterns for WS and mental-age matched control children, however, points to a substantial difference between the two subject groups: whereas the control children's errors affect infrequent irregular verbs, WS subjects have problems with frequent irregular verbs too. This difference between WS subjects and mental-age matched control subjects can already be observed in the youngest subjects. In addition, and contrary to the control children, the WS subjects' error rates for frequent irregular participles remain stable with increasing mental age. Based on this pattern of results we want to argue that the relatively low correctness scores for irregular participles obtained by the control children are due to the relatively high number of very infrequent participles included in our study. As these forms are acquired over time, correctness scores increase with age. The stable impairment of frequent irregular participles that can be observed in our WS subjects, in contrast, suggests that the production of irregular participles is impaired in these subjects. A general delay in the inflectional system of WS subjects as suggested by Thomas et al. can neither account for the normal performance on regular participles, nor for the error data on frequent irregular participles.

## 3.2 Elicitation of participles for novel verbs

The data of the first experiment have shown that our WS subjects display almost flawless performance with regular participle inflection and readily overregularize the regular affix *-t* to irregular verbs. This finding suggests that regular participle formation is intact in these subjects. In their study on English past tense formation, Thomas et al. however found that compared to mental-age matched controls "the WS group appeared to have an additional deficit in generalizing regular past tense formation to novel verbs" (p. 164). They argue that this reduced generalization to novel verbs is the consequence of a different developmental process followed by WS subjects where greater weight is placed on phonological information. According to Thomas et al., this results in lexical representations that are too specific to support generalization to novel verbs. Clahsen and Almazan, in contrast, did not report a deficit in generalizations to novel verbs for their WS subjects. To investigate this issue, we conducted a second elicitation task where subjects had to form participles for novel verbs.

### 3.2.1 *Method*

The experimental procedure and material was taken from an experiment conducted by Weyerts (1997). The experiment is designed as a board play. Subjects have to solve tasks to find a 'treasure'. The novel verbs are introduced as 'dinosaur-language'. Part of the child's task is to transform a given 2nd person singular imperative verb form into a participle (cf. (5)).

(5) "*Du bekommst die Aufgabe:* **Fupp** *die Segel. Wenn Du damit fertig bist, rufst Du dem Dinosaurier zu:* ***fertiggefuppt.***"
('Your task is: **Fupp** the sails. Once you are finished, tell the dinosaur: **fertiggefuppt** (participle).')

Test items consist of 14 novel verbs. Three of these novel verbs rhyme with existing irregular verbs, three rhyme with existing regular verbs, one rhymes with existing mixed verbs, and seven novel verbs do not rhyme with any existing verb.

Only four of the WS subjects participated in this experiment. Subject K. had moved out of the region and was no longer available for testing by the time we conducted this experiment. The data for the control children come from the original investigation of Weyerts (1997) and were kindly made available to us by Helga Weyerts. Because of the small number of verbs and subjects tested in this experiment, we present data that is collapsed for all WS subjects and all control children.

### 3.2.2 *Results and discussion*

Table 6 presents the relevant data for WS and control children. Rows 1 and 2 give the percentages of novel participles formed with *-t* or *-n* in relation to all 14 test items. The percentages of non-rhyming novel participles built with *-t* or *-n* are given in rows 3 and 4. Rows 5 and 6 present the percentages of *-t* and *-n* inflected participles for novel verbs that rhyme with existing irregular verbs.

As can be seen in rows 1 and 2 of the table, the adolescents with WS productively use the regular affix *-t* in forming participles for novel verbs. 49 out of a total of 56 produced participles (87.5%) are inflected with *-t*. This is virtually identical to the data of the control subjects who inflect 88.1% of the novel participles with *-t*. Irregular formations of novel participles occur only once in the WS data and six

**Table 6.** Participle forms of novel verbs

| | Results for: | Ending | WS subjects (groups I–III) | Control children (age 6–8)* |
|---|---|---|---|---|
| 1 | All test items | -t | 87.5% | 88.1% |
| 2 | | -n | 1.8% | 2.4% |
| 3 | Non-rhyming novel verbs | -t | 82.1% | 87.1% |
| 4 | | -n | 3.6% | 0.8% |
| 5 | Novel verbs rhyming with irregular verbs | -t | 91.7% | 96% |
| 6 | | -n | 0% | 0% |

*Data from Helga Weyerts (see Weyerts 1997).
Values missing from 100% are due to the production of forms with neither of the endings *-t* or *-n*.

times in the controls' data. A comparison of rows 3 to 6 of the table reveals that neither control nor WS subjects draw a clear distinction between non-rhyming novel verbs and novel verbs that rhyme with existing irregular verbs. Both types of verbs are generally inflected with *-t*.[4] Neither control children nor WS subjects produce any irregular participles of rhyming novel verbs that are formed in analogy to existing irregular verbs (see row 6).

The data do not provide evidence for a general deficit in the WS subjects' capacity to generalize to novel verbs as suggested by Thomas et al. (2001). Thomas et al. report a generalization rate for novel verbs which is only about 50%. This is in clear contrast to the generalization rate of 87.5% observed for our German WS subjects. The high generalization rate displayed by our WS subjects is however in line with the findings Clahsen and Almazan (1998) report for non-rhyming novel verbs. Our data and the data reported by Clahsen and Almazan suggest that the deficit in generalizing to novel verbs observed by Thomas et al. is not a characteristic feature of WS. Summarizing, the productive use of the suffix *-t* in novel verb participle formation further confirms that the WS subjects under study here, have no problems with regular inflection and readily apply it to form participles of novel verbs.

## 4. Regular and irregular inflection in German noun plurals

The German plural system consists of five different markers. Plural nouns can be marked by the markers *-s* (*Auto-Autos* 'car'), *-n* (*Blume-Blumen* 'flower'), *-e* (*Tisch-Tische* 'table'), *-er* (*Kind-Kinder* 'child'), or they can remain unmarked (*Ritter-Ritter* 'knight').

In contrast to the other plural markers, *-s* is special in several ways. It is the only marker that allows for monosyllabic plural forms such as *Parks* ('parks'), it is relatively free in its phonological distribution – blocked only after sibilants, and it occurs with nouns of any gender (see Marcus et al. 1995). All other plural forms are restricted to particular morphophonological contexts, show a dependency on gender, and are subject to a prosodic constraint that requires the plural form to end in a reduced syllable, i.e. an unstressed syllable with Schwa or a syllabic sonorant (Neef 1998; Golston & Wiese 1996; Wiese 1996). Moreover, the plural marker *-s* is very productive in German and freely occurs with all sorts of nouns which do not have a lexical entry such as derived nouns (*die Wenns* 'the ifs') or neologisms (Marcus et al. 1995). Finally, a range of psycho- and neurolinguistic studies has provided evidence that *-s* behaves differently from other plural markers (see Clahsen 1999 for a detailed review). Based on these differences between *-s-* and other German noun plurals, it has been suggested that *-s* is the default plural affix in German which applies when no stored irregular plural form is available and no other plural affix is applicable (e.g. Bornschein & Butt 1987; Janda 1990; Marcus et al. 1995; Wiese 1996; Clahsen 1999; Dressler 1999; Wunderlich 1999).

Theoretical considerations as well as results of psycho- and neurolinguistic testing indicate that although *-s-* is the default marker for German noun plurals, it is not the only regular plural affix in German. There is some agreement among researchers that the rather large group of *-n*-plurals on non-umlauting feminine nouns that end in Schwa in the singular (***die** Blume – Blume**n*** 'flower-fem') are regular too, because the *-n*-plural is completely predictable for these nouns (e.g. Bittner 1994; Dressler 1999; Wunderlich 1999, but see Clahsen 1999 for an opposing view). Wunderlich (1999) for instance has suggested a plural affix *-n* that applies when its input conditions [+noun, +feminine] are met by lexical entries.

In contrast to the predictable *-n*-marking on feminine nouns that end in Schwa in the singular form (henceforth $\textit{-n}^{\textit{fem}}$-plurals), it is largely unpredictable which masculine or neuter nouns will or will not take the *-n*-ending. Due to this unpredictability and because of their limited number, it is generally agreed that *-n*-plurals for masculine or neuter nouns that do not end in Schwa in the singular (***das** Hemd – Hemd**en*** 'shirt-neut.', henceforth called $\textit{-n}^{\textit{nonfem}}$-plurals) are irregular forms that are stored as fully inflected forms in the mental lexicon (e.g. Marcus et al. 1995; Wiese 1996; Sonnenstuhl et al. 1999; Clahsen 1999; Wunderlich 1999). In a recent series of experiments we could confirm this distinction between regular $\textit{-n}^{\textit{fem}}$- and irregular $\textit{-n}^{\textit{nonfem}}$-plurals (Penke & Krause 1999, 2002). We found that irregular $\textit{-n}^{\textit{nonfem}}$-plurals, but not regular $\textit{-n}^{\textit{fem}}$-plurals, produce frequency effects that are indicative of full-form storage.[5] Moreover, both types of *-n*-markers can be differently impaired in agrammatic Broca's aphasia. In addition to $\textit{-n}^{\textit{nonfem}}$-plurals, there is ample theoretical and experimental evidence for the assumption that noun plurals on *-er* are stored irregular forms too (e.g. Marcus et al. 1995; Wiese 1996; Clahsen 1999; Sonnenstuhl et al. 1999; Wunderlich 1999).

The status of the plural marker *-e* (*der Tisch-Tisch**e*** 'table-masc.') is however still controversial. Some researchers claim that *-e* is a regular plural marker (e.g. Bittner 1994; Dressler 1999; Indefrey 1999), while others state that noun plurals on *-e* are stored irregular forms (Marcus et al. 1995; Clahsen 1999). Moreover, it has recently been suggested that *-e* is not a plural marker at all, but is simply applied as last resort by the phonological operation of Schwa epenthesis to ensure that all native German plural forms leaving the lexicon meet the phonological constraint to end in a reduced Schwa syllable (Golston & Wiese 1996; Wunderlich 1999). In this respect, *-e* is complementary to masculine or neuter nouns that end in a Schwa syllable in the singular. As these nouns already fulfill the phonological constraint on the form of native German noun plurals, they generally remain unmarked in the plural form (*der Ritter-Ritter* 'knight-masc.').

Table 7. Overview on the theoretical status of the different plural markers

| Ending | Example: Singular – Plural | Plural form has to end in a reduced syllable | Status |
|---|---|---|---|
| *-er* | das Kind – Kinder ('child-neut.') | yes | stored irregular form |
| *-n*[nonfem] | das Hemd – Hemden ('shirt-neut.') | yes | stored irregular form |
| *-n*[fem] | die Blume – Blumen ('flower-fem.') | yes | regular affix |
| *unmarked* | der Ritter – Ritter ('knight-masc.') | yes | no affix, no stored form |
| *-e* | der Tisch – Tische ('table-masc.') | yes | no affix, no stored form, Schwa epenthesis |
| *-s* | der Park – Parks ('park-masc.') | no | regular default affix |

Analysis adopted from Wunderlich (1999).

Note that this short overview does not capture all the intricacies of the German noun plural system and is not meant as an extensive analysis of the German plural system. It can only highlight those areas of the German noun plural system where a certain consensus on the status of the different plural markers has been reached. Table 7 offers a summary on the discussed characteristics of the German noun plural system that are adopted in our study.

## 4.1 Method

Noun plurals were elicited with a simple completion task in which subjects had to provide the plural form for a given singular noun. Noun phrases were introduced by the numbers '1' and '2' to make the task clear to the subjects (cf. (6)).

(6)

| 1 Kind<br>2 ______ |
|---|

('1 child, 2 ______')

We elicited 20 plural forms for each of five different plural markers: (i) the regular default plural *-s*, (ii) the regular *-n*[fem]-plural for feminine nouns ending in Schwa in the singular, (iii+iv) irregular stored forms on *-er* and *-n*[nonfem], (v) and plurals ending in *-e*. This resulted in a total of 100 plural nouns elicited per subject. To control for frequency effects, the items of these five groups were closely matched for frequency between and within groups. The mean plural-form frequency for these five groups of test items ranged between 53.25 and 60.05 (frequency information based on the CELEX database). A complete list of the test items is given in the Appendix.

The noun phrases were presented visually on cards and read out aloud by the experimenter to avoid any reading problems. The children's responses were tape-recorded, transcribed and checked twice. Forms that were marked with endings that are not part of the German plural system and cases where subjects produced a noun plural for a different noun than the presented one were excluded from analysis. An inflectional error was counted if an incorrect plural marker or an unmarked form was produced.

Five WS subjects, 15 mental-age matched control subjects and six chronological-age matched controls participated in this experiment.

## 4.2 Results

Table 8 presents percentages of correctly produced noun plurals for each type of plural marker.

For the regular -*s*-plural, the WS subjects' correctness scores are slightly higher than for the mental-age matched control children ($\chi^2$-comparisons between each of the three subject and control groups n.s.). Moreover, correctness scores for the WS subjects in groups II and III are close to the mean correctness score for the chronological-age matched control group ($\chi^2$, n.s.).

A similar picture emerges for regular -$n^{fem}$-plurals. Correctness scores for WS subjects and mental-age matched controls are comparable and close to the adult

**Table 8.** Correctly inflected noun plurals

| % correct | | WS subjects | Mental-age matched controls | Chronological-age matched controls |
|---|---|---|---|---|
| Regular -*s*-plurals | group I | 79.5 | 71.7 | 91.7 |
| | group II | 87.5 | 75.3 | |
| | group III | 89.5 | 79.8 | |
| Regular -$n^{fem}$-plurals | group I | 92.5 | 93.9 | 100 |
| | group II | 86.8 | 100 | |
| | group III | 100 | 100 | |
| Irregular plurals on -*er* and -$n^{nonfem}$ | group I | 79.5<br>C.: 60.5<br>D.: 97.5 | 75 | 98.8 |
| | group II | 69 | 85.4 | |
| | group III | 90 | 82.3 | |

For the data on -*e*-plurals see Table 9 and Section 4.4.

level from early on ($\chi^2$-comparisons between each of the three subject and control groups n.s.). The relatively low correctness score obtained by WS subject group II for this marker is due to subject K. who produces a number of double plural markings where an additional plural marker *-s* is added to the correct *-n$^{fem}$*-inflected plural form (e.g. *1 Ratte – 2 *Rattens* 'rats'). This type of double-marking error was also reported by Clahsen and Almazan (1998). They observed that their English WS subjects produced past tense forms like **founds* in which the 3rd singular marker *-s* was incorrectly overapplied to a past tense form. Clahsen and Almazan interpret these errors as evidence for a strong tendency in WS subjects to overapply rules in contexts where rule application is prohibited. In any case, these errors of K. do not provide evidence for a deficit with regular plural marking, since in fact both regular plural markers are applied in these cases.

Summarizing, for the regular plural markers *-s* and *-n$^{fem}$* our WS subjects obtained high correctness scores which closely resemble the correctness scores of mental- and chronological-age matched control groups. This finding indicates that regular plural formation is intact in the German WS subjects under study here.

Compared to the high mean correctness score for regular noun plurals (88.2%) the mean correctness score for irregular noun plurals on *-er* and *-n$^{nonfem}$* is reduced for the WS subjects (77.3%). The individual data however show considerable variation between subjects. Three of the WS subjects (C. – group I, M. and K. – both group II) perform much worse on these irregular noun plurals than on the regular ones. For these three subjects, the mean correctness score for irregular noun plurals on *-er* and *-n$^{nonfem}$* is 66.1%. This is much lower than the 86.4% they obtain for regular noun plurals on *-s* and *-n$^{fem}$* ($\chi^2$, $p < .05$). A comparison between the mean correctness score for irregular plurals achieved by these three WS subjects (66.1%) and the mean score for the children of control groups I and II (80.4%) yields a clear difference between the two subject groups ($\chi^2$, $p < .05$). Moreover, all three WS children rarely overapply irregular noun plural patterns to produce plural forms for nouns that take other markers: only 5.1% of their errors are incorrect overirregularizations of the endings *-er* and *-n* (as in **Insekter* instead of *Insekten* 'insects' or **Hunden* instead of *Hunde* 'dogs'). This is in clear contrast to the 26% overirregularization errors observed for the mental-age matched control children of groups I and II ($\chi^2$, $p < .05$). The relatively high error rate for irregular plural forms and the low rate of overirregularizations indicate that irregular plural inflection is impaired for the three WS subjects C., K. and M..

In contrast to these three subjects, WS subjects D. (group I) and E. (group III) show no problems with irregular noun plurals. With a mean correctness score of 93.8% their performance is practically flawless and even comparable to the performance of the chronological-age matched control subjects. Whereas WS subject E. has no problems with regular or irregular plural formation, there is some evidence for a deficit in the plural system of WS subject D. The data suggest that D. has not acquired the distinction between stored irregular *-n*$^{nonfem}$-plurals and regular *-n*$^{fem}$-plurals, but has acquired a suffix *-n* which he uses as the regular default plural for German nouns. For one, D. is the only subject who shows error-free performance for *-n*$^{nonfem}$-plurals. All other control subjects – whether mental- or chronological-age matched controls – make at least one error in the plural formation of the 20 *-n*$^{nonfem}$ test items. Moreover, D. – in contrast to the WS subjects C., K. and M. – heavily overapplies *-n* to form plurals for other nouns. 72.7% of his errors are over-applications of *-n*, compared to an overapplication rate of 1.1% for the other four WS subjects and to a rate of 9.6% for all control subjects.

## 4.3 Discussion

Regular plural formation, just like regular participle inflection, is intact in all WS subjects under study here. This finding is in agreement with the results Clahsen and Almazan (2001) report for regular plural formation in English WS subjects.

With respect to overgeneralizations, however, the data display some differences to our data on German participle formation and to the data on English plural formation. Whereas the default participle affix *-t* is freely overapplied to irregular verbs by both WS and control subjects, this does not hold for the default plural affix *-s*. Only WS subject K. and one of the control children in group I overapply *-s* to a considerable extent: 79.3% of the plural errors for K. and 86.7% of the errors for control child L. are overregularizations of *-s*. The other WS and control subjects only rarely overapply *-s* to nouns that take other plural markers.[6] The overgeneralization rates for *-s* are 7.1% for the other four WS subjects, 5.5% for the other 14 mental-age matched control children, and 2.6% for the chronological-age matched controls respectively.[7] The low overgeneralization rates for the default plural *-s* observed in this experiment are in contrast to the results reported by Clahsen and Almazan (2001) for English WS subjects. They found that their WS subjects frequently overgeneralized *-s* to nouns that require irregular plurals and obtained overgeneralization rates that were sometimes more than twice as high as the overgeneralization rates of the control children. In our German WS subjects, high overapplication rates are only observed for K., who overgeneralizes *-s*, and for D., who overapplies *-n*.

Differences to the clear-cut results obtained for German participle inflection and English plural inflection do also show up in the data on German irregular plural inflection. Whereas all our WS subjects have difficulties with irregular German participles and all WS subjects of Clahsen and Almazan (2001) have problems with irregular plural formation in English, only three of the five WS subjects in our study show a parallel impairment of irregular German plural formation. For WS subject E. both regular and irregular noun plurals are unimpaired, whereas subject D. miscategorizes the plural marker *-n* as the default affix and thus exhibits an exceptionally good performance for the irregular *-n*$^{nonfem}$-plurals.

In sum, the WS subjects' data on German plural formation show a larger variation in performance patterns compared to the data on German participle and English plural inflection. This is, first and foremost, a reflex of the fact that the German system of noun plural inflection is much more complicated than the simpler systems of German participle and English noun plural inflection which consist of only one regular default affix besides stored irregular forms. In contrast to these systems, the system of German plural inflection hosts at least two regular affixes – the default affix *-s* and the regular *-n*$^{fem}$-affix, the application of which is restricted to feminine nouns ending in Schwa in the singular. Moreover, irregular forms come with different separable endings. This complexity and the range of available separable endings invite different pathways in acquisition that result in temporary miscategorizations of some of the plural markers. Bartke (1998), for instance, has observed that unimpaired children (aged between 3;10 and 8;10 years) acquiring the system of German noun plural formation may categorize each of the three plural markers *-s*, *-e*, or *-n* as the default affix for plural formation. The miscategorization of WS subject D. is thus in line with the findings for unimpaired German children of comparable mental age. Which marker is chosen as default affix is going to affect the performance in plural formation. Thus, D.'s performance with the irregular *-n*$^{nonfem}$-plurals is exceptionally good because he has categorized *-n* as the default affix for plural formation.

Although these individual pathways blur the overall picture, we can state the following two results: (i) Independent of which affix has been chosen as default affix, the data clearly show that regular plural formation is intact in German WS subjects. (ii) Due to different pathways in the acquisition of the German plural system, problems with irregular plural formation are probably not a sign to be observed in every German WS subject. They will, however, occur quite frequently.

## 4.4 Problems with the prosodic constraint on German noun plurals

Besides the problem with irregular noun plurals that affects three of our WS subjects, a closer look reveals yet another difference between WS and control subjects. This difference concerns the prosodic constraint that governs the shape of all native German plural nouns. As mentioned above, this constraint requires all native noun plurals to end in a reduced syllable, i.e. in a Schwa syllable or in a syllabic sonorant. If the plural form that is retrieved from the mental lexicon does not have the required prosodic shape, the phonological last resort operation of Schwa epenthesis applies, leading to *-e*-plurals.

Table 9. Data on the prosodic constraint on German noun plurals

| | | WS subjects | Mental-age matched controls | Chronological-age matched controls |
|---|---|---|---|---|
| % of correctly inflected noun plurals that take the ending *-e* | group I | 69.4 | 77.8 | 95.8 |
| | group II | 55.6 | 92.1 | |
| | group III | 83.3 | 97.7 | |
| % of overapplications of *-e* to nouns that take other plural endings* | group I | 15.8 | 27.3 | 50 |
| | group II | 15.7 | 48.1 | |
| | group III | 30 | 58.6 | |
| % of stress-final singular nouns produced without overt plural marking** | group I | 41.4 | 16.1 | 4 |
| | group II | 32.5 | 11.5 | |
| | group III | 37.5 | 10.4 | |

*Overapplication rates for *-e* were calculated in relation to the total number of incorrectly produced noun plurals.
**Overapplication rates for unmarked forms were calculated in relation to the total number of stress-final singular nouns that were incorrectly pluralized.

A look at Table 9 shows that the WS subjects' mean correctness score for *-e*-plurals is at only 66.7% and, thus, significantly lower than the mental-age matched controls' score of 89.2% ($\chi^2$, p < .05). In addition, control subjects frequently overapply *-e* to produce noun plurals for nouns that take other plural endings. As evident from the table, about half of the incorrectly inflected noun plurals of the control subjects are marked with the ending *-e* (e.g. **Neste* instead of *Nester* 'nests' **Hemde* instead of *Hemden* 'shirts'). This is in strong contrast to the data for our WS subjects who display a mean overapplication rate for the marker *-e* of only 17.2% ($\chi^2$, p < .05). In addition, a considerable amount of the noun plurals that are incorrectly produced by our WS subjects do not carry any overt plural marking. The bottom part of Table 9 gives the percentages of those stress-final singular nouns that were not overtly marked with any of the overt plural markers. Note, that all native stress-final singular nouns (such as for instance *Nest* 'nest-neut.' or *Insékt* 'insect-neut.') are subject to the prosodic constraint on the shape of noun plurals and have to end in a reduced syllable in the plural form (e.g. *Nester*, *Insekten*). Producing unmarked noun plurals for these stress-final nouns (e.g. *2 *Nest*, *2 *Insekt*) leads to a violation of this constraint. As can be seen in the table, in 36.4% of the cases where an incorrect plural form is produced for a stress-final singular noun, our WS subjects leave the noun unmarked. The corresponding figures for the mental-age and chronological-age matched control subjects are significantly lower, 13.3% and 4% respectively ($\chi^2$, p < .05).

The lower correctness scores and overapplication rates for *-e*-plurals and the higher percentage of unmarked noun plurals suggest that a core characteristic of the German noun plural system – namely the constraint on the prosodic shape of native plural nouns – is not operative in the WS subjects under study here. Note that with respect to this prosodic constraint, there is an important difference between noun plurals on *-n*$^{(fem\ or\ nonfem)}$ and *-er* on the one hand and noun plurals on *-e* on the other hand. For the former, obeying the prosodic constraint comes as a by-product of the long-term historic effect this constraint has exerted in the language system on the shape of noun plurals. Noun plurals on *-e*, in contrast, enable us to see the prosodic constraint while going into action. When a stress-final noun comes out of the lexicon without ending in a reduced syllable, this constraint sets off the last resort operation of Schwa epenthesis which applies in order to make it possible to pass the filter on the prosodic shape of plural nouns. It is exactly this filter which does not seem to be operative in our German WS subjects. As a consequence, in plural formation a large amount of stress-final nouns is not epenthesized with Schwa but remains unmarked. This is in sharp contrast to the mental-age matched control children who regularly apply Schwa epenthesis in plural formation of stress-final nouns.

These findings cannot be explained by the assumption that the inflectional system is generally delayed in WS as proposed by Thomas et al. (2001). First, the discussed differences between WS subjects and mental-age matched control subjects can already be observed for the first subject group (group I). Second, there is no clear age-trend discernible in the WS subjects' data. Under the assumption of a delayed development, we would expect the correctness scores for *-e*-plurals to increase and the number of unmarked noun plurals to decrease with increasing mental age. Contrary to this assumption, correctness scores for *-e* decrease but not increase from group I to group II, and the percentages of unmarked noun plurals increase but not decrease from stage II to stage III. Finally, a general delay in the inflectional system should affect all types of inflectional processes. This however does not hold true. For *-s*-plurals, for instance, our WS subjects achieve even higher correctness scores than the mental-age matched controls, whereas their scores for *-e*-plurals are worse than the scores of even the youngest control children.

## 5. Summary and conclusion

The aim of our study on the inflectional system in German WS was twofold. First, we wanted to investigate whether the findings reported for English WS subjects carry over to the different inflectional systems of German. Our second goal was to contribute to establishing a grammatical profile of intact and impaired language systems that are characteristic for this syndrome in German and across languages.

In three experiments on German participle and noun plural inflection we find that the production of regular inflected forms is unimpaired in the WS subjects under study here. This finding is in line with results reported by Clahsen and Almazan (1998, 2001) and Clahsen and Temple (2003) for past tense, plural and comparative inflection in English WS subjects.

In contrast to the intact performance with regular inflection, deficits show up for irregular inflection. All five WS subjects investigated here exhibit problems with irregular participle inflection. These become evident in their impaired performance with frequent irregular verbs, whereas errors for the mental-age matched control children affect infrequent irregular verbs. Three of the WS subjects (subjects C., K. and M.) also experience major problems with the production of irregular noun plurals. In addition, irregular plural markings are significantly less often overapplied by these subjects than by the control children. The impairment with irregular inflected forms observed in our WS subjects corresponds with the results reported by Clahsen and Almazan (1998, 2001), who found that performance on irregular English past tense and plural forms was significantly more impaired for their WS subjects than the performance with regular inflected forms.

## 5.1 Selective deficit or delay?

An important issue raised by Thomas et al. (2001) is whether these findings are to be interpreted as evidence for a selective deficit affecting irregular inflected forms or whether they merely result from a delayed development of the language system. According to Thomas et al., the data on English past tense formation are best to be explained as resulting from a slightly atypical and therefore delayed development affecting the inflectional system. The data on German WS subjects, however, provide no evidence for a delay that generally affects the inflectional system. First and in contrast to the findings reported by Thomas et al. (2001), we found no evidence for a delay in the acquisition of the regular inflectional system. For the WS subjects under study here, performance for regular inflected forms was always comparable to the performance of the mental-age matched control groups. Their performance with *-s*-plurals was even better than the performance of their respective mental-age matched control groups, and for *-n*$^{fem}$-plurals and regular participles they obtained scores that were even comparable to the scores of the chronological-age matched controls. A general delay in the inflectional system should however affect these regular forms, too.

Second, the problems our WS subjects experience with irregular inflected forms are worse than what would be expected by a delay. Thomas et al. are right in pointing out that to provide evidence for a selective deficit with irregular inflected forms it is not enough to show that irregular inflection is worse than regular inflection in WS. Instead, it must be shown that the WS subjects' performance with irregular forms is worse than what is to be expected considering their level of language development (p. 148). This however is the case in our German WS subjects. In each of the three areas where poor performance of the WS subjects was observed – in irregular participle inflection, irregular plural formation and with respect to the prosodic constraint on noun plurals – their performance was even worse than the performance of the youngest mental-age matched control subjects. Moreover, the WS subjects' results do not improve with time, as should be expected if their inflectional system was delayed in development (for further arguments against the proposal of Thomas et al. see Clahsen & Temple (2003)).

In sum, our results on German WS do not support the claim stated by Thomas et al. (2001) that the inflectional system is merely delayed in WS. In contrast, the pattern of impaired and intact inflectional capacities provides strong support for an impairment that selectively affects irregular inflected forms in German WS. Moreover, the close correspondence of our findings and the findings reported by Clahsen and Almazan (1998, 2001) – obtained for different languages, different inflectional systems and different WS subjects – suggest that the selective impairment of irregular inflectional morphology is a characteristic symptom of WS cross-linguistically. This does not preclude the possibility that the severity of this impairment may be variable across individuals, nor does it exclude the possibility that this impairment may not show up for some subjects in some inflectional systems, as observed in the German noun plural system.

### 5.2 On the nature of the observed deficits in WS

Clahsen and Almazan (1998) suggest an explanation for the selective deficit with irregular inflected forms that is based on the morphological theory of Wunderlich (1996). According to Wunderlich's account, irregular inflected forms are stored in subnodes of a structured lexical entry (see Section 3). Clahsen and Almazan (1998) propose that WS subjects have difficulties in accessing these subnodes – perhaps because lexical access is too fast and sloppy for these individuals (Clahsen & Temple 2003). If the irregular inflected form stored in a subnode of the respective lexical entry cannot be accessed, regular inflection will apply to produce a form with the required morphosyntactic feature specification. While this account explains the selective deficit with irregular inflected forms and the overregularization of regular affixes to irregular verbs and nouns, the data on German noun plurals indicate that there is more at stake in WS. A closer investigation of the WS subjects' data for noun plural production yields evidence for an atypical performance with respect to -*e*-plurals, unmarked forms and the overapplication of the ending -*e* to other nouns. This could be due to some problem with the phonological operation of Schwa epenthesis. Note, that the WS subjects have lower correctness scores and lower overapplication rates for the -*e*-ending and hence apply Schwa in significantly fewer cases than the control children. Alternatively, the prosodic constraint that governs the shape of native German plural nouns might not be operative in our German WS subjects. In this case, the phonological operation of Schwa epenthesis is available, the WS subjects however see no need to apply it in plural formation as the filter on the prosodic shape of German noun plurals is not operative.

Which of these two (or other alternative) explanations might hold has to be the topic of further research. Whatever the outcome, the data on German WS indicate that besides a deficit in accessing stored irregular forms in the mental lexicon the language system is affected by other deficits as well. A closer linguistic investigation of the intact and impaired language systems in WS cannot only help in determining a characteristic profile of this syndrome. A thorough evaluation of intact and impaired language functions against the background of the severe mental limitations typical for WS might also provide important insights into the relationships and dependencies that connect language and other cognitive capacities.

## Acknowledgements

The research reported in this paper was supported by German Science Foundation grant SFB 282/C8 to Martina Penke. We are grateful to Ulrike Janssen, Claudia Hegenscheidt and Eva Neuhaus for their assistance in data analysis. Thanks to Susanne Bartke and Ingrid Sonnenstuhl for their valuable comments.

## Notes

1. The data of WS subjects C. and M. have already been published in Krause and Penke (2002).

2. We are grateful to Dipl. Psych. Ralph Schliewenz for making the data accessible to us.

3. Due to the small number of WS subjects tested, running parametric group statistics did not seem advisable. To give an impression of the magnitude of the observed differences, we calculated non-parametric chi-square tests for each of the three different WS and mental-age matched control groups individually.

4. There might be a tendency for both WS and control subjects to produce more -*t*-inflected novel participles for rhyming novel verbs. Note however, that the test material contained only three of these novel verbs.

5. For further psycholinguistic results on the different status of German *-n*-plurals – albeit with a slightly different interpretation – see Sonnenstuhl and Huth (2002).

6. Whether this low overgeneralization rate might be due to neighbourhood effects that prevent overapplication of the default affix *-s* to nouns that rhyme with other irregular noun plurals, as suggested by one of the reviewers, has to be left to further investigation.

7. Overgeneralization rates for *-s* were calculated as follows: the number of *-s* overapplications was divided by the total number of all errors with plural formation.

## References


Baayen, R. H., Piepenbrock, R., & van Rijn, H. (1993). *The CELEX Lexical Database (CD-ROM)*. Philadelphia, PA: Linguistic Data Consortium, University of Pennsylvania.

Bartke, S. (1998). *Experimentelle Studien zur Flexion und Wortbildung*. Tübingen: Niemeyer.

Bellugi, U., Marks, S., Bihrle, A., & Sabo, H. (1988). "Dissociation between language and cognitive functions in WS". In D. Bishop & K. Mogford (Eds.), *Language Development in Exceptional Circumstances* (pp. 177–189). London: Churchill Livingstone.

Bellugi, U., Wang, P., & Jernigan, T. (1994). "Williams syndrome: An unusual neuropsychological profile". In S. Broman & J. Grafman (Eds.), *Atypical Cognitive Deficits in Developmental Disorders* (pp. 23–56). Hillsdale, NJ: LEA.

Bellugi, U., Lichtenberger, L., Mills, D., Galaburda, A., & Korenberg, J. (1999). "Bridging cognition, brain and molecular genetics: Evidence from Williams syndrome". *Trends in Neurosciences, 22*, 197–207.

Bittner, D. (1994). "Die Bedeutung der Genusklassifikation für die Organisation der deutschen Substantivflexion". In K.-M. Köpcke (Ed.), *Funktionale Untersuchungen zur Deutschen Nominal- und Verbalmorphologie* (pp. 65–80). Tübingen: Niemeyer.

Bornschein, M. & Butt, M. (1987). "Zum Status des -s-Plurals im gegenwärtigen Deutsch". *Linguistik in Deutschland*, W. Abraham and R. Arhammar (Eds.), 135–153. Tübingen: Niemeyer.

Capirci, O., Sabbadini, L., & Volterra, V. (1996). "Language Development in WS". *Cognitive Neuropsychology, 13*(7), 1017–1039.

Clahsen, H. (1999). "Lexical entries and rules of language". *Behavioral and Brain Sciences, 22*, 991–1060.

Clahsen, H. & Almazan, M. (1998). "Syntax and morphology in Williams syndrome". *Cognition, 68*, 167–198.

Clahsen, H. & Almazan, M. (2001). "Compounding and inflection in language impairment: Evidence from Williams Syndrome (and SLI)". *Lingua, 111*, 729–757.

Clahsen, H. & Temple, C. (2003). "Words and rules in children with Williams syndrome". In Y. Levy & J. Schaeffer (Eds.), *Language Competence across Populations: Towards a definition of specific language impairment in children* (pp. 323–352). Mahwah, NJ: LEA.

Dressler, W. U. (1999). "Why collapse morphological concepts?" *Behavioral and Brain Sciences, 22*, 1021.

Golston, C. & Wiese, R. (1996). "Zero morphology and constraint interaction: Subtraction and epenthesis in German dialects". *Yearbook of Morphology, 1995*, 143–159.

Gosch, A. & Pankau, R. (1996). "Longitudinal study of the cognitive development in children with Williams-Beuren syndrome". *American Journal of Medical Genetics, 61*, 26–29.

Indefrey, P. (1999). "Some problems with the lexical status of nondefault inflection". *Behavioral and Brain Sciences, 22*, 1025.

Janda, R. D. (1990). "Frequency, markedness, and morphological change: On predicting the spread of noun-plural -s in Modern High German and West Germanic". *Proceedings of the 7th Eastern States Conference on Linguistics*, 136–153.

Karmiloff-Smith, A., Grant, J., Berthoud, J., Davies, M., Howlin, P., & Udwin, O. (1997). "Language in Williams syndrome: How intact is 'intact'?" *Child Development, 68*, 246–262.

Krause, M. & Penke, M. (2002). "Inflectional morphology in German Williams syndrome". *Brain and Cognition, 48*, 410–412.

Marcus, G., Brinkmann, U., Clahsen, H., Wiese, R., & Pinker, S. (1995). "German inflection: The exception that proves the rule". *Cognitive Psychology, 29*, 189–256.

Mayer, M. (1969). *Frog, Where are You?* New York: Dial Books for Young Readers.

Neef, M. (1998). "The reduced syllable plural in German". In R. Fabri, A. Ortmann, & T. Parodi (Eds.), *Models of inflection* (pp. 244–265). Tübingen: Niemeyer.

Penke, M. (2002). Flexion im Mentalen Lexikon: Eine neuro- und psycholinguistische Perspektive. Unpublished postdoctoral thesis, University of Duesseldorf. http://www.phil-fak.uni-duesseldorf.de/sfb282/c8/Habil_Martina_Penke.pdf

Penke, M., Janssen, U., & Krause, M. (1999). "The representation of inflectional morphology: Evidence from Broca's aphasia". *Brain and Language, 68*, 225–232.

Penke, M. & Krause, M. (1999). "Broca's aphasia and German plural formation". *Brain and Language, 69*, 311–313.

Penke, M. & Krause, M. (2002). "German noun plurals: A challenge to the Dual-Mechanism Model". *Brain and Language, 81*, 303–311.

Rice, M., Mervis, C., Klein, B., & Rice, K. (1999). "Children with WS do not show an EOI stage". Paper presented at 24th Boston University Conference on Language Development, November 1999.

Sonnenstuhl, I., Eisenbeiss, S., & Clahsen, H. (1999). "Morphological priming in the German mental lexicon". *Cognition, 72*, 203–236.

Sonnenstuhl, I. & Huth, A. (2002). "Processing and representation of German -n plurals: A dual mechanism approach". *Brain and Language, 81*, 276–290.

Thomas, M. S. C., Grant, J., Barham, Z., Gsödl, M., Laing, E., Lakusta, L., Tyler, L. K., Grice, S., Paterson, S., & Karmiloff-Smith, A. (2001). "Past tense formation in Williams syndrome". *Language and Cognitive Processes, 16*(2/3), 143–176.

Volterra, V., Capirci, O., Pezzini, G., Sabbadini, L., & Vicari, S. (1996). "Linguistic abilities in Italian children with Williams syndrome". *Cortex, 32*, 663–677.

Wang, P. & Bellugi, U. (1994). "Evidence from two genetic syndromes for a dissociation between verbal and visual-spatial short-term memory". *Journal of Clinical and Experimental Neuropsychology, 16*, 317–322.

Weyerts, H. (1997). Reguläre und irreguläre Flexion: psycholinguistische und neuropsychologische Ergebnisse zu Erwerb, Verarbeitung und mentaler Repräsentation. Dissertation University of Duesseldorf.

Wiese, R. (1996). *The Phonology of German*. Oxford: OUP.

Wunderlich, D. (1996). "A minimalist model of inflectional morphology". In C. Wilder (Eds.), *The Role of Economy Principles in Linguistic Theory* (pp. 267–298). Berlin: Akademie-Verlag.

Wunderlich, D. (1999). "German noun plural reconsidered". *Behavioral and Brain Sciences, 22*, 1044–1045.

## Appendix

*List of tested verbs and nouns:*

| | |
|---|---|
| regular verbs | bellen, bremsen, fegen, heften, kleben, kneten, pellen, pressen, schleppen, schmecken, drehen, leben, legen, lernen, melden, rechnen, retten, stellen, trennen, glühen, klauen, knüpfen, löschen |
| irregular verbs | fechten, stechen, flechten, schmelzen, werben, nehmen, treffen, werfen, helfen, sprechen, sterben, essen, geben, lesen, sehen, treten, messen, pfeifen, schreien, schweigen, leiden, streichen, saufen, lügen, schwören, trügen |
| -*s*-plurals | Hotel, Auto, Streik, Foto, Tip, Büro, Zebra, Park, Detail, Brikett, Karton, Wrack, Labor, Schal, Opa, Moped, Taxi, Ballon, Bar, Krimi |
| -$n^{fem}$-plurals | Farbe, Flasche, Karte, Kerze, Nonne, Ehe, Stufe, Taube, Wange, Ware, Ratte, Achse, Kasse, Krise, Laune, Tulpe, Nase, Seife, Spitze, Suppe |
| -$n^{nonfem}$-plurals | Bauer, Fürst, Hemd, Muskel, Nerv, Ohr, Planet, Schmerz, Typ, Solist, Insekt, Pantoffel, Bär, Dorn, Fink, Komet, Narr, Pastor, Stachel, Vetter |
| -*er*-plurals | Licht, Rad, Feld, Gesicht, Blatt, Fach, Haus, Grab, Amt, Schild, Tuch, Gespenst, Lamm, Wurm, Mund, Korn, Biest, Kraut, Gemach, Nest |
| -*e*-plurals | Berg, Brief, Stuhl, Hund, Raum, Traum, Fluss, Film, Kuh, Brot, Braut, Beet, Bach, Elch, Dolch, Bus, Bauch, Ast, Bart, Tisch |

# Emergent linguistic competence in children with Williams syndrome*

## A study of Hebrew speaking toddlers

Yonata Levy
The Hebrew University, Israel

This chapter reports a longitudinal follow-up of two Hebrew speaking toddlers with Williams syndrome, whose linguistic profiles have been compared to the profiles of MLU matched typically developing children. The data suggested asynchrony between MLU and grammatical complexity in the first 2 years of the development of grammar. Error rates as well as percent of usage of certain variables differed from those observed in typically developing controls with respect to 50% of the variables on average. However, percent of complex clauses as well as percent of usage of noun+complement construction, which directly measure syntactic complexity, were mostly within the range of the controls. At no point in development were there unusual error types of the kind that are never encountered in typically developing children. It is suggested that this developmental pattern is related to issues of timing and should not be interpreted as deviance and atypicality.

Williams syndrome (WS; Williams, Barratt-Boyes, & Lowe 1961) is a rare autosomal genetic disorder (1:25,000 live births) characterized by typical facial dysmorphology, renal and cardiovascular anomalies, statural deficiencies, characteristic dental malformation and hypercalcemia (McKusick 1988). Most cases of WS are sporadic (but see recent findings, Osborne et al. 2001). A microdeletion on chromosome 7q11.23 has been identified in 98% of the individuals with WS. IQ in individuals with WS is typically within the 50–70 range and their cognitive profile has been described as uneven with spared auditory short term memory and spared linguistic and face recognition abilities, in the face of serious deficits in number, visuo-spatial cognition, motor behavior, planning and problem-solving (Bellugi, Marks, Bihrle, & Sabo 1993; Gosch, Stading, & Pankau 1994; Mervis et al. 1999; Udwin & Dennis 1995). Anatomical brain abnormalities have been documented from an early age (Reiss et al. 2000; Jones et al. 2002). A distinct behavioral phenotype and a relatively well-understood genotype have made WS a particularly good candidate for brain-behavior studies and as such it has attracted the interest of researchers in a number of domains.

For a long time WS has been the prime example within developmental studies of the modularity of language. Recent work however, has challenged this view. Most important in this regard has been the argument set forth by Karmiloff-Smith and colleagues against the adoption of static adult neuropsychological models as a framework for understanding developmental disorders. Karmiloff-Smith (1998) and Karmiloff-Smith, Sceriff and Thomas (2002) point to the role that development itself may play in shaping the end state knowledge. The authors claim that abnormal brains such as characterize congenital neurodevelopmental disorders, necessarily follow an abnormal developmental trajectory. Learning is affected by the initial neuro-computational impairments as well as by the way the initial state interacts with inner brain environments and external learning environments. It is argued that in cases of genetic disorders affecting brain structure, development proceeds under a different set of constraints that cause deviance from the normal rather than mere delay. The result may be an impaired knowledge state or a seemingly intact mature performance that serves to mask a changed acquisition route.

Is it necessarily the case that in congenital disorders that result in brain pathology language development is atypical? Brain development is a plastic process and the brain is more malleable than has been thought before both as a function of its internal status as well as of external influences and learning experiences. While pathology in brain development may alter the function of developing networks and affect cognitive development, the principles that explain such development remain the same as those that explain normal development (see Pennington 1999). It is possible that the behavioral consequences of the plasticity that is inherent in the brain throughout life and in young brains in particular, might mirror normal trajectories even in the face of structural abnormalities, at least during the early developmental phases. At a later stage however, plasticity may exhaust much of its resources.

Traditionally, brain plasticity has been defined as the capacity of the brain to diminish the impacts of lesions through structural functional changes (cf. Bach 1990). Because specific functional deficits often occur after injury to certain neuroanatomical locations, it has been tempting to suggest that, within the brain, structure equals function (Boyeson, Jones, & Harmon 1994). However, a structural approach does not offer sufficient developmental flexibility whereas evidence for brain maturation and experience dependent changes have been documented in many different structures (Hertz-Pannier 1999; Huttenlocher, de Courten, Garey, & Van der Loos 1982). Consider for example, the well-documented fact of a transient phase of synaptic over-abundance that is observed in the young normal brain. This period is followed by selective synaptic regression that occurs as a function of exposure to experience. This early synapse abundance is biologically driven and is likely to form the neurobiological correlates of both learning and individual variability of cortical anatomy and functional organization (Hertz-Pannier 1999).

Greenough, Black and Wallace (1987) suggest a linking between the period of excess of synaptic structures and what they refer to as learning effects produced by experience-expectant information. By experience-expectant information Greenough et al. (1987) mean the kind of experience that every member of the species is likely to encounter. The production of an excess of synapses, which are eventually selected by an experience-based process, seems to underlie what is being referred to as the sensitive period in young age. While later synapse formation is localized to regions where the type of information that the event presents is processed, early synapse formation has been observed in a number of areas in the brain (Karni & Bertini 1997; Karni et al. 1998). One may hypothesize that a similar mechanism could guarantee a normal course of language acquisition even under brain pathology such as is seen in congenital neurodevelopmental disorders.

In sum, whether genetic disorders affecting brain structure result in atypical developmental trajectories for language or whether the mechanism of brain plasticity can compensate for the anomaly and allow the brain to learn in the "right" way, is an empirical question that should be studied with respect to specific syndromes. An answer to this question requires a fine-grained analysis of the behavioral phenotype. It likewise requires a definition, or at least a discussion of what is meant by typicality.

Obvious cases of atypical development concern phenomena which are never attested in normal children. For example, Capirci, Sabbadini and Volterra (1996) report of an Italian speaking child with WS who, despite proficient syntax, made errors of agreement and of pronominalization that have never been attested in normal children. Note however, that this is the only report in the literature of such unusual language in WS nor has this been commonly reported in other disordered populations. Rather, what is commonly observed in disordered populations is atypical division of labor among acquisition strategies, for example, more extensive use of rote memorization in comparison with rule guided behavior than is seen in normally developing children (Karmiloff-Smith et al. 1997; Thomas et al. 2001). Developmental asynchrony between components of language has been likewise, frequently reported.

Does asynchrony indicate deviance from normalcy or is it an issue of timing and therefore an indication of delay rather than of atypicality? In its strong sense, normalcy predicts typical timing along with other characteristics. Under this interpretation delay of whatever kind would be a special case of deviation from the typical trajectory. Thus, the fact that language acquisition in children with neurodevelopmental disorders is typically late is sufficient in itself to deem it deviant. Developmental asynchrony within the language faculty becomes a special case of the latter. Note that such a strong sense of normalcy renders the claims of atypical learning trajectories under pathology, such as are expressed by Karmiloff-Smith (1998) and by Thomas et al. (2001), empirically trivial since delays in the onset of language characterize almost all of the neurodevelopmental disorders.

Based on considerations of modularity of linguistic sub-systems, and given the available knowledge concerning different timing of the development of brain areas (see Nelson & Luciana 2001), a weaker sense of "normal" may be more appropriate. On this weaker view one may talk about atypicality as a result of brain reorganization if indeed there are substantive differences in the way learning progresses that go beyond issues of timing. Delay in the emergence of language as well as asynchrony in the development of various linguistic components is the cost of reorganization which could nevertheless result in normal acquisition.

The current chapter will report of a study of emergent linguistic competence in Hebrew speaking toddlers with WS. It outlines developmental trajectories at the early stages of grammatical development. While the debate about the nature of WS underlying grammatical competence has centered on the nature of mature (or at least, fluent) linguistic knowledge, we believe that the focus should be on the early phases of development for this is when plasticity is most likely to take effect.

Before we consider findings that relate to the early phases of grammar acquisition in WS let us summarize the main empirical findings from older children and adults with WS that shed light on this controversy. This will be a brief summary since this work is referred to in great details in other chapters in the book. Karmiloff-Smith et al. (1997) report of impaired knowledge of grammatical gender agreement in French speaking children with WS whereas mental age matched controls were sensitive to gender agreement within noun phrases and extended their knowledge to nonce words as well, in which the noun ending did not match the gender of the noun. The individuals with WS did not demonstrate such knowledge of agreement. Levy and Hermon (2003) failed to replicate these findings with Hebrew speaking children. Surprisingly, the normal controls did not outperform the children with WS. All the groups in the study were equally poor in gender agreement when the phonological endings of the nouns did not match the noun gender.

Thomas et al. (2001) studied past tense formation in English speaking individuals with WS. Controlling for verbal mental age, the individuals with WS showed the same relation between performance on regular and irregular verbs as the typically developing (TD) children. However, deficits in generalization compared to performance on existing verbs, the effects of factors such as frequency and verb imageability produced unusual patterns of errors. The authors conclude that WS exhibit atypical developmental trajectory characterized by greater sensitivity and over-detailed phonological representations which are too specific to support robust generalizations.

Clahsen and Almazan (1998, 2001) and Clahsen and Temple (2003) reject this conclusion. Their findings suggest that individuals with WS have a selective deficit in irregular past tense formation pointing to deficient access or problems of memory, whereas their computational system is selectively spared, yielding good performance with regular verbs. Similarly, children with WS were as successful as the controls in compounding and in plural formation. Good performance in plurals and noun compounds is reported in Zukowski (2001) and in Bromberg, Ullman, Coppola, Marcus, Kelly and Levine (1994) as well. Krause and Penke (2002) too report of regular/irregular asymmetry in German participles and plurals, and argue for a spared grammatical system in individuals with WS. Finally, Lukács, Racsmány and Pléh (2001) found a similar regular/irregular asymmetry in the production of plurals in Hungarian speaking adolescents with WS.

Whereas morphosyntax in adolescents and adults with WS has been researched in depth, relatively little is known about the beginning phases of language development in children with WS. Examination of precursors to language in toddlers with WS showed reduced levels of pointing and impairments in triadic interactions (Laing et al. 2000). Pointing did not precede vocabulary development in the same way that it did in TD children (Mervis & Bertrand 1997). Overall delay was found in terms of the onset of canonical babbling, first words, as well as hand banging, which in normal children was found to be a consistent predictor of canonical babbling (Masataka 2001). Similar to children with other neurodevelopmental disorders, language in children with WS is delayed and development is slow. Singer-Harris, Bellugi, Bates and Rossen (1997) reported of a mean delay of two years. In a case study of a young child with WS, Capirci, Sabbadini and Volterra (1996) reported of a delay of one year. Below we report of a mean delay of two years in our subjects.

Vocabulary growth in WS was not correlated with joint attention (Mervis & Bertrand 1997). In a preferential looking task, toddlers with WS did not outperform toddlers with Down syndrome in matching words to pictures. Both groups performed at MA level and were significantly worse than CA normal controls (Patterson, Brown, Gsödl, Johnson, & Karmiloff-Smith 1999). As for expressive vocabulary, Mervis and Robinson (2001) reported of an advantage of two-year old toddlers with WS over age-matched controls with Down syndrome. The expressive vocabulary advantage was present even before any of the children began to combine words.

Thomas et al. (2001) argue that Clahsen and colleagues' work is problematic since it is based on four children with WS with a wide range of IQ levels. However, while case studies have limitations with respect to their generalizability and cannot characterize the syndrome as a whole, they can provide a plausibility argument in favor of one theoretical position over the other. With respect to the theoretical question under consideration in the current chapter, case studies are most relevant. If one can show that there are at least some individuals with WS who follow the normal course of language acquisition it would suggest that abnormal brain structure does not preclude the possibility of learning via normal developmental trajectories.

To the best of my knowledge, Capirci, Sabbadini and Volterra (1996) is the only published longitudinal case study of language development in a child with WS. Observations of this Italian-speaking girl began when she had about 20 words and no syntax. Apart from delay in the onset of language, the study reports of similarities between the acquisitional course followed by this child and the developmental course observed in normal children. However, some differences were noted as well. In particular, while the child had good vocabulary and proficient syntax she made agreement errors and errors of pronominalization of the kind not documented in normally developing Italian children. By the age of 4;10, the child's cognitive profile as measured on normative tests was typical of WS, with linguistic abilities better than visuo-spatial ones, although the latter were less impaired than one often sees in children with WS.

We report of a longitudinal study of two Hebrew speaking children with WS – Y and BT – whose linguistic profiles at various points in their development have been compared to the profiles of MLU matched TD children Below is a short summary of the linguistic phenomena in Hebrew that are relevant to the current study. Related acquisitional facts, describing typical development of the features that were investigated in Y and BT are summarized as well.

## A brief description of relevant aspects of Hebrew grammar and related acquisitional facts

Hebrew has the characteristics of Semitic languages, i.e. words are composed of consonantal roots cast in vocalic word patterns. The roots are usually triconsonantal while the patterns are in the form of vocalic infixes, prefixes and suffixes. There are seven verb-patterns – *binyanim* – and about three-dozen noun patterns – *mishkalim*. All verbs are analyzable into root+pattern. With respect to nouns, however, this generalization is only partial since some nouns do not have a recognizable root.

It is generally the case in Hebrew that the roots convey core meanings, while the derivational paradigms may partially introduce meaning modulations. While the formal paradigms are highly systematic and well-formedness is clearly defined, the semantics that the derivational patterns convey is only partially predictable from their forms. Hebrew has a rich inflectional morphology. Generally, verbs are inflected for tense, number, person and gender. Hebrew nouns are classified for gender. Agreement with respect to gender, number and person is obligatory between subjects and predicates as well as within noun phrases. Subject- complement constructions that are without verbs, traditionally called "nominal sentences", are well formed in Hebrew. An accusative marker *et* is obligatory. Note 1 gives examples of agreement, noun+complement constructions and the use of accusative *et*.[1]

The acquisition of Hebrew morphology has been studied extensively in recent years. Berman (1985, 1994) investigated the development of verb morphology. She argues that early verb use is rote-learned and thus, item based. Typically, the child has one verb form per root. Once the child begins to vary verb forms, each root will appear in many patterns and in a variety of inflectional endings.[2] Hebrew speaking children start out with *semantically* unanalyzed forms of verbs yet at the same period they can effectively control the necessary formal manipulations of the various root+pattern combinations. For quite some time children continue to use a rich variety of verbs in appropriate contexts, not knowing that these formal manipulations may be systematically used to achieve modulations of meanings. It is only around age 4, a long time after they have been using most verb patterns productively, that children's errors indicate that they begin to appreciate the semantics of the system (Berman 1985, 1994).

Previous studies of the acquisition of gender in a variety of languages, including Hebrew, show that children master the formal-morphological parts of this system relatively early (Levy 1988; Mulford 1985; Smoczynska 1985). Thus, even under age 3, errors of linguistic gender on inanimate nouns, which mark gender morphologically, are rare. In cases of animate nouns in which linguistic gender is determined by the semantic notion of gender, errors are common and learning is a more protracted process. These findings hold across all languages studied so far, among them Hebrew (Levy 1988).

In a cross-sectional survey of productive syntax in Israeli children ages 1;0–5;6, Dromi and Berman (1986) found an increase in the use of polyclause utterances and a decrease in the use of one-clause utterances, documented up to age 4. A decrease was observed in the production of nominal and copular clauses as well, along with an increase in the use of clauses with finite verbs. This is in line with the view that an increase in the use of sentences with finite verbs characterizes more advanced grammatical stages (Berman 1994; Rice & Wexler 1996).

Previous studies have shown that at or around MLU 3, children control agreement and errors become minimal. Crucial parts of the verb morphology are likewise acquired around this stage. A reduction in errors of morphology along with a wealth of derivational and inflectional forms suggests that the core structures of Hebrew morphology have been acquired at this developmental stage.[3] At about the same time, use of accusative marker *-et-* is almost error free and the proportion of complex clauses increases (Berman 1985; Dromi & Berman 1986; Levy 1988).

However, unlike errors of morphology, the amount of errors of syntax and meaning at this stage does not decrease in a similar fashion. In other words, while morphology has been largely mastered, the child's syntactic and lexical repertoires grow richer and more complex but her performance with respect to those aspects is not as yet error free (Levy et al. 2000).

In sum, the grammatical variables – listed below – that entered the profiles presented in the current study were chosen according to the following facts concerning normal development of Hebrew: similar to other languages, increased use of tensed verbs indicates that functional categories have developed. Reduced proportions of noun+complement clauses that are a common grammatical construction in Hebrew, along with increased proportions of complex clauses signal improved syntax. Gender marking on inanimate nouns is a formal morphological marker that is acquired prior to or around MLU 3. Agreement is a syntactic operation that children master when MLU is about 3 and the Hebrew accusative marker *et* is likewise acquired at that time.

## A longitudinal follow-up of two Hebrew speaking children with WS

The linguistic profiles of Y and BT, when MLU (in morphemes) grew from 1.8 to 2.8, were compared to profiles of TD children. These are naturalistic, longitudinal case studies in the tradition of the classical work on early language development (Brown 1973). BT – a girl, and Y – a boy, were studied in naturalistic play situations in their respective homes. The children had a confirmed genetic diagnosis of WS (FISH; Mervis et al. 1999). In both cases pregnancy and birth were uneventful. WS was diagnosed during the first months of the child's life. The children came from monolingual, middle class, well-educated families.

Data collection started when the children were beginning to combine two words.[4] Every three months three, one-hour sessions were held with Y and BT. All three sessions took place in the course of one week. The experimenter was instructed to interact with the child in a natural way, focusing on activities that encouraged conversation. Specific manipulations were not attempted. The sessions were audio-recorded and later transcribed by the person who collected the data. The same experimenter saw both children for the whole period of data collection. The analysis below is based on 18 hours of recorded conversations with Y and BT, divided into five periods covering the duration of the study.

Y was 3;9–5;3 years old and BT was 4;2–5;8 years old. Both children had an MLU of 1.8 when data collection started. MLU rose to 2.8 at the end of the study. The children were equated on proportion of utterances with MLU longer than 5 as well. This procedure controls for potential biases that are inherent in central

**Table 1.** Age, number of coded utterances, MLU and % of utterances of length 5 and above for Y and BT

| Period | AGE | | Size of corpora | | MLU | | % utterances 5 and longer | |
|---|---|---|---|---|---|---|---|---|
| | Y | BT | Y | BT | Y | BT | Y | BT |
| I | 4;3 | 3;10 | 601 | 652 | 1.8 | 1.8 | 7.7 | 6 |
| II | 4;8 | 4;2 | 532 | 407 | 2.4 | 2.2 | 13.5 | 9.8 |
| III | 4;10 | 4;7 | 509 | 642 | 2.4 | 2.1 | 13.9 | 11.2 |
| IV | 4;12 | 5;1 | 486 | 646 | 2.5 | 2.3 | 14.4 | 10.7 |
| V | 5;8 | 5;4 | 604 | 438 | 2.8 | 2.8 | 16.8 | 18.7 |

measures such as the mean. For Y the proportion of utterances of length 5 and above was 7.7%–16.8%. For BT this proportion was 6%–18.7%. Table 1 gives ages, sizes of analyzed corpora, MLU and percent of utterances of length 5 and above for Y and BT for the duration of the study.

Twenty TD children, ages 2;0–2;4, MLU 2:2–2:8 (mean = 2:6; SD = 0:16) served as controls. Percent of utterances of length 5 and above in the controls was 8.4%–15%. This percentage is higher than what has been reported in Dromi and Berman (1986) for their sample of Hebrew speaking two year olds. Note that the lowest MLU in the control children is higher than MLU in Y and BT's earliest recordings. Thus, the controls are matched to Y and BT on MLU and on percent of utterances longer than 5 for period II–V, yet not for period I. While there were TD children in our sample with an MLU under 2, they were not matched to Y and BT on percent of sentences longer than 5. This is an intriguing fact that will be discussed later in the chapter.

Each control child was seen twice on consecutive days, for a total of 1–1/12 hours. A similar procedure for obtaining speech samples to those described above was applied. Thus the control data was cross sectional rather than longitudinal, yet it was drawn from a group of children whose MLU and percent of sentences longer than 5 covered most of the period of data collection for Y and BT. This will be further elaborated in the section on Coding and analysis. For each developmental period a profile was constructed for the children, composed of 12 linguistic variables, and compared to the profile of TD children of equivalent language age.

## Coding and analysis

The complete corpora were coded twice, by two independent coders. Child utterances were coded according to the CHILDES system (MacWhinney 1995), supplemented by a special coding system for Hebrew texts (Levy 1995). Excluded from the coding were imitations, repetitions, game-like utterances as well as utterances in which there were problems of articulation. The files were later compared and disagreements over coding were resolved by discussion. Utterances for which agreement could not be reached were discarded from the analysis. Those constituted 0.8% of Y's entire corpus and 0.6% of BT's entire corpus. Thus the analysis presented below is based on instances for which there were complete agreement between the coders.

Coding referred to correct usage as well as to errors, and concerned all aspects of morphology, syntax, lexical choices and pragmatics. The coding of grammatical errors is problematic because of the non-standard use that may be found in colloquial speech and the central role that extra-linguistic context plays in the interpetation of utterances within discourse. Since the level of education of the children's parents was comparable to that of the researchers who did the coding, the coders' standard of colloquial speech was adopted as the baseline for coding decisions.

The errors found in the children's productions were divided into three main categories: syntactic, morphological and meaning. This broad division offered a first-pass impression of the children's performance, although dividing errors into these three categories involved some controversial decisions since certain errors related to more than just one linguistic aspect. Syntactic errors (**syn**) related to diverse syntactic phenomena such as subordinate constructions and the relevant functors, agreement, use of accusative marker *et*, prepositions and ungrammatical subject omissions which are cases of omissions of third person as well as of subject pronoun with present tense verbs.[5] Errors of morphology (**mor**) included formal errors involving root consonants, word patterns and inflections. Recall that in Hebrew one can often distinguish formal morphological from semantic errors.

Errors of meaning (**mean**) related to lexical, semantic and pragmatic aspects of utterances. For example, errors in word choice, use of incompatible terms and problems of reference were considered as tapping lexical-semantic problems. Utterances in which the child used a negative term and immediately contradicted it by using a positive term that reversed the meaning of the statment, or instances in which reference could not be determined from what was actually said were coded as meaning problems. Errors of gender marking on animate nouns, inappropriate marking of tense, person and number, and lack of definite marker when definiteness was required, were likewise counted among the meaning errors. Errors of tense, number, person and gender were coded as meaning errors when the focus was on the correct marking of the semantic concept rather than on agreement or on problems of morphological form.

As for the specific variables, those were chosen from among the variables studied in TD children, as summarized in the section on Hebrew. Based on the above, the following 12 variables were investigated: error types – **syn**, **mor**, and **mean**, percent of use of Hebrew noun+complement clauses (**hc**), percentage of complex sentences (**coj+rel**), errors of syntactic agreement (**agr**), errors of direct object marker (**et**), errors in gender marking on inanimate nouns (**gi**), errors of gender on animate nouns (**ga**), use of past tense verbs (**past**), errors of word choice (**wc**) and pragmatic infelicity (**prg**).[6] Note that all of the specific errors are also included in the overall count of the respective error category, i.e. **syn**, **mor** or **mean**. While gender marking on animate nouns, errors of word-choice and pragmatic infelicity as well as the combined count of meaning errors code for semantic and pragmatic aspects of the children's speech, the other variables are more clearly formal-grammatical.

Percentages were calculated in the following way: Percent of the different error types – **syn**, **mor**, and **mean** – was calculated out of the total number of errors committed by the child Percent of noun+complement (**hc**) and complex (**coj+rel**) clauses were calculated out of the total number of coded utterances for each child. Percent of use of accusative marker (**et**) and of agreement (**agr**) were calculated relative to obligatory contexts of usage. That is, **et** was calculated relative to the number of utterances in which an accusative marker was required, while agreement was calculated relative to instances of noun (or pronoun)-verb combinations.[7] Errors of gender on animate (**ga**) and inanimate (**gi**) nouns were calculated out of the total number of errors of morphology. Percent of past tense (**past**) was calculated out of the total number of verbs used by the child. Errors of word-choice (**wc**) and errors of pragmatics (**prg**) were calculated out of the total number of errors of meaning committed by the child.

The mean and standard deviation (SD) of the control group provide measures of the performance and the variance seen in TD children from period II through V. Y and BT were considered similar to the controls with respect to a given variable if their achievements were within one SD from the normal mean. In such cases Y and BT's performance was marked ^. If Y and BT's error rates were above one SD or their correct performance was below one SD, they were considered below the level of the controls, marked as –. If their performance was above one SD and their error rates were below one SD, they were considered better than the average normal child and their performance was marked +. A similar analysis was adopted in Levy et al. (2000) in which language in children with various neurodevelopmental syndromes was compared to the profile of TD controls. Conti-Ramsden (1998) and Johnson and Carey (1998) use a comparable approach in their respective studies. Note that our focus is on a child's whole profile and the way it compares with the profiles of the controls, rather than on performance on individual variables. Furthermore, by considering the distribution around the group mean, rather than the mean itself, we are picking up the variance across TD children within the same language levels as Y and BT throughout the period of the study. Thus, the comparison covers the range of performance seen in TD children who are MLU matched to Y and BT, correcting for the fact that data from the controls was cross-sectional, rather than longitudinal.

## Findings

Growth in MLU for BT and for Y over the period of the study is presented in Figure 1. As can be seen in Figure 1, both children show an increase in MLU of about 1 point on average during the 18 months of the study. Both reached MLU 2.8 in the final session. This level of MLU is achieved by TD children in the first half of their third year, whereas Y and BT were in the fourth and fifth year when MLU was nearing 3. Note that MLU for the first period of the study for both Y and BT is 1.8, which is outside the range of the MLU of the TD controls. A comparison can therefore be drawn between Y and BT and the TD controls in relation to four out of the five periods of the study.

Table 2 gives the performance of Y on the 12 variables for each of the five periods of the study along with the means and SD of the control group. Table 3 gives the scores achieved by BT. A dividing line is drawn in Tables 2 and 3, between the eight grammatical variables and the last four variables, which are primarily semantic. The latter are likely to be affected by the children's lower than normal IQ. Recall that a ^ sign indicates that the score achieved by the children is within one SD of the mean of the controls. A + sign indicates that Y or BT are better than the controls (they make less errors or show more usage). A – sign indicates that Y and BT are performing worse than the controls (they make more errors or show less usage).

Since period I is outside the range of MLU of the controls, the comparison will focus on periods II–V with occasional reference to period I. In periods II–IV, Y and BT have a similar percent of noun+complement clauses (**hc**) as well as a similar percent of complex clauses (**coj+rel**) as do the controls. This suggests that the combined measure of MLU along with percent of sentences longer than MLU 5 is not just measuring length but in fact captures knowledge of syntax as it is

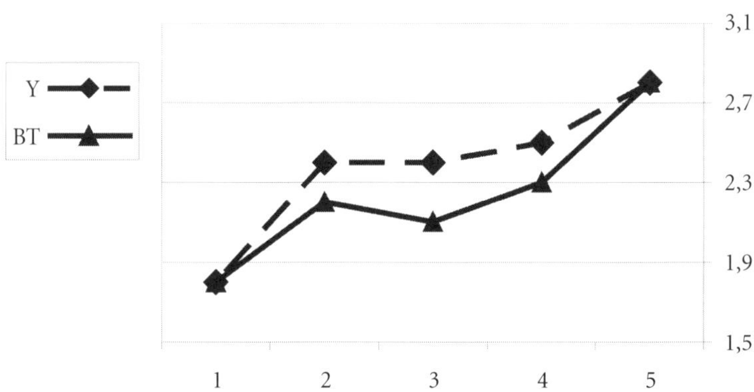


**Figure 1.** MLU for Y and BT for periods I–V

**Table 2.** Language profiles of Y measured on 12 linguistic variables and their status relative to the mean performance (+/– SD) of typically developing controls

| variables | Controls mean % (SD) | 1 | 2 | 3 | 4 | 5 |
|---|---|---|---|---|---|---|
| syn | 29.5 | 22.9 | 17.9 | 17.9 | 17.9 | 31.5 |
| | SD = 9.56 | ^ | + | + | + | ^ |
| mor | 13.6 | 20.5 | 12.8 | 11.9 | 11.0 | 8.5 |
| | SD = 8.64 | ^ | ^ | ^ | ^ | ^ |
| hc | 12.3 | 14.1 | 6.6 | 6.2 | 6.0 | 6.8 |
| | SD = 6.8 | ^ | ^ | ^ | ^ | ^ |
| coj+rel | 5.5 | 4.2 | 3.3 | 5.5 | 7.7 | 13.5 |
| | SD = 4.9 | ^ | ^ | ^ | ^ | + |
| past | 21.4 | 3 | 30 | 21 | 13 | 16 |
| | SD = 7.65 | – | + | ^ | – | ^ |
| et | 6.6 | 6.1 | 11.1 | 11.8 | 12.5 | 3.3 |
| | SD = 2.2 | ^ | – | – | – | + |
| gi | 3.1 | 0 | 0.5 | 0.4 | 0.4 | 1.5 |
| | SD = 2.3 | + | + | + | + | ^ |
| agr | 8.5 | 16.7 | 0 | 0 | 0 | 7.9 |
| | SD = 4.04 | – | + | + | + | ^ |
| mean | 58.2 | 56.6 | 69.4 | 70.2 | 71.1 | 60.1 |
| | SD = 11.2 | ^ | ^ | – | – | ^ |
| ga | 10.6 | 7 | 5.4 | 4.9 | 4.4 | 0.7 |
| | SD = 5.4 | ^ | ^ | + | + | + |
| wc | 3.7 | 2.4 | 10.2 | 11.3 | 12.4 | 9.7 |
| | SD = 1.2 | + | – | – | – | – |
| prg | 8.9 | 17.1 | 14.3 | 11.0 | 7.8 | 12.1 |
| | SD = 3.1 | – | – | ^ | ^ | – |

^ = within one SD from the mean
–/+ = below/above one SD from the mean
syn = percent of syntactic errors
mor = percent of errors of morphology
mean = percent of meaning errors
hc = percent of verbless clauses
coj+rel = percent of complex clauses
past = percent of past tense verbs
ct = percent errors of use of direct object marker
gi = percent of errors of gender in inanimate nouns
agr = percent of errors of agreement
ga = percent of errors of gender in animate nouns
wc = percent of errors of word choice
prg = percent of errors of pragmatics

**Table 3.** Language profiles of BT measured on 12 linguistic variables and their status relative to the mean performance (+/– SD) of typically developing controls

| variables | Controls mean % (SD) | 1 | 2 | 3 | 4 | 5 |
|---|---|---|---|---|---|---|
| syn | 29.5 | 15.9 | 40.4 | 17.4 | 18.5 | 19.6 |
| | SD = 9.56 | + | – | + | + | + |
| mor | 13.6 | 12.7 | 27.9 | 13.2 | 10.2 | 10.1 |
| | SD = 8.64 | ^ | – | ^ | ^ | ^ |
| hc | 12.3 | 13.9 | 5.1 | 8.1 | 6.3 | 6.9 |
| | SD = 6.8 | ^ | + | ^ | ^ | ^ |
| coj+rel | 5.5 | 2.4 | 3.1 | 4.2 | 5 | 10.8 |
| | SD = 4.9 | ^ | ^ | ^ | ^ | + |
| past | 21.4 | 24 | 22 | 13 | 17 | 26 |
| | SD = 7.65 | ^ | ^ | – | ^ | ^ |
| et | 6.6 | 11.8 | 8.7 | 10.5 | 0 | 0 |
| | SD = 2.2 | – | ^ | – | + | + |
| gi | 3.1 | 0.5 | 0 | 0 | 0.4 | 0.9 |
| | SD = 2.3 | + | + | + | + | ^ |
| agr | 8.5 | 0 | 7.7 | 3.9 | 0 | 10.2 |
| | SD = 4.04 | + | ^ | + | + | ^ |
| mean | 58.2 | 71.3 | 31.7 | 69.4 | 71.4 | 70.3 |
| | SD = 11.2 | – | + | ^ | – | – |
| ga | 10.6 | 2.9 | 7.3 | 2.6 | 3.2 | 1.8 |
| | SD = 5.4 | + | ^ | + | + | + |
| wc | 3.7 | 11.5 | 4.8 | 15.6 | 17 | 15.9 |
| | SD = 1.2 | – | ^ | – | – | – |
| prg | 8.9 | 15.3 | 5.8 | 15 | 12.1 | 12.3 |
| | SD = 3.9 | – | ^ | – | ^ | ^ |

^ = within one SD from the mean
syn = percent of syntactic errors
mor = percent of errors of morphology
mean = percent of meaning errors
hc = percent of verbless clauses
coj+rel = percent of complex clauses
past = percent of past tense verbs
et = percent errors of use of direct object marker
gi = percent of errors of gender in inanimate nouns
agr = percent of errors of agreement

–/+ = below/above one SD from the mean
ga = percent of errors of gender in animate nouns
wc = percent of errors of word choice
prg = percent of errors of pragmatics

reflected in the use of sentence types. In period V complex clauses in both children *exceed* the percent seen in the controls.

A consideration of the eight grammatical variables in Table 1 reveal + or – signs for Y in 50% of the cells. Table 2 shows 47.5% of the cells for BT with + or – signs. That is, the grammatical profiles of Y and BT differ from profiles of language matched TD controls on ~ 50% of the variables x points in time. Interestingly, 37.5% and 32.5% of the cells respectively, are marked as +, that is, Y and BT were doing *above* one SD of the performance of the TD children in over one third of the cases examined. Note that the +/– signs are not confined to certain profiles. However, both children do not have a single – sign in the final period of the study in any of the grammatical variables, and BT does not have – signs in the period IV either.

Within the eight grammatical variables, accusative *et*, gender of inanimate nouns and agreement are strictly formal and do not involve semantics to the extent that, for example, marking past tense does. Throughout the period of the study the children are either within one SD or above the performance of the controls on those variables, except Y, whose errors on accusative *et* exceed one SD during periods II–IV.

The differences between the profiles of Y and BT and the controls were recalculated relative to an interval of 1½ SD. This interval is more traditionally used to define non-normative performance (Leonard 1998). For Y, 22.5% of the cells are still outside the normal range, with 10% being above the performance of the controls. For BT too, 22.5% of the cells are outside the normal range, with 12.5% above the performance of the controls.[8]

## Summary and discussion

Y and BT are two Hebrew speaking preschoolers with WS. Their language development was studied longitudinally, since the emergence of word combinations. Linguistic profiles were drawn for the children at five points in time, when MLU was 1.8–2:8. MLU increased very slowly during the period of the study. In their fourth and fifth year, Y and BT were at an MLU level typical of 2;0–2;4 years old. Thus, similar to other studies (Capirci et al. 1996; Mervis & Robinson 2000; Singer-Harris et al. 1997), onset of language in our subjects was delayed and growth in MLU was slow. Note that delay is very common in children with other neurodevelopmental disorders, as well. In fact, it is the hallmark of language development in disordered populations.

The comparison drawn between Y and BT and the controls takes into consideration the variability seen in normal development by looking at a group of language-matched children and considering the distribution around the mean. We asked whether at any point during a given developmental phase (as measured by MLU and percent of sentences longer than 5), the profiles of Y and BT were similar to profiles of TD children. Thus, the focus of the study was the entire profile rather than individual variables.

Interestingly, we did not find TD children with MLU lower than 2, yet with percent of sentences longer than 5 that was equivalent to the percentage seen in Y and BT. This was the first indication that MLU may not be a reflection of linguistic complexity for Y and BT in the same way that it is in TD children.

Despite low MLU, percent of noun+complement constructions and complex clauses in Y and BT during period I was within the normal range, and performance on most of the variables was either within or above the range seen in the controls, whose MLU was higher. As for periods II–V, while the differences in performance between the children with WS and the controls were in both directions, the children outperformed the normal controls on 35% of the variables, whereas they were poorer on just 15% of the variables. Marking gender on inanimate nouns (**gi**) and agreement (**agr**), which are formal-grammatical variables, were among the variables that Y and BT performed the best on. These data suggest that MLU may underestimate Y and BT's grammatical development.

This conclusion does not hold however, in the case of the linguistic variables that are semantic-conceptual, where higher than normal error rates have been observed. This is not surprising given the children's general cognitive handicap. The increased number of errors in word choice is nevertheless unexpected in view of the reported good vocabularies in children with WS (Mervis & Robinson 2000). It is possible that these conflicting results are due to the different methodologies used in the respective studies. Mervis and Robinson (2000) were based on parental reports, which, while noting usage, are presumably less sensitive to the accuracy and appropriateness in context of the words that the children use. The findings of the current study show that when *correct* usage is the focus of the analysis, the children performed less well then language matched normal controls.

When grammatical as well as meaning variables are considered, the profiles show that during periods II through V the performance of Y and BT differed from the performance of the controls on 50% of the variables on average. Recalculating the differences with respect to 1½ SD resulted in a difference in performance on 22% of the measured variables.

Returning to the theoretical question at the focus of this chapter: did our study uncover atypical trajectories en route to mature linguistic performance? The longitudinal follow up of Hebrew speaking toddlers with WS suggests asynchrony between MLU and grammatical complexity in the first 2 years of the development of grammar. Error rates as well as percent of usage of certain variables differed from those observed in typically developing controls with respect to 50% of the variables on average.[9] Note however, that percent of complex clauses as well as percent of usage of noun+complement construction, which directly measure syntactic complexity, are mostly within the range of the controls. Since percent of sentences longer than 5 was controlled for, it follows that the relatively low MLU of Y and BT is a function of more usage of very short utterances and fewer utterances of length 3–4 relative to the controls. Thus, proportion of shorter vs longer utterances in discourse and amount of errors and correct use of specific variables are not synchronized in Y and BT in the same way that they are in TD children. Throughout the period of data collection, there were no unusual error types of the kind that are never encountered in TD children. I suggest that this developmental pattern is related to issues of timing and should not be interpreted as deviance and atypicality.

As reviewed in the Introduction to this chapter, many studies have found problems resulting from atypical timing in the language of WS. Thomas et al. (2001) report of an overall delay in the acquisition of past tense seen in regular as well as irregular verbs. The authors however, offer a different theoretical interpretation of these findings to the one discussed here. Studies of early language development in WS agree that there is delay in the onset of language as well as slow progression. Note however, that progress is typically measured with respect to MLU, which was shown to be problematic in the current work. Patterson et al.'s (2000) study showed a lack of advantage of toddlers with WS in word learning over MLU matched children with Down syndrome. These unexpected findings reflect an issue of timing of vocabulary development relative to the expected WS linguistic phenotype. Finally, Jarrold et al. (1998) argued that verbal abilities in WS develop at a higher rate than visual-perceptual abilities and this difference in rate of development predicted that differences in performance between those abilities will be seen in older persons and in particular, in individuals who have reached a higher level of verbal abilities. Differences among various sub-tests are minimal in individuals with WS who have low levels of achievements. This conclusion has recently received support in a longitudinal study of the individuals in Jarrold et al.'s (1998) original study (Jarrold, Baddeley, Hewes, & Phillips 2001).

In conclusion, in the early phases of the development of language, children with WS show asynchronous development, yet without any other signs of deviant language. Asynchrony in itself is insufficient to support the claim that the developmental trajectories that the children follow are atypical (Karmiloff-Smith 1998) but rather points to issues of timing that are related to the developmental pace of various components of language (Tager-Flusberg 1999). Disorders of timing are most clearly seen in the over all delay in the onset of language which is common in other neurodevelopmental disorders as well (Levy et al. 2000). What has been documented in the current longitudinal study with respect to individual variables is of the same nature.

Nevertheless, the statement that "development itself is the key to understanding developmental disorders" (Karmiloff-Smith 1998) is important, in that it shifts the theoretical focus from static adult models to dynamic developmental frames. From this perspective, a most important factor in development is the fantastic potential of the young brain to reorganize when there is pathology such that learning will occur in as optimal a way as possible. The data suggest that when there are congenital brain abnormalities, of the kind seen in WS, the reorganization will be such that while there are likely to be delays, the typical developmental trajectory will be followed, at least during the early phases.

## Notes

* This work was supported by grant no. 795/97 from the Israel Science Foundation. The author would like to thank the Israeli Williams Syndrome Association for their help in carrying out this research.

1. Examples (1)–(4) illustrate agreement patterns in Hebrew. Examples (5)–(7) demonstrate noun+complement constructions and the use of accusative *et*.

| (1) | ha-yeled | nixnas | la- | kit*a* | ha-xadash*a* |
|---|---|---|---|---|---|
| | the-boy | entered-sg/m | to(def)-class/f | | the-new/f |
| | 'The boy entered the new class' | | | | |

| (2) | ha-yald*a* | nixnes*a* | la- | kit-*ot* | ha-xadash-*ot* |
|---|---|---|---|---|---|
| | the-girl | entered-sg/f | to(def)-classes/f/pl | | the-new/f/pl |
| | 'The girl entered the new classes' | | | | |

| (3) | ha-yelad*im* | nixnesu | la- | xadar*im* | ha-xadash*im* |
|---|---|---|---|---|---|
| | the-boys | entered-pl | to(def)-room/m/pl | | the-new/m/pl |
| | 'The boys entered the new rooms' | | | | |

| (4) | ha-yelad*ot* | nixnesu | la- | xadar*im* | ha-xadash*im* |
|---|---|---|---|---|---|
| | the-girls | entered-pl | to(def)-rooms/m/pl | | the-new/m/pl |
| | 'The girls entered the new rooms' | | | | |

| (5) | ha-yeled | xaxam |
|---|---|---|
| | the-child | clever |
| | 'The child (is) clever' | |

| (6) | ima | ba- | bayt |
|---|---|---|---|
| | mother | in(def)-home | |
| | 'Mother (is) at home' | | |

| (7) | ima | ra'ata | et | ha-yeled |
|---|---|---|---|---|
| | mother | saw-past/f/sg | (acc.marker) | the(def)-boy |
| | 'Mother saw the boy' | | | |

2. For example, the root G-D-L may appear in the child's speech in the following forms: GaDaL 'he grew up'; hiGDiL 'he increased'; GuDaL 'he was grown-passive'; GiDeL 'he grew-causative'.

3. The full derivational system of Hebrew is not mastered by children until they are well into the school years.

4. In fact, the experimenter visited the children for nearly 6 months *prior* to the first session reported here. During that time there were no word combinations and the children spoke only single words. These sessions are therefore not included in the current report.

5. Hebrew has a 'mixed' pattern of subject omission. While subjects can be freely omitted in 1st and 2nd person past and future, omission is ungrammatical in 3rd person past and future as well as in all persons in the present tense.

6. Pragmatic infelicity relates to cases in which the child's choice of words or construction was such that, had the *general context* been different, that same word or construction would have been appropriate. Discourse exchanges in which the child does not respond to the investigator's questions and changes the topic inappropppriately, exchanges in which the child's response indicates lack of understanding of the requirments of the conversation are likewise coded as pragmatically inappropriate. The following are examples of pragmatically appropriate and inappropriate uses:

| | | | | |
|---|---|---|---|---|
| Ch: | ve-ima | ve-aba | yiknu | lanu |
| | and-mom | and-dad | will buy-pl.3rd | to-us |
| | 'And mom and dad will buy us' | | | |
| Res: | ma? | | | |
| | 'what?' | | | |

Omission of the direct object results in a grammatical, yet, referentially opaque and thus pragmatically unacceptable sentence. The following is an example of a pragmatically appropriate exchange:

| | | | | |
|---|---|---|---|---|
| Ch: | tavi | li | uga | kazot |
| | bring-3rd.fem.sg | me | cake | like-this |
| | 'get me a piece of this cake' | | | |
| Res: | ze nigmar, mictaeret | | | |
| | 'It's finished, sorry' | | | |
| Ch: | az | kazoti | | |
| | then | like-this-fem.sg | | |
| | 'so, like this one' | | | |

7. In Hebrew, adjectives and certain prepositions likewise agree with the head noun. However, there were no such instances in the children's productions.

8. For a comparison of Y and BT to children with other neurodevelopmental disorders see Levy (in press).

9. The coding system includes the option of 'comments' which allowed the coders to note exceptional errors. As stated in the text, no such errors were found.

## References

Bach, R. P. (1990). "Brain plasticity as a basis for recovery of function in humans". *Neuropsychologia, 28*, 547–554.

Bellugi, U., Marks, S. Bihrle, A., & Sabo, H. (1993). "Dissociations between language and cognitive functions in Williams syndrome". In D. Bishop & K. Mogford (Eds.), *Language Development in Exceptional Circumstances* (pp. 177–189). Hillsdale, NJ: LEA.

Berman, R. A. (1985). "The acquisition of Hebrew". In D. I. Slobin (Ed.), *The Cross-Linguistic Study of Language Acquisition* (pp. 255–372). Hillsdale, NJ: LEA.

Berman, R. A. (1994). "Developmental perspectives on transitivity: A confluence of cues". In Y. Levy (Ed.), *Other Children, Other Languages* (pp. 189–242). Hillsdale, NJ: LEA.

Boyeson, M. G., Jones, J. L., & Harmon, R. L. (1994). "Sparing of motor function after cortical injury: A new perspective on underlying mechanisms". *Archives Neurology, 51*, 405–414.

Bromberg, H., Ullman, M., Coppola, M., Marcus, G., Kelly, K., & Levine, K. (1994). "A dissociation of lexical memory and grammar in Williams syndrome: Evidence from inflectional morphology." Paper presented at the Sixth International Professional Conference of the Williams Syndrome Association, San Diego, CA.

Brown, R. (1973). *A First Language*. Cambridge, MA: Harvard University Press.

Capirci, O., Sabbadini, L., & Volterra, V. (1996). "Language development in William's syndrome: A case study". *Cognitive Neuropsychology, 13*(7), 1017–1039.

Clahsen, H. & Almazan, M. (1998). "Syntax and morphology in Williams syndrome". *Cognition, 68*, 167–198.

Clahsen, H. & Almazan, M. (2001). "Compounding and inflection in language impairment: Evidence from Williams syndrome (and SLI)". *Lingua, 111*, 729–757.

Clahsen, H. & Temple, C. (2003). "Words and rules in Williams syndrome and SLI." In Y. Levy & J. Schaeffer (Eds.), *Language Competence across Populations: Toward a definition of SLI* (pp. 323–352). Hillsdale, NJ: LEA.

Conti-Ramsden, G. (1998). "What is the nature of specific language impairment? Is SLI really specific?" In A. Baker, M. Beers, G. Bol, J. de Jong, & G. Leemans (Eds.), *Child Language Disorders in a Cross-linguistic Perspective* (pp. 47–64). *ASCLD, 6*, Universiteit van Amsterdam, Nr. 71.

Dromi, E. & Berman, R. A. (1986). "Language general and language specific in developing syntax". *Journal of Child Language, 14*, 371–387.

Gosch, A., Stading, G., & Pankau, R. (1994). "Linguistic abilities in children with Williams-Beuren syndrome". *American Journal of Medical Generics, 52*, 291–296.

Greenough, W. T., Black, J. E., & Wallace, C. S. (1987). "Experience and brain development". *Child Development, 58*, 539–559.

Hertz-Pannier, L. (1999). "Brain plasticity during development: Physiological bases and functional MRI approach". *Journal of Neuroradiology, 26*(1), 66–74.

Huttenlocher, P. R., de Courten, C., Garey, L. J., & Van der Loos, H. (1982). "Synaptogenesis in human visual cortex – evidence for synapse elimination during normal development". *Neuroscience Letters, 33*, 247–252.

Jarrold, C., Baddeley, A., & Hewes A. K. (1998). "Verbal and nonverbal abilities in the Williams syndrome phenotype: Evidence for Diverging developmental trajectories". *Journal of Child Psychology and Psychiatry, 39*, 511–523.

Jarrod, C., Baddeley, A., Hewes, A. K., & Phillips, C. (2001). "A longitudinal assessment of diverging verbal and non-verbal abilities in the Williams syndrome phenotype". *Cortex, 37*(3), 423–432.

Jones, W., Hesselink, J., Courchesnes, E., Duncan, T., Matsuda, K., & Bellugi, U. (2002). "Cerebellar abnormalities in infants and toddlers with Williams syndrome". *Developmental Medicine and Child Neurology, 44*(10), 688–694.

Johnson, S. C. & Carey, S. (1998). "Knowledge enrichment and conceptual change in folk biology: Evidence from Williams syndrome". *Cognitive Psychology, 37*(2), 156–200.

Karmiloff-Smith, A. (1998). "Development itself is the key to understanding developmental disorders". *Trends in Cognitive Sciences, 2*, 389–398.

Karmiloff-Smith, A., Scerif, G., & Thomas, M. (2002). "Different approaches to relating genotype to phenotype in developmental disorders". *Developmental Psychobiology, 40*(3), 311–322.

Karmiloff-Smith, A., Grant, J., Berthoud, I., Davies, M., Howlin, P., & Udwin, O. (1997). "Language and Williams syndrome: How intact is "intact"?" *Child Development, 68*, 274–290.

Karni, A. & Bertini, G. (1997). "Learning perceptual skills: Behavioral probes into adult cortical plasticity". *Current Opinions in Neurobiology, 7*(4), 530–535.

Karni, A., Meyer, G., Rey-Hipolito, C., Jezzard, P., Adams, M. M., Turner, R., & Ungerlieder, L. G. (1998). "The acquisition of skilled motor performance: Fast and slow experience-driven changes in primary motor cortex". *Proc. Nat. Acad. Science, 95*(3), 861–868.

Krause, M. & Penke, M. (2002). "Inflectional morphology in German Williams syndrome". *Brain and Cognition, 48*(2–3), 410–413.

Laing, E., Butterworth, G., Ansari, D., Gsödl, M., Longhi, E., Panagiotaki, G., Paterson, S., & Karmiloff-Smith, A. (2002). "Atypical development of language and social communication in toddlers with Williams syndrome". *Developmental Science, 2*, 125–143.

Leonard, L. B. (1998). *Children with specific language impairment*. Cambridge, MA: The MIT Press.

Levy, Y. (1988). "On the early learning of formal grammatical systems: Evidence from studies of the acquisition of gender and countability". *Journal of Child Language, 15*, 179–187.

Levy, Y. (1995). "Coding manual for Hebrew texts-Revised". *Publications in Developmental Psychology* 2. Jerusalem: Levin Institute, The Hebrew University.

Levy, Y. (in press). "Longitudinal follow-up of two children with Williams syndrome". *Journal of Child Language*.

Levy, Y., Tennebaum, A., & Ornoy, A. (2000). "Spontaneous language of children with specific neurological syndromes". *Journal of Speech, Language and Hearing Research, 43*, 351–365.

Levy, Y. & Hermon S. (2003). "Grammar in Hebrew speaking adolescents with WS". *Developmental Neuropsychology* (*Special Issue on Williams syndrome*), *23*(1–2), 61–85.

Lukács, A., Racsmány, M., & Pléh, C. (2001). "Vocabulary and morphological patterns in Hungarian children with Williams syndrome: A preliminary report". *Acta Linguistica Hungarica, 48*(1–3), 243–269.

MacWhinney, B. (1995). *The CHILDES Project.* Hillsdale, NJ: LEA.

Masataka, N. (2001). "Why early linguistic milestones are delayed in children with Williams syndrome: Late onset of hand banging as a possible rate-limiting constraint on the emergence of canonical babbling". *Developmental Science, 4*(2), 158–164.

McKusick, V. (1988). *Mendelian Inheritance in Man: Catalog of autosomal dominant, autosomal recessive and X-linked phenotypes.* Baltimore, MD: Johns Hopkins University Press.

Mervis, C. B. & Bertrand, J. (1997). "Relations between cognition and language: A developmental perspective". In L. B. Adamson & M. A. Romski (Eds.), *Research on Communication and Language Disorders: Contributions to theories of language development.* New York, NY: Brooks.

Mervis, C. B., Morris, C. A., Bertrand, J., & Robinson, B. F. (1999). "Willliams syndrome: Findings from an integrated program of research". In H. Tager-Flusberg (Ed.), *Neurodevelopmental Disorders* (pp. 65–110). Cambridge, MA: The MIT Press.

Mervis, C. B. & Robinson, B. F. (2000). "Expressive vocabulary ability in toddlers with Williams syndrome or Down syndrome: A comparison". *Developmental Neuropsychology, 17*(1), 111–126.

Mulford, R. & Morgan, J. L. (1983). "On learning to assign gender to new nouns in Icelandic". Paper presented at the Ninth Annual Minnesota Regional Conference on Language and Linguistics, Minneapolis, May 13–14, 1983.

Nelson, C. A. & Luciana, M. (2001). *Handbook of Developmental Cognitive Neuroscience.* Cambridge, MA: The MIT Press.

Osborne, L. R., Li, M., Pober, B., Chitayat, D., Bodurtha, J., Mandel, A., Costa, T., Grebe, T., Cox, S., Tsui, L.-C., & Scherer S. (2001). "A 1.5 million-base pair inversion polymorphism in families with Williams-Beuren syndrome". *Nature Genetics, 29, November 2001.*

Patterson, S. J., Brown, J. H., Gsödl, M. K., Johnson, M. H., & Karmiloff-Smtih, A. (1999). "Cognitive modularity and genetic disorders". *Science, 286*, 17 Dec. 1999.

Pennington, B. F. (1999). "Dyslexia as a neurodevelopmental disorder". In H. Tager-Flusberg (Ed.), *Neurodevelopmental disorders* (pp. 307–330). Cambridge, MA: The MIT Press.

Reiss, A. L., Eliez, S., Schmitt, J. E., Strauss, E., Lai, Z., Jones, W., & Bellugi, U. (2000). "Neuroanatomy of Williams syndrome: A high resolution MRI study". *Journal of Cognitive Neuroscience, supplement 1*, 65–73.

Rice, M. L. & Wexler, K. (1996). "A phenotype of specific language impairment: Extended optional infinitives". In M. Rice (Ed.), *Toward a Genetics of Language* (pp. 215–237). Hillsdale, NJ: LEA.

Singer-Harris, N., Bellugi, U., Bates, E., Jones, W., & Rossen, M. (1997). "Contrasting profiles of language development in children with Williams and Down syndromes". *Developmental Neuropsychology, 13*(3), 345–370.

Smoczynska, M. (1985). "The acquisition of Polish". In D. I. Slobin (Ed.), *The Cross linguistic Study of Language Acquisition, Vol. 1* (pp. 595–686). Hillsdale, NJ: LEA.

Tager-Flusberg, H. (1999). "Language development in atypical children". In M. Barrett (Ed.), *The Development of Language* (pp. 311–348). Hove, Sussex: Psychology Press.

Thomas, M. S. C., Grant, J., Gsödl, M., Laing, E., Barham, Z., Lakusta, L., Tyler, L. K., Grice, S., Patterson, S., & Karmiloff-Smith, A. (2001). "Past tense formation in Willliams syndrome". *Language and Cognitive Processes, 16*, 143–176.

Udwin, O. & Dennis, A. (1995). "Psychological and behavioral phenotype in genetically determined syndromes: A review of research findings". In G. O'Brien & W. Yule (Eds.), *Behavioral Phenotypes* (pp. 90–208). London: MacKeith.

Williams, J. C. P., Baratt-Boyes, B. G., & Lowe, J. B. (1961). "Supravalvular aortic stenosis". *Circulation, 24*, 1311–1318.

Zukowski, A. (2001). Uncovering Grammatical Competence in Children with Williams Syndrome. Unpublished dissertation, Boston University, Graduate School of Arts and Sciences.

# Wh-questions in Greek children with Williams syndrome

## A comparison with SLI and normal development*

Stavroula Stavrakaki
University College London

This study investigates the performance of Greek children with Williams syndrome (WS) on the production of referential and non-referential wh-questions and compares it to the performance of Specifically Language Impaired (SLI) children and normally developing (ND) children. The WS and ND children showed a high level of performance on the production of wh-questions whereas the SLI children's performance dropped significantly especially on object-wh questions. Error analysis indicated that WS and ND children produced mainly non-grammatical errors, i.e. conversion of referential into non-referential wh-questions, whereas the SLI children produced many grammatical errors. Based on the above results, I suggest that the WS children resemble ND children in terms of syntactic abilities, whereas the SLI children have severe deficits with wh-question formation.

## 1. Introduction

Developmental disorders are often considered to be those where there has never been evidence that a skill was previously mastered and has been lost (Temple 1997). Recently, subtle developmental disorders of higher cognitive functions, e.g. memory and language, have received great attention by neuroscientists, psycholinguists, and neuropsychologists. Specifically, the question of whether impaired/unimpaired linguistic performance reflects selective deficits/selective sparing in language development in developmental disorders (Clahsen & Temple 2003; Temple 1997; van der Lely 1999) or it reflects abnormal development of the entire cognitive system (Thomas et al. 2001; Thomas & Karmiloff-Smith 2003) has motivated a number of studies on atypical populations that exhibit asymmetries between linguistic and other cognitive abilities. Consequently, the study of Williams syndrome (WS) and Specific Language Impairment (SLI) has received significant interest since these developmental disorders could provide crucial evidence for the way in which cognitive functions develop due to their specific characteristics.

On the one hand, individuals with Williams syndrome exhibit a relative sparing of language abilities (Clahsen & Temple 2003; Clahsen & Almazan 1999; Pléh et al. 2003; Volterra et al. 1996) despite mental retardation. The bulk of research on linguistic abilities in WS is concerned with the question of whether morphosyntactic and/or lexical abilities in WS subjects can be described as intact or not (Karmiloff-Smith 1998; Clahsen & Temple 2003). Based on findings from investigations into morphosyntactic and lexical abilities of English speaking children with WS (Clahsen & Almazan 1998, 2001; Clahsen & Temple 2003; Clahsen, Ring, & Temple 2003; Temple et al. 2002), Clahsen and colleagues have suggested that lexical representations and/or their access procedures are impaired in WS whereas the computational system for language is selectively spared. However, the above proposal has been challenged by Karmiloff-Smith and colleagues who call into question the intact status of the relatively good – compared to other cognitive abilities – grammatical abilities in individuals with WS (Karmiloff-Smith 1998; Thomas et al. 2001; Thomas & Karmiloff-Smith 2003). Alternatively, they suggest that language abilities in WS reflect the abnormal development of the entire cognitive system; hence, there is no evidence for 'residual normality' in WS (Thomas & Karmiloff-Smith 2003).

On the other hand, the language development of children with SLI is characterized by severe problems whereas their cognitive, motor, and social development falls within the normal range (on criteria setting, cf. Stark & Tallal 1981). SLI in children is not a homogeneous disorder; there is much heterogeneity across SLI children with respect to the extent of the linguistic impairment they exhibit, the range of the linguistic subsystems involved (e.g. phonology, syntax, semantics, pragmatics) and the modality affected (e.g. expressive vs. receptive deficits) (Watkins 1994). However, relatively homogeneous subgroups of SLI have been identified (cf. Bishop & Adams 1989; van der Lely 1998, 1999). Research findings indicate that some SLI children have primary deficits in morphosyntactic abilities (Clahsen 1991; Clahsen et al. 1997; Rice et al. 1995; Rice et al. 1998; Stavrakaki 2001a, 2001b; van der Lely 1998, 1999; van der Lely & Battell, in press). Grammatical errors are a hallmark of these SLI children (Bishop 1994). These children, who over and above any secondary impairment in, for example, lexical or pragmatic development, have impaired grammatical abilities can be characterized as children with grammatical SLI (van der Lely 1998, 1999).

Due to the unusual dissociation between linguistic and other cognitive abilities in WS and SLI, direct comparisons between the linguistic performance of WS and SLI children may advance our understanding of the linguistic abilities/disabilities in both developmental disorders (cf. Clahsen & Almazan 1998). Previous comparisons of the results from the WS subjects to those of the SLI studies using the same experimental tasks indicated differences in morphosyntactic skills (Clahsen & Almazan 1998, 2001). The issue of whether the grammatical profile of children with SLI can extend to children with WS is quite crucial for the current debate on residual normality in developmental disorders (cf. Clahsen & Temple 2003; Temple & Clahsen 2003; Thomas & Karmiloff-Smith 2003). If developmental disorders such as SLI and WS are characterized by an ultimate abnormal functional architecture (Thomas & Karmiloff-Smith 2003), then linguistic performance on the surface regardless of whether it is good or bad, should result from abnormal functions in the underlying mechanisms. Although this account does not make a precise prediction with respect to the grammatical performance of individuals with superficially different profiles, e.g. individuals with SLI and WS, it can make a general prediction: Due to the ultimate abnormal functional architecture in both developmental disorders, some similarities in the grammatical performance of both disorders should be expected. Alternatively, if residual normality holds, then grammatical abilities should be intact while other cognitive abilities are severely impaired; specifically, grammatical abilities should be selectively spared in WS and consequently quite different from those in SLI (Clahsen & Temple 2003).

Adopting a comparative perspective to the grammatical profile of WS, in this study I investigate the performance of Greek children with WS on the production of wh-questions and compare it to the performance of SLI children and normally developing children. Furthermore, I report on similarities and/or differences between all groups' performance. Finally, I discuss the implications of this study for current theoretical approaches to WS; I particularly focus on whether the syntactic ability of producing wh-questions in Greek with WS can be described in terms of residual normality or an abnormal functional system.

## 2. The experimental study: Eliciting wh-questions from Greek children with WS, SLI and normal development

### 2.1 Subjects

The performance of three groups of subjects is presented here: one group of WS children, one group of SLI children and one control group of normally developing children. Information on the selection processes and details on the profiles of these groups are presented below.

#### 2.1.1 *WS subjects*

3 Greek children who were independently diagnosed with WS by multidisciplinary teams in Greek hospitals in Thessaloniki participated in this study. The diag-

**Table 1.** Chronological age, verbal and non-verbal IQ

| | CA | VERBAL IQ (verbal age) | NON VERBAL IQ (non-verbal age) |
|---|---|---|---|
| Filio | 14:10 | 51 (7:6) | 42 (6:2) |
| Giorgos | 10:5 | 83 (8:2) | 56 (6:2) |
| Eleni | 9:2 | 54 (4:9) | 48 (3:6) |
| Mean | 11:5 | 62.6 (6:9) | 48.6 (5:3) |
| (SD) | (2.5) | (17.6) (1.7) | (7.023) (1.5) |

nosis has been confirmed on the basis of the fluorescent in situ hybridization (FISH) technique, i.e. a specialized chromosome analysis utilizing specially prepared elastin probes. Details of subjects' profiles are given in Table 1. WS children's IQ was calculated on the basis of the Greek version of WISC-III test (Georgas et al. 1997). It should be noted that exact calculation of verbal and non-verbal mental ages was made only for Giorgos (verbal age: 8;2, non-verbal age: 6;2) and Filio (verbal age: 7;6, non-verbal age: 6;2). Eleni's exact verbal and non-verbal age was not calculated due to the fact that the Greek standardized version of WISC-III (Georgas et al. 1997) which was used in this study allows calculation of mental ages from 6;2 to 16;10; her scores on the Greek version of WISC-III indicated that her verbal and non-verbal age was definitely below 6;2. A pilot application of the WISC-III$^{GR}$ in 4 preschool children indicated that the normally developing children that reached Eleni's scores for verbal and non-verbal IQ were 4;9 and 3;6 years old respectively.[1]

### 2.1.2 *SLI subjects*

8 SLI children[2] participated in this experiment. All children were selected from child centers in Greece and met the exclusion criteria proposed by Stark and Tallal (1981), i.e. normal non-verbal IQ performance, normal hearing acuity, absence of motor impairment, absence of autistic symptoms, absence of otitis media history, neurological impairment and psychoemotional disorders. Details on their chronological ages and non-verbal IQ performance on the WISC-III are presented in Table 2.

There was no exact matching between children with SLI and WS; with respect to chronological age, the WS children are older than SLI children, whereas with respect to the non-verbal age, the WS children ranged between 3;6 to 6;2 whereas the SLI children performed normally (in accordance with their chronological age).

The linguistic abilities of the SLI children were assessed on the basis of the Diagnostic Verbal IQ test for Greek children (Stavrakaki & Tsimpli 1999). The performance of these children on the part of the test examining lexical and grammatical abilities is presented in Table 3.

These SLI children performed significantly better on that part of the test examining the lexical abilities than examining grammatical (morphosyntactic) abilities

**Table 2.** SLI children: chronological age and non-verbal IQ

| Subjects | CA | NON-VERBAL IQ |
|---|---|---|
| Nikos | 10 | 89 |
| Marios | 9:5 | 112 |
| Agni | 9 | 86 |
| Antonis | 8:6 | 102 |
| Manolis | 8:5 | 110 |
| Linos | 7 | 98 |
| Maria | 6:1 | 103 |
| Akis | 6:3 | 105 |
| Mean (SD) | 8:1 (1.4753) | 100.625 (9.2572) |

**Table 3.** Lexical vs. morphosyntactic abilities in SLI children: correct performance (%) on the lexical and morphosyntactic part of the language test

| Language test | Mean correct performance (SD) |
|---|---|
| Lexical part | 74.375 (8.6344) |
| Morphosyntactic part | 39.8763 (17.0638) |

[$t(7) = -9.192$ $p < .0001$]; hence, they were characterized as SLI children with grammatical deficits (cf. van der Lely 1999).

### 2.1.3 *Normally developing children*

16 normally developing children were also tested on the production of wh-questions. The chronological age of children is presented in Table 4.

As shown in Table 4, the children's mean chronological age was 4;4 (range 3;6–5;6, SD: 0.73). Therefore, the percentage of correct performance of these children on the production of wh-questions can constitute a measure of their abilities to produce wh-questions at this age. These children constituted the language age control group for the SLI children in Stavrakaki's studies on SLI (Stavrakaki 2001a, 2001b, 2002a, 2002b) The matching procedure between SLI and normally developing children was as follows. Each SLI child was matched to two control children on the basis of individual raw scores from the Diagnostic Verbal IQ test for Greek children (Stavrakaki & Tsimpli 1999). This group of normally developing children will also be used as the control group for the WS children. Recall that the non-verbal age of the WS children ranged from 3:6 to 6:2 (years:months); there were two children whose non-verbal age was 6:2 and one child whose non-verbal age was 3:6. The performance of the youngest WS child will be compared to that of the normally developing children aged 3:6 and 3:7. Due to the fact that normally developing children aged 5:6 performed at ceiling on all question types, normally developing children older than 5:6 were not included in the control group. On the

Table 4. Normally developing children: chronological age

| Subjects | CA |
|---|---|
| Maria | 5:6 |
| Thodoris | 5:6 |
| Stavroula | 4:8 |
| Anastasis | 4:8 |
| Dimitris | 4:7 |
| Markos | 4:6 |
| Angelos | 4:5 |
| Anna | 4:4 |
| Maria B. | 4:1 |
| Filio | 4 |
| Takis | 4 |
| Tasos | 4 |
| Konstantinos | 3:11 |
| Nikos | 3:11 |
| Vagelis | 3:7 |
| Petros | 3:6 |
| Mean | 4:4 |
| (SD) | (0.73) |

basis of their non-verbal age, the older WS children of the group are expected to perform at ceiling.

## 2.2 Experimental material and procedure

The experimental material consisted of subject and object *which-NP* and *who* questions. It should be noted that the formation of both subject and object wh-questions require two kinds of movement:

i. Wh-operator movement, that is overt raising of a wh-operator to a clause initial position (Chomsky 1986).
ii. V-to-C movement. This movement is obligatory in Greek and follows from the assumption that interrogatives have an abstract Q morpheme which occupies the C position (Chomsky 1991) and has the effect of attracting the verb to C obligatorily (Tsimpli 1990).

These two movements satisfy the well-formedness constraint on question formation, that is, the wh-criterion (Rizzi 1990), which is given in (1) below:

(1) Wh-criterion

a. A wh-operator must be in a Spec-head relation with a head carrying the wh-feature.

b. A head carrying the wh-feature must be in a Spec-head relation with a wh-operator.

Although both kinds of movement, i.e. wh-operator movement and V-to-C movement take place in both subject and object wh-questions only in object wh-questions the word order is OVS[3] whereas in subject wh-questions the word order is SVO, as shown in the examples in (2a, b) below:

(2) a. Pios htipise ton elefanta?
Who-nom-hit-past-3s-the-elephant-acc
Who hit the elephant?
b. Pion htipise o elephantas?
Who-acc-hit-past-3s-the-elephant-nom
Who did the elephant hit?

Referential (which-NP questions) and non-referential (who-questions) subject and object questions were included in the test material. There is a clear difference between referential and non-referential questions with respect to discourse presuppositions. The former but not the latter are Discourse-linked (D-linked) (Pesetsky 1987) in the sense that in those questions (*which-NP* questions) the speakers are required to introduce a set of presupposed discourse entities to which the *which*-phrase could refer.

In sum, 4 types of wh-questions were tested: referential subject questions, referential object questions, non-referential subject and non-referential object questions. Examples of the test material are presented in (3a–d) below:

(3) a. Pios pithikos kinigise ton elefanta? (referential subject question)
who-monkey-nom-chased-3s-the-elephant-acc
Which monkey chased the elephant?
b. Pion pithiko kinigise o elefantas? (referential object question)
Who-monkey-acc-chased-3s-the-elephant-nom
Which monkey did the elephant chase?
c. Pios kinigise ton elefanta? (non-referential subject question)
Who-nom-chased-3s-the-elephant-acc
Who chased the elephant?
d. Pion kinigise o elefantas? (non-referential object question)
Who-acc-chased-3s-the-elephant-nom
Who did the elephant chase?

To elicit wh-questions, games were designed in which the child asked a puppet a question about a scenario acted out with toys (cf. Thornton 1990). With respect to normally developing children and SLI children, six exemplars for each question type were tested giving a total of 24 responses per child. With respect to WS children, eight exemplars for each question type were tested[4] giving a total of 32 responses per child. For *which-NP* questions there were three animals, of which two were identical. In particular, suppose there were two monkeys in the workplace and a dog was chasing one of them. Then the experimenter proceeded as follows:

(4) Experimenter: *S afti tin istoria, o rinokeros kinijise enan apo tus pithikus*
In this story, the rhino chased one of the monkeys.
*Rotise tin kukla pion pithiko*
Ask the puppet which one.
Child: *Pion pihtiko kinijise o rinokeros*
Who-monkey-acc-chase-3s-the-rhino-nom
Which monkey did the rhino chase?

For the elicitation of who-questions, there were used three different animals in each story. Consider the example below:

(5) Experimenter: *S afti tin istoria, o rinokeros kinijise ton pithiko*
In this story, the rhino chased the monkey.
*Rotise tin kukla pion*
Ask the puppet who
Child: *Pion kinijise o rinokeros?*
Who-acc-chase-3s-the-rhino-nom
Who did the rhino chase?

## 2.3 Results

### 2.3.1 *Normally developing children*

The correct performance of normally developing children on all types of wh-questions is presented in Table 5.

As shown in Table 5, Greek children around the age of four exhibit mastery of wh-questions. The lowest correct performance was attested on *which*-O questions. It should be noted that even the youngest children of the group aged 3;6, and 3;7 showed a high level of performance on the production of wh-questions, especially on the production of who-object questions.

In Table 6, the error types attested in the data from normally developing children are presented.

The above error types were classified as non-grammatical and grammatical. The former included two kinds of errors: (i) Errors that do not indicate grammatical problems. (ii) Errors that were ambiguous as to whether they reflect a strategic, pragmatically motivated choice for avoiding syntactic complexity or difficulties with grammatical operations.[5] The latter included errors that indicated grammatical violations. It should be noted that two normally developing children

**Table 5.** Correct performance on the production of wh-questions

| Subjects | CA | Subject wh-questions | | Object wh-questions | |
|---|---|---|---|---|---|
| | | Who-S questions | Which-S questions | Who-O questions | Which-O questions |
| Maria | 5:6 | 6 (100%) | 6 (100%) | 6 (100%) | 6 (100%) |
| Thodoris | 5:6 | 6 (100%) | 6 (100%) | 6 (100%) | 6 (100%) |
| Stavroula | 4:8 | 6 (100%) | 6 (100%) | 6 (100%) | 6 (100%) |
| Anastasis | 4:8 | 6 (100%) | 6 (100%) | 6 (100%) | 6 (100%) |
| Dimitris | 4:7 | 6 (100%) | 6 (100%) | 6 (100%) | 6 (100%) |
| Markos | 4:6 | 6 (100%) | 6 (100%) | 6 (100%) | 5 (83.33%) |
| Angelos | 4:5 | 6 (100%) | 6 (100%) | 6 (100%) | 5 (83.33%) |
| Anna | 4:4 | 6 (100%) | 6 (100%) | 6 (100%) | 6 (100%) |
| Maria B. | 4:1 | 6 (100%) | 6 (100%) | 6 (100%) | 6 (100%) |
| Filio | 4 | 6 (100%) | 5 (83.33%) | 4 (66.66%) | 4 (66.66%) |
| Takis | 4 | 6 (100%) | 5 (83.33%) | 5 (83.33%) | 4 (66.66%) |
| Tasos | 4 | 6 (100%) | 4 (66.66%) | 5 (83.33%) | 4 (66.66%) |
| Konstantinos | 3:11 | 6 (100%) | 4 (66.66%) | 5 (83.33%) | 4 (66.66%) |
| Nikos | 3:11 | 6 (100%) | 5 (83.33%) | 4 (66.66%) | 4 (66.66%) |
| Vagelis | 3:7 | 6 (100%) | 6 (100%) | 6 (100%) | 3 (50%) |
| Petros | 3:6 | 6 (100%) | 5 (83.33%) | 6 (100%) | 3 (50%) |
| Mean | 4:4 | 100 % | 91.67% | 92.71% | 81.25% |
| (SD) | (0.73) | (0) | (12.17) | (12.13) | (19.13) |

**Table 6.** Error types produced in the obligatory contexts of wh-questions out of the total responses (96 responses for each question type)

| Error type | Which-S | Which-O | Who-O |
|---|---|---|---|
| NP omission in wh-phrase | 8 (8.33%) | 15 (15.626%) | |
| Yes/no question | | 3 (3.125%) | 3 (3.125%) |
| Who-S | | | 2 (2.083%) |
| No response | | | 2 (2.083%) |

did not respond to one of the questions the experimenter asked. In particular, they answered 'I do not know' and 'I do not remember'. This error type has been classified neither as non-grammatical nor as grammatical error.[6] The other attested error types were classified into these general classes, i.e. non-grammatical vs. grammatical in the following way:

(A) Non-grammatical errors

i. The omission of NP in which-S and which-O questions. This is the main error type in which-subject and which-object questions (8.33% and 15.62% respectively). Omitting NPs, children produced who-object questions instead of which-object questions. It should be noted that *which* (=pios) and *who* (=pios) are phonologically identical in Greek; hence, the omission of the NP in which-questions results in the production of who-questions. These responses cannot be characterized as ungrammatical; they are rather inappropriate in the sense that they do not constitute the expected adult responses. Note that the omission of the NP phrase occurred mainly in obligatory contexts of object rather than of subject wh-questions. Therefore, the slight drop[7] of children's performance on object D-linked questions is due to the omission of the NP in which-NP questions. A possible explanation should take into account processing factors. First, in which-object questions the A-bar chains are referential (Pesetsky 1987) and thus related to a pre-established set of discourse entities. Due to the discourse-linked status of *which*-object questions discourse related knowledge is required for their interpretation; in addition, syntactic knowledge of wh-movement is required as is the case for object questions (Avrutin 2000). Syntactic knowledge of wh-question formation has been acquired by normally developing children, as shown by their high level of correct performance on who-object questions; hence, the slight drop in the normal performance on which-object questions can be attributed to the discourse-linked status of wh-questions. In this way, the omission of the NP phrase can be explained. Consider the example in (6) below:

(6) a. *Pios rinokeros kinijise ton elefanta?* (target response)
Who-rhino-nom -chased-3s-the-elephant-acc
Which rhino chased the elephant?

b. *Pios kinijise ton elefanta?* (ND child's response)
Who-nom-chased-3s-the-elephant-acc
Who chased the elephant?

ii. Subject-for-object question. The normally developing children turned a target object who-question into a subject question. In other words, they applied the SVO word order strategy and produced subject instead of object wh-questions with OVS word order. Recall that the formation of object wh-questions requires application of syntactic operations (e.g. movement) whereas the formation of subject wh-questions can be achieved through the application of the default word order, i.e. the SVO word order. This error type may indicate problems with the wh-operator movement and V-to-C movement. It may also be due to a simple processing preference for the SVO word order to avoid extra computational processes. This error type cannot be considered as indicative of normal performance since few instances have been attested (2.083%).

(B) Grammatical errors

i. Yes/no questions with SVO word order were produced instead of who-object questions. This error type indicates difficulties with the wh-operator movement and V-to-C movement. First, no movement of the wh-operator takes place. Second, there is no evidence for the V-to-C movement at least in overt syntax. This is so because yes/no questions with SVO word order in Greek differ from declarative sentences in intonation only and they do not trigger movement to CP.[8] Consider the examples in (7) below:

(7) a. Pion esprokse o elefantas? (target response)
who-acc-push-3s-the-elephant-nom
Who did the elephant push?

b. o elefantas esprokse? (ND child's response)
The-elephant-push-3s-past
Did the elephant push?

This error type was produced by the youngest children of the study (aged 3:6–4). The few instances of yes/no questions that were produced instead of the target *who* and *which* object-questions (3.125% for each question type) cannot be interpreted as indicative of any problems with the object wh-questions due to the overall high level of performance of normally developing children on object wh-questions.

In sum, the performance of normally developing children indicates that Greek children aged 4 have already acquired the syntactic processes required for the formation of wh-questions. The few incorrect responses are mainly due to non-grammatical rather than to grammatical errors.

### 2.3.2 *SLI children*

The correct production of wh-questions by SLI children is depicted in Table 7.

As can be seen, the SLI children's performance drops on object-questions, especially on who-object questions. This pattern of performance indicates severe problems with producing wh-questions. The significantly better performance of SLI children on subject than object wh-questions – as shown by a paired-samples T-Test [$t(7) = -4.245$ $p = .004$ and $t(7) = -8.776$ $p < .001$ for which- and who-questions respectively] – can be attributed to the fact that subject-questions are produced by applying the least complex SVO word order, whereas producing object-questions requires the application of a syntactic procedure, i.e. the wh-operator movement.

Table 7. The correct production (%) of wh-questions by SLI children

| | Subject questions: Mean (SD) | | Object questions: Mean (SD) | |
|---|---|---|---|---|
| | Who-S questions | Which-S questions | Who-O questions | Which-O questions |
| Nikos | 3 (50%) | 5 (83.33%) | 0 | 0 |
| Marios | 4 (66.66%) | 6 (100%) | 0 | 1 (16.66%) |
| Agni | 3 (50%) | 4 (66.66%) | 2 (33.33%) | 4 (66.66%) |
| Antonis | 4 (66.66%) | 4 (66.66%) | 1 (16.66%) | 3 (50%) |
| Manolis | 3 (50%) | 4 (66.66%) | 0 | 0 |
| Linos | 3 (50%) | 2 (33.33%) | 0 | 0 |
| Maria | 3 (50%) | 2 (33.33%) | 0 | 0 |
| Akis | 2 (33.33%) | 3 (50%) | 0 | 0 |
| Mean | 52.08 % | 62.5% | 6.25 % | 16.66% |
| (SD) | (10.68) | (23.15) | (12.4) | (26.73) |

Table 8. Error types produced in the obligatory contexts of subject and object wh-question out of the total responses (48 for each question type)

| Error type | Question type | | | |
|---|---|---|---|---|
| | Which-S | Which-O | Who-S | Who-O |
| Who-S question | | | | 2 (4.16%) |
| Which-S question | | 4 (8.33%) | | 13 (27.08%) |
| Yes/no question | | | | 2 (4.16%) |
| Which-O question | | | | 7 (14.58%) |
| Case error | | 10 (20.83%) | 6 (12.5%) | 11 (22.916%) |
| Which-object question with case errors | | | | 2 (4.16%) |
| Wh-pronoun (or wh-phrase) | 23 (47.91%) | 23 (47.916%) | 12 (25%) | 8 (16.66%) |
| Gap-filling | | 3 (6.25%) | | |

Error analysis indicated that the SLI children produced many error types, especially in the obligatory contexts of object wh-questions. Consider Table 8.

The errors above have been classified as non-grammatical or grammatical.

## Non-grammatical errors

i. Subject-for-object question. This error type has also been produced by normally developing children. Few such errors have been attested (4.16%).
ii. Which-subject-for-who-object-question. This is the most frequent error type attested in the obligatory contexts of who-object questions (27.08%). The SLI children turned a target who-object question into a which-subject question; in other words, apart from turning object-questions into subject questions,

they converted non-referential questions into referential ones, as shown by the example in (8b) below:

(8) a. *pion esproxe i kamila?* (target response)
Who-acc-push-3s-past-the-camel-nom
Who did the camel push?

b. *pia kamila esproxe ton rinokero?* (SLI response)
Who-camel-nom-push-3s-past-the-rhino-acc
Which camel pushed the rhino?

iii. Which-object questions-for-who-object-questions. The SLI children turned a non-referential who-object question into a referential which-object question. It seems that the formation of a wh-object question is supported by the introduction of a referential NP. This preference for referential wh-questions may indicate difficulties with using the wh-pronouns in who-object questions. Being function words, the interpretation of wh-pronouns especially in the context of who-object questions requires pure syntactic procedures. By introducing a referential NP while producing wh-questions, SLI children seem to get help from pragmatic cues.

iv. Wh-pronouns for both subject and object questions: This was a very frequent error (47.91, 47.91, 25%, and 16.66% for which-subject, which-object, who-subject, and who-object respectively). The SLI children produced a wh-pronoun instead of the whole wh-question. For example, they produced the pronoun *pion(=who-acc)* instead of the target question *pion htipise o elefantas? (=who-acc-hit-3s-past-the-elephant-nom)*. This error type can be interpreted in the following ways. Consider first the possibility of methodological problems, i.e. the child did not understand the test instructions, as pointed out by an anonymous reviewer. However, if this were the case then the child should not produce any wh-questions at all. As the data indicates, the SLI children produced some wh-questions and especially subject wh-questions, which means that they understood the instructions. Another possible interpretation of the data is that the SLI children produced a wh-pronoun instead of the whole wh-question due to extraordinary difficulty with the computational component of language. Therefore, this error type may indicate extreme economical preferences by SLI children.

Grammatical errors

i. Case errors were found in the obligatory contexts of object and subject questions. This error type was a frequent one (20.83%, 12.5%, and 22.9% in which-object questions, who-subject questions, and who-object questions respectively). Case errors indicate problems with checking operations in terms of current syntactic theory (Chomsky 1995).

(9) **pion xtipise ton rinokero?*
Who-acc-hit-3s-past-the rhino-acc

ii. Yes/no questions with SVO word order instead of who-object questions (4.16%). This error type was also produced by normally developing children.
iii. Gap-filling errors (6.26%). These errors show problems with operator movement, as shown by the split between the wh-pronoun and the NP. Consider the example in (10) below:

(10) a. pion pithiko htipise o andras? (target response)
who-monkey-acc-hit-3s-past-the-man-nom
Which monkey did the man hit?
b. o andars pion htipise ton pithiko? (SLI response)
the-man-nom-who-acc-hit-3s-past-the-monkey-acc
Which did the man hit the monkey?

It should be noted that there was an error type that was a combination of grammatical and non-grammatical problems. Specifically, which-object questions with case errors were produced in the obligatory contexts of who-object questions (4.16%). The children made the following error types: (i) They produced a referential instead of a non-referential wh-question (ii) They made case errors: Look at the example in (11) below:

(11) pion kinigise o pithikos? (target question)
who-acc-chased-3s-the-monkey-nom
Who did the monkey chase?
Pion rinokero kinigise ton pithiko? (SLI response)
Who-rhino-acc-chased-3s-the-monkey-acc

In sum, the SLI performance is characterized by severe deficits in the production of wh-questions (cf. van der Lely & Battell, in press). SLI children showed low level of correct performance on object questions and especially on who-object questions; besides the non-grammatical errors produced by SLI children, errors indicating problems with grammatical operations, e.g. case checking errors, gap-filling errors and no operator movement errors (yes/no questions) were also attested.

#### 2.3.3 *WS children*

The correct performance of the WS children is presented in Table 9.

Table 9. Correct production of wh-questions by WS children

| | Subject wh-questions | | Object wh-questions | |
|---|---|---|---|---|
| | Who-S questions | Which-S questions | Who-O questions | Which-O questions |
| Filio | 8 (100%) | 8 (100%) | 8 (100%) | 8 (100%) |
| Giorgos | 8 (100%) | 8 (100%) | 8 (100%) | 8 (100%) |
| Eleni | 5 (62.5%) | 5 (62.5%) | 6 (75%) | 2 (25%) |

Table 10. Error types produced by Eleni in the obligatory contexts of subject and object wh-questions out of the total responses (8 for each question type)

| Error type | Who-S questions | Which-s questions | Who-O questions | Which-o questions |
|---|---|---|---|---|
| Object questions | 3 (37.5%) | 2 (25%) | | |
| Omission of NPs | | 1 (12.5%) | | 4 (50%) |
| Case error | | | | 1 (12.5%) |
| Wh-word | | | 1 (12.5%) | 1 (12.5%) |
| Wh-phrase | | | | |
| Subject | | | 1 (12.5%) | |
| Wh-question | | | | |

As shown in Table 9, 2 out of the 3 children with WS exhibited ceiling performance on the formation of wh-questions; this was not the case for the youngest child of the group, whose performance dropped especially on the production of object which-NP questions.[9] Let us compare the performance of the youngest WS child to that of normally developing children aged 3;6, and 3;7. These children performed at ceiling (100%) on who-object and -subject questions. Both of them showed a high level of correct performance on which-subject questions (100% and 83.33% for Vagelis (3:7) and Petros (3:6) respectively) and performed correctly half of the times on which-object questions (50%). Therefore, the performance of the WS child is lower than that of the control children; but the WS child shows a high level of performance on who-object questions and her performance drops on which-object questions, as is the case with normal children. Let us now look at the error types produced by Eleni. They are presented in Table 10.

The above error types have been classified in three categories. The first one included responses that were syntactically more complex than the target ones and so have been coded as errors indicating overuse of pure grammatical rules/processes. The other two categories included grammatical and non-grammatical errors, as was the case with normally developing and SLI children.

Errors indicating overuse of pure grammatical rules/process

i. Object-for-subject-questions. Eleni turned the subject into object questions. This is the most frequent error type in the obligatory contexts of who-S and which-S questions (37.5% and 25% respectively). It should be noted that the formation of object wh-questions requires knowledge of syntactic movement, i.e. wh-operator movement and V-to-C movement, as it cannot be achieved through the use of the SVO word order strategy.[10] Therefore, this error type indicates that Eleni exhibited sophisticated knowledge of wh-questions formation. Consider an example of this error type below:

(12) a. *Pia katsika filise ti gata?* (target response)
Who-goat-nom-fem-kissed-3s-the-cat-acc
Which goat kissed the cat?
b. *Pia filise i katsika?* (WS child's response)
who-acc-kissed-3s-the-goat-nom
Who did the goat kiss?

Non-grammatical errors

i. The omission of NP in which-S and which-O questions (12.5% and 50% respectively); in this way, who-object questions were produced instead of which-object questions. This error type produced by normally developing children.
ii. The wh-pronoun and wh-phrase (which-NP) instead of the whole question in the obligatory contexts of who-O and which-O questions (12.5% and 12.5% respectively). Since this error type has not been produced systematically, it cannot be taken as indicative of the WS child's performance. The same error type was also produced by SLI children.
iii. Subject-for-object wh-question. Just 1 subject who-question instead of the target who-object question was produced (12.5%). This error type was produced by both normally developing and SLI children.

Grammatical errors

i. Just one case error (12.5%) was produced; hence, this error type cannot be considered as indicative of the WS child's performance. This error type was also produced by SLI children.

In sum, Eleni exhibited sophisticated knowledge of wh-question formation. First, she showed high level of correct performance on who-object questions. Second, she overused the syntactic operations required for the formation of object wh-questions and produced object-for-subject wh-questions; the reverse pattern of performance, that is, the production of subject-for-object wh-questions was attested once. Third, her low performance on the obligatory contexts of which-object questions does not reflect grammatical limitations, as the main the error type attested in these contexts, i.e. omission of the NP in the which-NP phrase, is not a grammatical error. This pattern of performance is in agreement with that of normally developing children whose main error type was the omission of NP in the which-NP phrase. Forth, pure grammatical errors have not been attested with the exception of just one case error. This pattern of performance is also similar to that of the young normally developing children (aged 3:6–4) who produced few grammatical errors, i.e. yes/no questions instead of object wh-questions.

## 3. General discussion

In the present study, I have investigated the linguistic ability of producing wh-questions in Greek children with WS, SLI, and normal development. The aims were to determine whether there were any similarities and/or differences between the performance of individuals with WS, SLI and normal development. Furthermore, I was interested in determining whether the performance of children with WS on the production of wh-questions can be described in terms of residual normality or not.

Consider first the syntactic abilities required for the production of wh-questions in children with WS. The crucial test of assessing these abilities is provided by the correct performance on object wh-questions. Producing object wh-questions requires use of computational abilities as no default word order strategy, i.e. the SVO word order strategy, can be applied. The children with WS participated in this study exhibited full knowledge of wh-questions formation. This is so because the overall correct performance of WS children on object wh-questions is very high. Recall that the older children with WS performed at ceiling. However, there is heterogeneity in the performance of the WS children since the correct performance of the youngest WS child (Eleni) dropped especially on which-object questions. This drop cannot be taken to indicate any problems with the syntactic operations required for the production of wh-questions. Detailed error analysis indicated that the drop of the youngest WS child's performance on which-object questions is related to the D-linked status of these questions, as shown by the error type attested, that is, the omission of the NP. Therefore, the low level of Eleni's correct performance of object wh-questions cannot be attributed to difficulties with syntactic processes. Further evidence for Eleni's ability to apply the operation of syntactic movement comes from the fact that she produced object instead of subject wh-questions. In other words, Eleni appeared to apply complicated syntactic procedures to produce object wh-questions excessively, even in contexts in which unimpaired children did not use them (cf. Clahsen & Temple 2003).

Let us now compare the performance of the WS children to that of normally developing children. Such comparisons are very crucial because they can indicate whether atypical children have residual intact skills alongside selective deficits or generalized disorders affecting the entire system. The older children with WS performed at ceiling as predicted by their non-verbal age. Recall that ceiling performance was shown by normally developing children aged 5:6. Comparing the performance of the youngest WS child whose non-verbal age is estimated at 3:6 to that of normally developing children is very important. This is so because she produces some error types and her performance drops on which-object questions. As mentioned before, the drop of her performance on which-object questions is mainly related to the omission of NP in the which-NP phrase. This error is not a grammatical error in nature but may be related to the D-linked status of referential questions as argued before. Therefore, the WS child converted the which-NP object questions into who-object questions and showed preference for using strictly syntactic processes in the formation of wh-questions, that is, processes required for the formation of who-object questions. Interestingly, the control children showed exactly the same pattern of performance with respect to the main error type as they omitted the NP phrase in which-object questions. The control children showed a high level of performance on who-object questions. All in all, both the control children and the WS children have acquired the syntactic operation of wh-question formation.

Except for the above similarities between the normal and WS performance, there was a striking difference: the production of object questions in the obligatory contexts of subject ones. This error type was produced by the younger WS child. It can be interpreted as an overuse of complicated syntactic procedures required for object-wh-questions. This preference for grammatical processes and rules (required for object wh-questions) over simple heuristic strategies (e.g. the SVO word order strategy in order to produce subject wh-questions) is compatible with the profile of WS children as referred in the literature. Specifically, WS children overuse grammatical rules for past tense formation in English (Clahsen & Almazan 1998) as shown by the overgeneralization of the regular suffix both to existing regular forms and to novel words rhyming with existing irregulars.

In contrast to WS children, the SLI children had severe problems with wh-questions formation. Except for exhibiting low performance on object wh-questions, they produced a high percentage of errors indicating deficits in syntactic operations, e.g. case checking errors. A striking difference between SLI and WS performance was also found with respect to the non-grammatical errors. Specifically, the SLI children resorted to the SVO word order strategy and to referentiality to produce wh-questions, hence they produced referential subject wh-questions instead of non-referential object questions; the WS child (and normally developing

**Table 11.** Summary of the WS, SLI, and normal performance on wh-questions

| SLI | WS | Normal performance |
|---|---|---|
| Low performance on wh-questions especially on object wh-questions | *High level of correct performance | *High level of correct performance |
| Preference for referential representations (preference for which-NP questions over who-questions) | *Omission of NP in which-NP questions | *Omission of NP in which-NP questions |
| Case checking errors | | |
| Subject instead of object wh-questions | Object instead of subject wh-questions | |

children) showed the reverse pattern, i.e. they produced non-referential instead of referential wh-questions.

Despite the completely different linguistic profile of children with SLI and WS, there were some common error types attested in both SLI and WS data. For example, case errors and conversion of object wh-questions into subject ones. However, it should be noted that such errors were attested once in the WS child's responses. Therefore, as mentioned before, these errors cannot be considered as indicative of the WS child's performance and thus they cannot constitute a reliable basis to compare with the SLI performance. Crucially, the grammatical profile of children with WS syndrome does not extend to children with SLI and vice versa.

In addition to the clear-cut differences between the SLI and WS performance, there were major differences between the SLI and normal performance. Specifically, the SLI performance indicates difficulties with the computational component of language (cf. van der Lely 1999) whereas normally developing children exhibit sophisticated knowledge of syntax. It should be noted that the normally developing children have been matched to the SLI children on the basis of linguistic abilities. However, there were striking differences between the performance of both groups not only in quantitative terms, i.e. the level of correct performance but also in qualitative terms, i.e. the attested error types. Crucially, some error types that indicate severe problems with producing object wh-questions, e.g. referential subject questions instead of non-referential object questions, case errors, and gap filling errors, have not been attested in the errors produced by normally developing children. Therefore, it can be concluded that the SLI children have severe deficits in the syntactic processes required for the production of wh-questions.

In Table 11 the main points of WS, SLI, and normal performance on wh-questions are summarized.[11] Similarities across populations are indicated by asterisk (*).

In general terms, the SLI performance appears to be quite different than the normal, whereas the WS performance appears to be close to it. In other words, the SLI children have severe difficulties with the syntactic operation of wh-movement, whereas the WS children do not, despite mental retardation. As far as the WS performance is concerned, it should be noted that there are three points that show evidence for residual normality (cf. Clahsen & Almazan 2003; Temple & Clahsen 2003). First, the high level of correct performance by all WS children on who-object questions indicates that core syntactic processes, i.e. syntactic movement, are intact in the grammar of the WS children. Second, the omission of the NP in which-NP questions by both Eleni (the WS child) and normally developing children indicate that the WS child and the normally developing children produced the same kind of errors, i.e. pragmatic rather than syntactic errors. Finally, the production of object-for-subject wh-questions indicates that the WS child has acquired the syntactic processes required for wh-formation and used them excessively.

All in all, in this paper I studied the production of wh-questions by Greek children with WS compared to SLI and normally developing children. I argued that the WS children are able to use the syntactic processes of wh-question formation and in this sense they resemble normal children, whereas the SLI children have severe deficits with the syntactic operations required for wh-question formation.

## Notes

* I thank Harald Clahsen who brought this paper to the editors' notice. I am also grateful to all the children who participated in this study. Many thanks go to M.-A. Chrysomalli, G. Darili, E. Darili, E. Lefkou, A. Makridou-Timotheidou, K. Taze, K. Thomaidi, A. Varlamis, and M. Vlassopoulou, for their help with the identification of subjects and their great support to my work throughout the years. I also thank two anonymous reviewers for comments and suggestions. Parts of this paper have been presented at the 23rd annual meeting of the Linguistics Department at the University of Thessaloniki, 2002 and at the Euresco conference on Theoretical and Experimental Linguistics in Corinth, 2002. Thanks also go to the audiences of these conferences for comments and suggestions, especially, Marcel den Dikken and Yosef Grodzinksy. Part of the work included in this paper has been supported by a research grant from the Greek State Scholarship Foundation (IKY) awarded to the author; the preparation of this chapter has been completed while the author has been supported by a Marie-Curie fellowship from European Commission (MCFI-2001-01891).

1. This procedure was followed, due to the absence of a standardized IQ test for preschool children in Greek.

2. For details on the cognitive and linguistic abilities of these SLI children see Stavrakaki (2000, 2001a, 2001b, 2002a, 2002b, in press).

3. It is pointed out by an anonymous reviewer that the order OVS does not necessarily imply V to C movement; since Greek is a relatively free word order language, there are structures

with OVS word order which are not analyzed as CPs. However, the derivation of the OVS word order in Greek in structures other than wh-questions is out of the scope of this paper, which focuses on subject and object wh-questions in Greek.

4. We increased the number of trials in the WS group, since fewer WS than SLI children participated in the study.

5. I adopt this definition of non-grammatical errors from van der Lely and Battell (in press).

6. This error may reflect children's reduced attention for a few moments.

7. It should be noted that this drop is compatible with recent studies on wh-questions' development (Avrutin 2000); however, Greek children still show a high level of performance on the production of which-object questions.

8. It is pointed out by an anonymous reviewer that there are yes/no questions with VSO word order:

> klotsise o elefantas tin kamilopardali?
> Kick-3s-the-elephant-nom-the-giraffe-acc
> Did the elephant kick the giraffe?

It should be underlined that only yes/no questions with SVO word order were attested in our data. In both yes/no questions with SVO and VSO word order the verb moves to T but not to C; the difference between them is that only in the SVO word order the subject occupies a Topic position.

9. It has been pointed out by an anonymous reviewer that the drop of Eleni's performance on which-object questions can be explained in terms of Cinque's (1990) analysis of D-linked phrases; according to this analysis D-linked phrases do not involve A-bar movement but are base-generated in their surface position and are coindexed with a *pro* in the object position. The implications of the above analysis for the performance of the WS child are as follows: Eleni's performance on object who-questions which involve movement is very high whereas Eleni's low performance on object which questions which may not involve movement is very low. It is further suggested by the anonymous reviewer that the above observations might indicate that Eleni's difficulties with wh-questions lie in the domain of pragmatics or discourse rather than in the domain of syntax. However, the non-movement analysis of which-questions as suggested by Cinque (1990) is not supported by the SLI data of this study. Recall that the SLI children showed low level of performance on the production of which-object questions; if the non-movement analysis of which-questions held, than SLI children would show a high level of performance on which-object questions.

10. Recall that the word order in object wh-questions in Greek is OVS.

11. In this summary, the main error types produced by each group of children are included.

## References

Avrutin, S. (2000). "Comprehension of discourse-linked and non-discourse-linked questions by children and Broca's aphasics". In Y. Grodzinsky, L. Shapiro, & D. Swinney (Eds.), *Language and the Brain* (pp. 295–313). New York, NY: Academic Press.

Bishop, D. & Adams, C. (1989). "Conversational characteristics of children with semantic-pragmatic disorder. What features lead to a judgment of inappropriacy?" *British Journal of Disorders of Communication, 24*, 241–264.

Bellugi, U., Bihrle, A., Neville, H., Jernigan, T., & Doherty, S. (1992). "Language, cognition and brain organisation in a neurodevelopmental disorder". In M. Gunnar & C. Nelson (Eds.), *Developmental Behavioral Neuroscience: The Minnesota symposium on child psychology* 24 (pp. 201–232). Hillsdale, NJ: LEA.

Bishop, D. (1994). "Grammatical errors in Specific Language Impairment: Competence or performance limitations?" *Applied Psycholinguistics, 15*, 507–550.

Cinque, G. (1990). *Types of A-bar Dependencies*. Cambridge, MA: The MIT Press.

Clahsen, H. (1991). *Child language and developmental dysphasia: Linguistic Studies of the acquisition of German*. Amsterdam: Benjamins.

Clahsen, H. & Almazan, M. (1998). "Syntax and morphology in children with Williams syndrome." *Cognition, 68*, 167–198.

Clahsen, H. & Almazan, M. (2001). "Compounding and inflection in language impairment: Evidence from Williams syndrome (and SLI)." *Lingua, 111*, 729–757.

Clahsen, H., Bartke, S., & Göllner, S. (1997). Formal features in impaired grammars: a comparison of English and German SLI children. *Journal of Neurolinguistics, 10*(2/3), 151–171.

Clahsen, H. & Temple, C. M. (2003). "Words and rules in Williams syndrome". In Y. Levy & J. Schaeffer (Eds.), *Language Competence across Populations* (pp. 323–352). Hillsdale, NJ: LEA.

Clahsen, H., Ring, M., & Temple, C. (this volume). "Lexical and morphological skills in English-speaking children with Williams syndrome".

Chomsky, N. (1986). *Knowledge of Language: Its nature, origin and use*. New York, NY: Praeger.

Chomsky, N. (1991). "Some notes on the economy of derivation and representation". In R. Freidin (Ed.), *Principles and Parameters in Comparative Grammar* (pp. 417–454). Cambridge, MA: The MIT Press.

Chomsky, N. (1995). *The Minimalist Program*. Cambridge, MA: The MIT Press.

Georgas, D., Paraskevopoulos, I., Bezevengis, I., & Giannitsas, N. (1997). *Guidelines for the Greek WISC III*. Athens: Ellinika Grammata.

Karmiloff-Smith, A. (1998). "Development itself is the key to understand developmental disorders". *Trends in Cognitive Sciences, 2*, 389–398.

Pesetsky, D. (1987). "Wh-in-situ: Movement and unselective binding". In E. Reuland & A. ter Meulen (Eds.), *The Representation of (in)Definiteness* (pp. 98–129). Cambridge, MA: The MIT Press.

Pléh, C., Lukács, A., & Racsmány, M. (2003). "Morphological patterns in Hungarian children with Williams syndrome and the rule debate". Ms. Budapest University of Technology and Economics.

Rice, M., Wexler, K. & Cleave, P. (1995). "Specific Language Impairment as a period of Extended Optional Infinitives". *Journal of Speech and Hearing Research, 38*, 850–863.

Rice, M., Wexler, K., & Hershberger, S. (1998). "Tense over time: The longitudinal course of tense acquisition in children with Specific Language Impairment." *Journal of Speech Language, and Hearing Research, 41*, 1412–1431.

Rizzi, L. (1990). "Residual verb-second and the Wh-criterion." *Technical Reports in Formal and Computational Linguistics* 2. Universite de Geneve.

Stark, R. & Tallal, P. (1981). "Selection of children with specific language deficits". *Journal of Speech and Hearing Disorders, 46*, 114–122.

Stavrakaki, S. (2000). "Verb lexicons in SLI: Some experimental data from Modern Greek." *Journal of Greek Linguistics, 1*, 95–131.

Stavrakaki, S. (2001a). Specific Language Impairment in Greek: Aspects of syntactic production and comprehension. Ph.D. thesis, University of Thessaloniki.

Stavrakaki, S. (2001b). "Comprehension of reversible relative clauses in specifically language impaired and normally developing Greek children." *Brain and Language, 77*, 419–431.

Stavrakaki, S. (2002a). "Sentence comprehension in Greek SLI children". In N. Hewlett, L. Kelly, & F. Windsor (Eds.), *Investigations in Clinical Linguistics and Phonetics* (pp. 57–72). Hillsdale, NJ: LEA.

Stavrakaki, S. (2002b). "A-bar movement constructions in Greek children with SLI: Evidence for deficits in the syntactic component of language". In E. Fava (Ed.), *Clinica Linguistics: Theory and applications in speech pathology and therapy* [Current Issues in Linguistic Theory 227] (pp. 131–155). Amsterdam: John Benjamins.

Stavrakaki, S. (in press). "Aspects of theory of mind: Evidence from Greek children with Specific Language Impairment". *Selected papers from the 8th Conference of Greek Psychologists*. Athens: Ellinika grammata.

Stavrakaki, S. & Tsimpli, I. M. (1999). "Diagnostic verbal IQ test for Greek preschool and school age children". Poster presented at the 5th European Conference on Psychological Assessment, August, 25–29, University of Patras.

Temple, C. M. (1997). *Developmental Cognitive Neuropsychology*. Hillsdale, NJ: LEA.

Temple, C. M. & Clahsen, H. (2003). "How connectionist simulations fail to account for developmental disorders in children?" Commentary to appear in *Behavioral and Brain Sciences.*

Temple, C. M., Almazan, M., & Sherwood, S. (2002). "Lexical skills in Williams syndrome: A cognitive neuropsychological analysis". *Journal of Neurolinguistics, 15*, 462–495.

Thomas, M. & Karmiloff-Smith A. (2003). "Are developmental disorders like cases of adult brain damage: Implications from connectionist modeling". To appear in *Behavioral and Brain Sciences.*

Thomas, M. S. C., Grant, J., Barham, Z., Gsadl, M., Laing, E., Lakusta, L. Tyler, L. K., Grice, S., Paterson, S., & Karmiloff-Smith, A. (2001). "Past tense formation in Williams syndrome." *Language and Cognitive Processes, 16*, 143–176.

Thornton, R. (1990). Adventures in Long Distance Moving: The acquisition of complex wh-questions. Ph.D. thesis, University of Connecticut.

Tsimpli, I. M. (1990). "The clause structure and word order of Modern Greek". *UCL Working Papers in Linguistics, 2*, 226–255.

van der Lely, H. (1998). "SLI in Children: Movement, economy and deficits in the computational-syntactic system". *Language Acquisition, 7*(2–4), 161–193.

van der Lely, H. (1999). "Learning from grammatical SLI". *Trends in Cognitive Sciences, 3*(8), 286–288.

van der Lely, H. & Battell, J. (in press). "Wh-Movement in children with Grammatical SLI: A test of the RDDR hypothesis". *Language*.

Volterra, V., Capirci, O., Pezzini, G., Sabbadini, L., & Vicari, S. (1996). "Linguistic abilities in Italian children with Williams syndrome". *Cortex, 32*, 663–677.

Watkins, R. (1994). "Specific Language Impairment in children: An introduction". In R. Watkins & M. Rice (Eds.), *Specific Language Impairment in Children* (pp. 1–15). Baltimore, MD: Brookes.

# The comprehension of complex wh-questions in German-speaking individuals with WS

## A multiple case study

Julia Siegmüller and Jürgen Weissenborn
University of Potsdam / Humboldt University, Berlin

Studying the comprehension of complex wh-questions in 9-to-22-years-old individuals with Williams-Syndrome (WS) matched to unimpaired controls we investigated the question whether WS-individuals can achieve adult-like grammatical competence, and whether it is reached along the same developmental paths as in unimpaired language development. We found that their performance corresponded to the stages of unimpaired linguistic development in non-verbal-mental-age matched controls, except for two WS-individuals showing adult-like behavior although they had not reached the corresponding mental age. The particular difficulties the WS-individuals displayed with adjunct-questions as compared to the controls are explained in terms of a sensitivity of the learning mechanisms of the WS-individuals greater than in unimpaired learners to predictible patterns in the input like the ones constituted by the verb and its syntactically and thematically related complements.

### Introduction

The aim of this study is to investigate the similarities and differences in linguistic behavior between individuals with Williams syndrome (WS) and unimpaired controls. With respect to linguistic development in children with WS it has been argued that it is delayed compared to unimpaired development (Clahsen & Almazan 1998, 2001; Krause & Penke 2001; Zukowski 2001, also see Bartke this volume). Furthermore it has been suggested that it may also be qualitatively different, i.e. showing linguistic behavior which is not observed in language-unimpaired children (Karmiloff-Smith et al. 1997; Thomas et al. 2001). A further question not independent of these issues, and which can only be answered on the basis of focused investigations into particular areas of linguistic knowledge, is in which of these areas individuals with WS do or do not reach adult linguistic competence. This may help us to gain a better understanding of the nature of the limitations of the linguistic capacities in these individuals. This is especially desirable with respect to the question to which extent the linguistic performance of individuals with WS depends on their non-linguistic cognitive capacities, a question which bears on the issue of the modular nature of linguistic knowledge. So far evidence concerning this issue has been controversial: there are findings which support the view that linguistic knowledge in individuals with WS may be below, equal to, or above mental age (above mental age: Clahsen & Almazan 1998; equal and below mental age: Volterra et al. 1996; Mervis et al. 1999; equal to mental age: Zukowski 2001).

Recent work on the linguistic abilities of individuals with WS suggests that rule driven core morphological and syntactic knowledge and its use are basically intact whereas more irregular, lexically based knowledge and processing may be impaired. The reasons for these impairments have been attributed to representational and/or information processing deficits, like memory processes (e.g. Barisnikov et al. 1996). Thus it has been found that regular plural and past tense formation are adult-like, whereas deficits are observed with irregular plurals and past tense (e.g. Clahsen & Almazan 1998, 2001; for a different view see Thomas et al. 2001; Karmiloff-Smith et al. sub.). Similarly, the interpretation of passives and binding relations have been shown to be adult-like. It is in this domain that WS subjects performed even better than mental age matched (i.e. 5–7 years) controls (e.g. Clahsen & Almazan 1998). A slightly different picture with respect to the syntactic capacities of WS subjects arises from the work of Zukowski (2001). When investigating language competence in 8–16 year-old WS subjects and mental age matched controls (4–7 years) in the area of the production of embedded relative clauses, affirmative and negative wh-questions, and of grammaticality judgments of correct and incorrect sentences containing the negative polarity item *any* and its affirmative counterpart *some*, she found that WS subjects never performed better than age-matched controls. Furthermore she found that the performance profile of WS subjects and controls in the different tasks was very similar, and that differences between the two groups were rather quantitative than qualitative in nature; that is the WS subjects' linguistic behavior exaggerated patterns seen in children of typical development. These findings are strong evidence for dissociation between and within different areas of linguistic knowledge, and thus support the modularity hypothesis.

Additional evidence for this view comes from the comparison between subjects with WS and with Specific Language Impairement (SLI) who in some of the morphological and syntactic domains previously mentioned, display the opposite pattern of impaired and intact linguistic behavior. That is to say, they perform better with irregular past tense than with regular past tense formation, and they have problems with verbal passives and binding principles for pronouns and anaphors (Clahsen & Almazan 1998; van der Lely in press).

An area of linguistic knowledge which recently has been identified as presenting particular difficulties for children with SLI in production as well as in comprehension are operator – variable constructions such as simple wh-questions, i.e. the wh-questions *What did Peter read?* as opposed to complex wh-questions such as *What did Peter say (that) he read?* in which the initial wh-pronoun asks a question about the embedded clause (e.g. for German, comprehension: Penner & Kölliker Funk 1998; for English, production only: van der Lely in press; van der Lely & Battell 2003). The findings of Zukowski (2001) concerning the production of affirmative and negative simple wh-questions in WS subjects showing that they perform as do mental-age matched controls, suggest that the same opposite performance of WS and SLI subjects might be found in this area too.

The aim of our study in pursuing this line of research was to investigate whether the finding that WS subjects can reach adult-like performance in particular language areas (i.e. the comprehension of verbal passives and binding, Clahsen & Almazan 1998), or that they perform at least as well as controls matched for mental age (i.e. the production of simple affirmative and negative wh-questions, Zukowski 2001) could be extended to the comprehension of complex wh-questions in German speaking WS subjects. Furthermore, we wished to find out whether non-adult-like linguistic behavior in WS subjects would be qualitatively different from non-adult-like linguistic behavior in unimpaired individuals. Complex wh-questions are particularly interesting for the issue, of whether adult or mental-age related performance can be reached in this area, and whether it is reached along the same developmental path, i.e. showing the same intermediate profiles of performance before reaching the adult stage, for two reasons. Firstly, overall adult-like comprehension of complex wh-questions seems to be a relatively late development in languages of similar structures. There is evidence that unimpaired children do not reach adult-like behavior before 7–9 years of age. Secondly, adult-like behavior is not reached at the same time for all particular types of complex wh-questions but some types are acquired earlier than others, thus giving rise to a specific developmental profile in typical language development (e.g. De Villiers et al. 1990; Weissenborn et al. 1990, 1995; for the development of the production of complex wh-question, see e.g. McDaniel et al. 1995).

With respect to the question of whether individuals with WS can reach adult linguistic performance in the domain under investigation we will endeavor to show that two of our WS subjects have indeed attained the adult level, even with a lower non-verbal mental age. In one case we will show that this level is reached at the same chronological age as in the controls. With respect to the question whether non-adult-like profiles of performance in subjects with WS and controls are similar or different, we will see that these profiles are very similar, and that any differences found are quantitative and not qualitative in nature thus supporting the findings of Zukowski (2001). We will argue that these differences may be related to differences in specific aspects of the learning and information processing mechanisms of WS subjects.

## Constraints on the interpretation of complex wh-questions in German

In the following we will sketch the constraints on the interpretation of the different types of complex wh-questions in German which are to be tested in our study.

I. The initial wh-pronoun is an argument (iARG) or an adjunct (iADJ). The embedded clause is also introduced by an argument or an adjunct wh-pronoun albeit a different one.

(1) *Wem zeigt die Erzieherin, was man reparieren kann?* (=*iARG*)
Whom does the kindergarden teacher show what to repair?

(2) *Wie fragt Peter, wem er helfen soll?* (=*iADJ*)
How does Peter ask whom to help?

II. The initial wh-pronoun is an argument or an adjunct. The embedded clause is introduced by a lexically one (COPY).

(3) *Wem sagt Peter, wem er Bescheid geben will?* (=*COPY*)
Whom does Peter tell whom he will let it know?

III. The initial wh-pronoun is the so-called scope marker *was* (what). The wh-pronoun in the embedded clause is any other wh-pronoun (SCOPE).

(4) *Was sagt Jan, wem er helfen will?* (=*SCOPE*)
*What does John say who to help?*

IV. There is only an initial wh-pronoun. The embedded clause is verb initial, followed by the subject (INVersion).

(5) *Wem sagt Jan möchte er nachlaufen?* (=*INV*)
To whom does Jan say he wants to run after?

These questions differ with respect to whether the initial wh-pronoun must, can, or cannot be interpreted in relation to the matrix clause or the embedded clause. Which one of these alternatives is the case, depends basically on the properties of the initial wh-pronoun in the matrix clause and the properties of the embedded clause. There are regional differences with respect to the possible interpretations of these sentences.[1] In the following we focus on the northern variety of German which is the target variety of the participants in our study. Thus, in (1)–(2), the question can only be answered with respect to the matrix clause. That is, for example, in (1) the initial wh-pronoun could not be interpreted as the indirect object of the verb "to repair" in the embedded clause, i.e. "…what to repair *to whom*". In the generative framework the relation of the wh-pronoun to the position where it has to be interpreted forms a so-called wh-chain (see e.g. Haegeman 1994). That means sentences with two referentially different wh-rponouns like (1) and (2) contain two chains. The unavailability of the interpretation of (1) just mentioned is now explained by the presence of an initial wh-pronoun in the embedded clause which blocks the formation of a wh-chain between a constituent of the embedded clause be it an argument or an adjunct. This is the so-called "wh-island constraint" (see e.g. Ross 1967; Bayer 1990). Question (3) which has identical wh-pronouns in the matrix and the embedded clause is ambiguous for some German speakers: Besides the interpretation within the matrix clause an interpretation within the embedded clause can also be observed (Bayer 1990; Weissenborn et al. 1990, 1995). (4) can only be answered with respect to the embedded clause. The initial wh-pronoun '*was*' (what) has no specific lexical-semantic content. That is to say, there is no subcategorised argument position which could be filled by *was*, i.e. it is an expletive element. Its function is to mark the whole sentence as a [+WH-question] which has to be answered with respect to the wh-pronoun in the embedded clause. In this sense we may consider the initial wh-pronoun '*was*' (what) as a lexicalized copy of the feature [+WH-question] of the embedded wh-pronoun. This means that *was* (what) can be considered part of a wh-chain of the embedded wh-pronoun. An explanation along these lines would also account for the reading of (3), in which the embedded question is answered; here it is the entire wh-pronoun which has been copied to the sentence initial position. Similarly, the interpretation of question (5) would be obtained by successively moving the embedded wh-pronoun from its base position in the embedded clause to the front of the matrix clause, e.g. "Wem$_i$ sagt Jan möchte er ($t_i$) nachlaufen?" Whom$_i$ does Jan say he wants to run after ($t_i$)?

Given that the control part of our study replicates with a subset of the test items and with an extended age range of subjects – the study by Weissenborn et al. (1995) with German children which was based on a study by De Villiers et al. (1990) with English children – we expect to find the same developmental picture for our controls. Therefore, it is that questions involving one wh-pronoun, and thus one wh-chain, i.e. INV and SCOPE (see above the discussion of the question types) are acquired earlier than the other question types, i.e. iARG, iADJ, and COPY, which involve two different wh-pronouns, and thus two wh-chains. Furthermore we predict an advantage regarding argument-questions over adjunct-questions which has also been found in the earlier studies (for more details see De Villiers et al. 1990). Based on the findings concerning the syntactic abilities of subjects with WS discussed above, we would expect to find a profile of performance for them, possibly depending on their mental age, which would correspond to one of the profiles found in the controls.

## Methods

### Participants

*WS subjects*

The WS subjects were between 9 and 22 years old. Six WS subjects participated in the study, four were female and two male. All of them are monolingual German speakers and live with their families. They have been clinically diagnosed as having WS and the diagnosis genetically confirmed at a later date (FISH). The non-verbal mental age was determined with the CFT 20 (Weiß 1998); for the subject JF the CFT 1 was used (Cattell et al. 1997).

In the following some additional information concerning the linguistic and non-linguistic cognitive profile of the WS subjects will be provided. The data have been collected through parental reports and language tests. More detailed clinical data of the WS subjects will be provided in Table 1.

JF (9;0) For JF no language disorders were reported until age 6;00. By then morphological errors such as regularisation of irregular forms were noticed which lasted until the time of the investigation. She did not receive language therapy. Her non-verbal mental age is 5;8.

PL (9;8) For PL no language disorders were reported. She attends a school for mentally handicapped children where she is taught reading and writing. Her non-verbal mental age is 7;6.

PM (12;0) PM showed a severe language disorder in early childhood and had already received language therapy for eight years, when the investigation started. At about age 6;00 his syntactic age was 2;6 (Penner 1999; Kauschke & Siegmüller 2002). At the time of the study his speech no longer showed syntactic errors. His non-verbal mental age is 6;6.

GC (13;2) GC produced her first words around her first birthday, but then stagnated on the one-word stage for two years. The acquisition of more complex sentences advanced very slowly. At the time of the investigation, she suffered from severe word-finding difficulties (Glück 1998). Her non-verbal mental age is 6;0.

MA (18;2) MA produced his first words at 18 months of age. No language disorders have been reported. He is able to read and write in a slow manner. MA's non-verbal mental age is 7;6.

SJ (22;0) SJ began to produce words at 18 months. She stagnated on the one-word stage until the age of five. She did not receive professional language therapy. At school she learned to read and write. She is able to use arithmetical and orthographic training programs on a PC. Her non-verbal mental age is 7;6.

*Controls*

120 children from 3;6 to 9;0, and 12 adults (between 20 and 40) participated in the experiment (see Table 2 for the distribution across age groups). All were monolingual German speakers of the same regional variety of German as the WS subjects, and had no known developmental disorders. The age range was chosen so that the controls covered the development of complex wh-questions from the beginning to the adult stage. The adult stage is reached at age 9;0. Given the assumption that in the controls chronological and mental age coincide, our control group covers the range of mental ages found in the WS subjects. This allows us to control for the factor of mental age in the performance of the WS subjects. The 12 adult controls were added in order to have close to chronological age matched controls also for the two oldest WS subjects, and thus to control for a possible age effect.

## Experiments

*Pretest*

In order to make sure that all the participants had the necessary linguistic knowledge to process the complex wh-questions to be tested, a pretest was run with the candidates for the study. It first tested whether the subject had acquired the verb-second rule which is a necessary prerequisite to understanding wh-question in German (Penner & Kölliker Funk 1998; Weissenborn 2000), and secondly, whether the subject was able to process sentences of the length of the test items. For the first part of the pretest the diagnostic material of two German SLI tests were used (Penner 1999; Kauschke & Siegmüller 2002), the second part was constructed especially for this study. All the WS subjects included scored at ceiling in the pretest.

*Materials and procedure*

The test items were constructed from the 5 different types of complex wh-questions discussed above, i. e. iARG, iADJ, COPY, SCOPE, INV, constituting the five main conditions of the study. Table 3 illustrates the different question types.

**Table 1.** Clinical data of the WS subjects

| **Subjects** | **JF** | **PL** | **PM** | **GC** | **MA** | **SJ** |
|---|---|---|---|---|---|---|
| Chronological age | 9;0 | 10;4 | 12;0 | 13;2 | 18;2 | 22;0 |
| Non-verbal IQ | 55 | 85 | 76 | 62 | 66 | 75 |
| Non-verbal mental age | 5;8 | 7;6 | 6;6 | 6;0 | 7;6 | 7;6 |
| AWST[a] (mental age matching) | PR* 42 | PR 56 | PR 40 | PR 32 | PR 67 | PR 76 |
| LeMo[b] | 95% | comprehension: 95%<br>production: 75% | comprehension: 80%<br>production: 65% | comprehension: 75%<br>production: 75% | 100% | comprehension: 100%<br>production: 80% |
| PDSES[c] (mental age matching) | normal | –1 SD below average (morphology) | –2 SD below average (morphology) | –1 SD below average in wordproduction | normal | normal |
| FEW[d] (mental age matching) | ∅ –** | ∅ – | ∅ – | ∅ – | normal | normal |

* PR = Percent rank; ** ∅ – = below average; a = Aktiver Wortschatztest, German Naming Test, Kiese and Kozielski (1979); b = LeMo (Lexical Assessment Battery, phonological processing only), De Bleser et al. t.a.; c = Patholinguistische Diagnostik bei Sprachentwicklungsstörungen (Assessment auf language disordes in children, SLI), Kauschke and Siegmüller (2002); d = Frostig Entwicklungstest der visuellen Wahrnehmung (Test of the development of visual perception), Frostig (1968).

Table 2. Control subjects per age group

| Age group | Number of participants |
|---|---|
| 3;0–3;11 | 11 |
| 4;0–4;11 | 13 |
| 5;0–5;11 | 28 |
| 6;0–6;11 | 29 |
| 7;0–7;11 | 18 |
| 8;0–8;11 | 11 |
| 9;0–9;11 | 10 |
| Sum | 120 |
| Adults | 12 |

Table 3. Conditions of the experiment

| Question type | |
|---|---|
| iARG | *Wem zeigt die Erzieherin, was man reparieren kann?*<br>Whom does the kindergarden teacher show, what to repair? |
| iADJ | *Wo fragt Peter, wem er helfen soll?*<br>Where does Peter ask, whom to help? |
| COPY | *Wem verspricht Peter, wem er Bescheid sagen will?*<br>Whom does Peter promise, whom he will let it know? |
| Scope | *Was sagt Jan, wem er helfen will?*<br>What does Jan say, whom he will help? |
| INV | *Wem sagt Jan möchte er nachlaufen?*<br>To whom does Jan say he wants to run after? |

The total number of test sentences was 30, constituting 6 tokens per condition. For each of the test items a story was constructed, accompanied by two or three additional black-and-white drawings (see Figure 1), which altogether provided necessary contextual information so that the test question could either be answered with respect to the matrix or to the embedded clause. During the experiment the subject was told to watch the pictures and listen to the story. At the end of the story the experimenter asked a question to which the subject was prompted to answer. The stories presented three children (Lisa, Peter and Jan), who had been equipped with typical tools in order to facilitate the identification (for more details concerning the experimental method, see De Villiers & Roeper 1996).

Sample story and test question (all stories and questions are listed in the Appendix):

(6) *Jan besucht Lisa. Lisa möchte nicht, dass Jan mit ihrer neuen Puppe spielt und versteckt sie. Abends fragt die Mama, wo die Puppe ist. Lisa sagt: "Ich*

*habe sie vorhin hinter meinem Schrank versteckt."*
**Test question:** *Wann sagt Lisa, wo sie die Puppe versteckt hat?*

Jan visits Lisa. Lisa does not want Jan to play with her new doll. Therefore she hides the doll. In the evening, her mother asks her, where she put her new doll. Lisa answers: "I have hidden my new doll behind my wardrobe."
**Test question:** When does Lisa say, where she had hidden her doll?

## Results and discussion

### Control data

We will first briefly present the results for the control subjects to which the results of the WS subjects are then to be compared. Figure 2 shows that adult performance in the domain of complex wh-questions, all conditions considered, is attained at about age 9;00. A statistical analysis, using the Mann-Whitney U-Test reveals no significant difference between 9-year-olds and adults for overall correct behavior (U = 144; p > .09)

Notice that Figure 2 is misleading, in the sense that it suggests a steady overall development, whereas when the performance in the different conditions were compared over time, as shown in Table 4 and then grouped into three developmental groups, as shown in Figure 3, as well as in Tables 5 and 6, we observe important

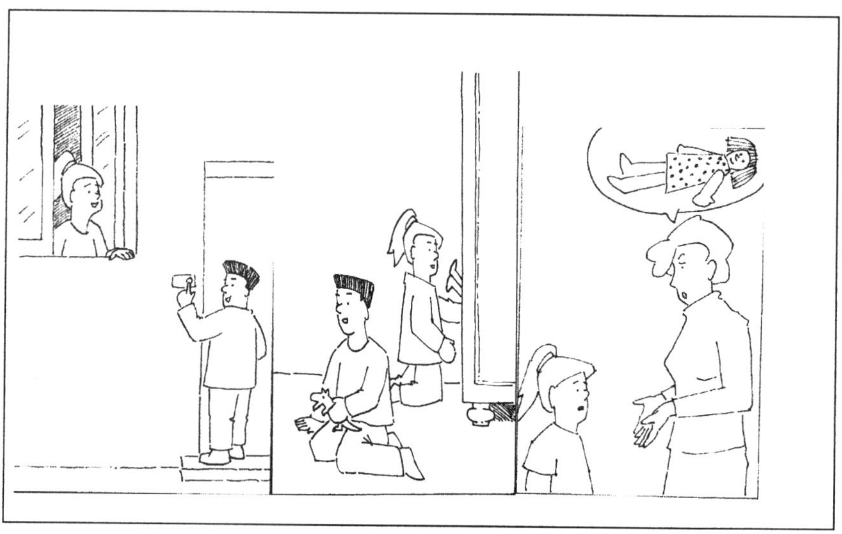

**Figure 1.** Example of a picture set for a story, followed by a complex wh-question

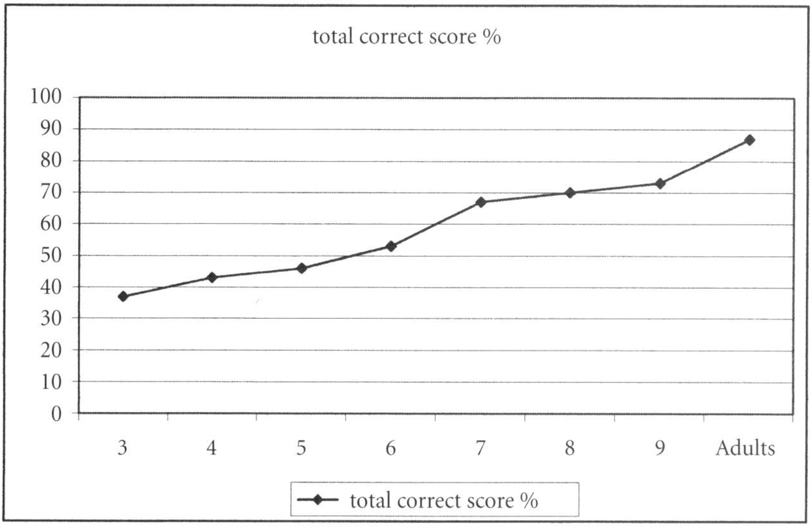


**Figure 2.** Total correct scores of normal controls (per age group)

differences with respect to the different conditions. Thus in the conditions SCOPE (*Was sagt Jan, wem er helfen will?* What does Jan say, whom he will help?) and INV (*Wem sagt Jan möchte er nachlaufen?* To whom does Jan say he wants to run after?) we find near adult performance almost from the beginning.

There is no statistically significant difference between the different developmental groups for these two conditions SCOPE and INV (Mann-Whitney U-Test, see Table 6). To the contrary, in the COPY condition (*Wem verspricht Peter, wem er Bescheid sagen will?* Whom does Peter promise, whom he will let it know?), the iARG (*Wem zeigt die Erzieherin, was man reparieren kann?* Whom does the kindergarden teacher show, what to repair?), and the iADJ conditions (*Wo fragt Peter, wem*

**Table 4.** Mean correct scores for the different conditions per age group

| | | | Main conditions | | | Sub conditions (n = 6) | | | |
|---|---|---|---|---|---|---|---|---|---|
| Age | N | Corrects | Argument | Adjunct | Scope | COPY | INV | iARG | iADJ |
| 3 | 11 | 11.45 | 6.18 | 5.27 | 4.55 | 0.27 | 5.36 | 0.73 | 0.36 |
| 4 | 13 | 13.38 | 7.85 | 5.54 | 5.23 | 0.54 | 5.08 | 2.08 | 0.38 |
| 5 | 28 | 14.54 | 8.25 | 6.29 | 5.57 | 1.07 | 4.38 | 2.5 | 1.04 |
| 6 | 29 | 16.66 | 9.21 | 7.45 | 5.48 | 1.45 | 4.72 | 3.17 | 1.65 |
| 7 | 18 | 20.83 | 11.22 | 9.61 | 5.89 | 2.17 | 4.61 | 4.72 | 3.39 |
| 8 | 11 | 21.91 | 11.45 | 10.45 | 5.72 | 2.82 | 4 | 5.27 | 4.18 |
| 9 | 10 | 23.9 | 13.3 | 11 | 6 | 4.2 | 3.8 | 5.7 | 4.3 |
| Erw. | 12 | 26.08 | 13 | 13 | 6 | 4.42 | 3.75 | 6 | 5.92 |

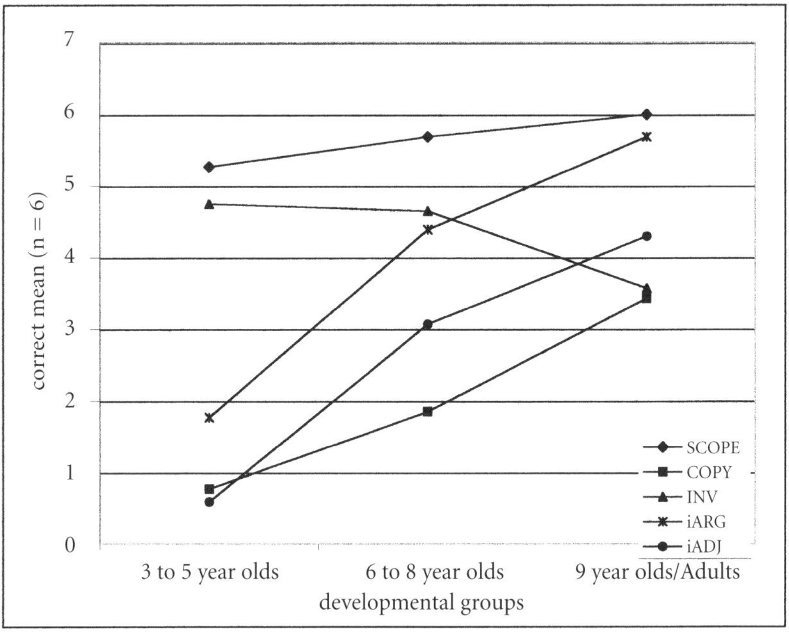


**Figure 3.** Behavior of the control children, grouped per different developmental phases in the different conditions

*er helfen soll?* Where does Peter ask, whom to help?) we find significant increases in performance between the age groups (Mann-Whitney U-Test, see Table 6).

Therefore, as predicted, we observe a difference between the performance with the structures with an obligatory embedded clause interpretation in which only one overt lexically subcategorised wh-pronoun is involved, and consequently only one wh-chain, i.e. SCOPE and INV, – remember that *was* (what) in the SCOPE condition has to be analysed as a non-subcategorised, expletive question-marker –, and the performance in the other conditions in which two subcategorised wh-pronouns, and thus two wh-chains are involved, not allowing an embedded clause reading in the adult language because of the wh-island constraint.

**Table 5.** Mean correct scores for the different conditions per developmental phase

| Group | Total correct | iARG | iADJ | Scope | COPY | INV |
|---|---|---|---|---|---|---|
| Age 3–5 | 13,6 | 1,77 | 0,59 | 5,27 | 0,77 | 4,75 |
| Age 6–8 | 18,8 | 4,39 | 3,07 | 5,69 | 1,85 | 4,65 |
| Age 9 | 22 | 5,69 | 4,3 | 6 | 3,43 | 3,57 |
| Adults | 26 | 6 | 5,92 | 6 | 4,53 | 3,92 |
| Age 9 and Adults | 24,45 | 5,72 | 5,09 | 6 | 3,91 | 3,77 |

Table 6. Group comparisons of the different conditions (Mann Whitney U-Test)

| | Age 3–5 (n = 52) vs. age 6–8 (n = 54) | Age 6–8 (n = 54) vs. age 9 & Adults (n = 22) |
|---|---|---|
| Total correct score | U = 552; p < .0000 | U = 224,5; p < .0000 |
| Subconditions: | | |
| SCOPE | U = 1065; p < .0322 | U = 462; p < .1306 (n.s.) |
| COPY | U = 879; p < .0009 | U = 231; p < .0000 |
| INV | U = 1310,5; p < .5394 (n.s.) | U = 488,5; p < .2269 (n.s.) |
| iARG | U = 685; p < .0000 | U = 235; p < .0000 |
| iADJ | U = 652,5; p < .0000 | U = 175; p < .0000 |

Table 7. Within group effects in selected subconditions (Wilcoxon Test, per developmental phase)

| | Age 3–5 (n = 52) | Age 6–8 (n = 54) | Age 9 & Adults (n = 22) |
|---|---|---|---|
| Conditions | | | |
| COPY vs. iARG | .0000 | .0000 | .0001 |
| COPY vs. iADJ | .8022 | .0011 | .0021 |
| iARG vs. iADJ | .0000 | .0000 | .0125 |
| Within conditions | | | |
| COPY-ARG vs. COPY-ADJ | .009 | .0008 | .7583 |
| iARG-ARG vs. iARG-ADJ | .893 | .1215 | .1159 |
| iADJ-ADJ vs. iADJ-ARG | .0366 | .0000 | .3525 |

This means that up to age 5;00 the children are not systematically obeying this constraint. At age 6;00–8;00 they start to obey it in the iARG and the iADJ conditions, whereas in the COPY condition it is still not obeyed (see Table 5).

As an explanation for these findings following the approach taken in Weissenborn et al. (1990, 1995) we propose that in the case of the double wh-constructions, i.e. iARG, iADJ, and COPY, the child does not yet fully lexically analyse the initial wh-pronoun, i.e. she ignores its case features, and only retains its wh-feature basically treating the wh-pronoun as the scope marker *was* (what). This explanation predicts an even stronger SCOPE-reading effect in the case of the identity of the two wh-pronouns such as in the COPY-condition if we assume that the features of the initial wh-pronoun are collapsed with the ones of the medial, embedded wh-pronoun. This is exactly what we find as shown in Table 6 and particularly in Table 7: performance for COPY is significantly worse than for iARG in iADJ in children between six and eight years of age.

An additional explanation which is not incompatible with the one given above, is following a suggestion proposed by De Villiers et al. (1990), that, speaking in terms of chain formation, children, up to this point are not able to keep apart, or to compute in parallel the A-bar-chain related to each of the two wh-pronouns which are subcategorised by two different verbal heads, i.e. the verb of the matrix and the embedded clause. Only when the child starts to analyse the two wh-pronouns as two referentially unrelated lexical items which are subcategorised in two different syntactic positions, i.e. the complement position of the verb of the matrix and the embedded clause respectively, can the correct reading be attained. At about age 9;00 adult performance in all conditions is reached (see Tables 4, 5 and 6).

### WS data

Comparing the results for the individuals with WS with the results for the controls taking all conditions into consideration, we find that two subjects, JF (CA 9;00, MA 5;8) and MA (CA 22;00, MA 7;6) out of the six subjects reach adult performance, although their non-verbal mental age is below the mental age at which adult performance is reached in unimpaired children, i.e. 9;00 (see Tables 4, 5 & 8).

The good results of MA and JF become more transparent in the translation of their raw scores into T-Scores. See Table 9 for the comparison of the T-Scores of the WS-single cases and the chronologically matched children. MA and JF score as or above their chronologically matched controls, indicated by the T-Scores 53 (equal to controls, MA) and 78.5 (two SD better than controls, JF).

If we look at the subjects who do not reach adult performance, although their chronological age is in all cases above the one at which adult performance is reached, (see Tables 4 and 5) we observe, in unimpaired children, the following: With respect to the conditions SCOPE, INV, COPY and iARG these individuals are basically similar to the 6;00–8;00 years old controls (see Table 10).

Consequently, their linguistic performance corresponds to the performance of the controls matched according to their non-verbal mental age. But there is a striking difference with respect to the iADJ condition in which we find a significant difference between the control children and the WS individuals.

**Table 8.** Results of the WS subjects ordered by chronological age

| | | All correct conditions (n = 6) | | | | | |
|---|---|---|---|---|---|---|---|
| Subject | CA/MA | (n = 30) | Scope | COPY | INV | iARG | iADJ |
| JF | 9;0/5;8 | 28 | 6 | 5 | 6 | 6 | 5 |
| PL | 10;4/7;6 | 17 | 6 | 3 | 4 | 5 | 1 |
| PM | 12;0/6;6 | 17 | 4 | 4 | 5 | 3 | 1 |
| GC | 13;2/6;0 | 21 | 6 | 1 | 6 | 5 | 3 |
| MA | 18;2/7;6 | 27 | 6 | 6 | 4 | 6 | 5 |
| SJ | 22;0/7;6 | 19 | 6 | 2 | 6 | 4 | 1 |
| MEAN | | 21.5 | 5.67 | 3.5 | 5.16 | 4.83 | 2.67 |
| SD | | 4.89 | 0.82 | 1.87 | 1.0 | 1.87 | 2.0 |

**Table 9.** T-Score-Transformation of the total correct score of the Williams syndrome subjects, compared to the chronological control groups

| Subject | Number of cont-rols | Age of controls | More than 2 SD's T < 30 | 2 SD T = 30–40 | 1 SD T = 40–50 | Mean score of control group T = 50 | 1 SD T = 50–60 | 2 SD T = 60–70 | More than 2 SD's T > 70 |
|---|---|---|---|---|---|---|---|---|---|
| JF | 14 | 8;6–9:5 | | | | | | | 78.5 |
| PL | 14 | 8;6–9:5 | 23.5 | | | | | | |
| PM | 12 | Adults | 22.7 | | | | | | |
| GC | 12 | Adults | | 34.8 | | | | | |
| MA | 12 | Adults | | | | | 53 | | |
| SJ | 12 | Adults | 28.8 | | | | | | |

**Table 10.** Comparisons of means: controls age 6–8 and 4 WS subjects

| | Controls age 6–8 | WS subjects PL, PM; GC, SJ | Mann-Whitney U-Test between Controls and WS |
|---|---|---|---|
| SCOPE | 5.69 | 5.5 | U = 156; p > .892 |
| INV | 4.65 | 5.25 | U = 123; p > .336 |
| COPY | 1.85 | 2.5 | U = 90; p > .076 |
| iARG | 4.39 | 4.25 | U = 129.5; p > .423 |
| iADJ | 3.07 | 1.5 | U = 1; p > .000 |

Thus, all other things being equal, it seems to be the case that the WS individuals have greater difficulties in interpreting structures with adjunct questions than with argument questions. This predicts that in the WS subjects' data we should find for the COPY-condition with adjunct wh-pronoun a less good performance than with an argument question word. This seems to be the case: for COPY-ADJ we find mean correct 0.5 answers whereas for COPY-ARG we find 2, although the difference does not appear significant.

It is of note that although overall, we also find a better level of performance for argument questions in the controls, the difference in the performance for adjunct questions nowhere reaches the same proportion as in the individuals with WS.

## Discussion

How can we explain this 'weakness' in the processing of complex adjunct questions? We would like to propose the following explanation, which is compatible with the findings concerning specific aspects of the linguistic performance of WS subjects in other areas of grammar. It has been claimed that the acquisition of regular past-tense formation presents no difficulty to WS subjects but that they have problems with irregular past tense formation (e.g. Clahsen & Almazan 1998, 2001;

for a different view see Karmiloff-Smith et al. 1997; Thomas et al. 2001; Karmiloff-Smith et al., submitted). In analogy to this finding we wish to argue that the relation between a verb and its subcategorised complements is a regular, i.e. predictable one, in the sense that each time an argument of a given verb is realised as a wh-pronoun in a particular syntactic function it will take the same phonological form, realising the same grammatical features such as case, e.g. *Wer gab wem was?* (Who did give what to whom?). Thus a learning and processing mechanism which is especially sensitive to co-occurrence patterns and their underlying regularities should more readily relate a given verb to its syntactic complements than to information syntactically realised as non-subcategorised constituents, i.e. adjuncts.

This predicts that when the WS subjects listen to the story on the basis of which they will then have to answer the test question, the information which is coded in the form of arguments of the verb should be more salient, i.e. *visible* to the WS subject; and thus more readily available as an interpretation for the question operator, i.e. the argument wh-pronoun than information in the forms of adjuncts which are not syntactically related to the verb in the question sentence. An additional factor which may strengthen the differences in the accessibility of the information necessary to answer the test question may be related to possible weaknesses in memory processes in WS (Barisnikov et al. 1996; Vicari et al. 1996a; Vicari et al. 1996b). Thus the information coded as an argument in the story may be primed by the corresponding argument wh-pronoun in the test question in combination with the verb of which it is a complement. It is this priming effect, which may compensate in the iARG-condition for a possible memory deficit; whereas in the case of information coded as adjuncts, no such compensating priming mechanisms can be drawn on. Obviously one would expect that this priming effect should also influence the performance of the controls. We would like to suggest that the better performance of the controls in the argument condition supports this view (see Table 5). Our explanation also predicts that the few errors which occur in the two WS individuals who overall perform like adults, should occur with adjunct questions. This is indeed what we find. But these two subjects also show that some individuals with WS seem to be able to overcome the observed weakness in processing adjunct-questions to the same extent as unimpaired subjects do. Whether, as this explanation predicts, the sub-group of WS subjects which performed worse than their 6–8 year-old controls in the processing of iADJ do indeed show memory deficits as compared to their controls, and whether the two adult-like performing WS subjects do not, has to be the object of future investigation.

## Summary and conclusion

With respect to our initial questions we have found that two of our individuals with WS do reach adult performance in the comprehension of complex wh-questions although they have not reached the corresponding mental age. With respect to the other four WS subjects we found that their linguistic performance largely corresponded to their mental age with the exception of one specific type of complex wh-question, i.e. iADJ-questions (e.g. *Wann sagt Lisa, wo sie die Puppe versteckt hat?* When does Lisa say where she has hidden the doll?), where their performance was below that of the controls matched for mental age.

This was explained in terms of a specific sensitivity of the learning and processing mechanisms of the WS subjects to regular, i.e. predictible patterns in the linguistic input such as ones constituted by the verb and its syntactically, i.e. case marked, and thematically related complements. We assumed that this results in an advantage in the accessibility – and consequently also in the recall of information in the story – necessary in order to answer the test question which is syntactically encoded as arguments over information syntactically coded as an adjunct. Thus we would like to argue that the difference in the linguistic performance between the WS subjects and the controls matched for mental age is not due to a difference in linguistic knowledge but that it is a result of the interaction between the strengths, i.e. pattern detection and recognition, and the weaknesses, i.e. certain aspects of memory processes in the learning and processing mechanisms of the WS subjects. Further research will have to show whether our findings which are based on the investigation of only a few individuals with WS can be generalised in the sense of being part of the general characterisation of the linguistic phenotype of the Williams syndrome.

It is an interesting question for further research whether the relative rarity of adverbial modification, or adjuncts in our terms, which has been reported for the speech production of individuals with WS may also be accounted for along the lines of our explanation for the comprehension of complex wh-questions (see e.g. Rubba & Klima 1991 for adverbial modification).

Another open question, which also has to be the subject of future research, is whether the weakness in the interpretation of complex adjunct questions which were observed in some individuals with WS of widely different age constitutes the end stage of the development or whether it could improve with growing age or with the help of appropriate training programs.

## Acknowledgements

We would like to thank all the participants in our study for their patient co-operation. Thanks also to Barbara Höhle and Marita Böhning for help with the statistical analysis and various comments. Comments were also provided by Tom Roeper, Susanne Bartke and Christine Erb. We thank them all. Earlier versions of this paper have been presented at the International workshop on "Separability of cognitive functions: What can be learned from Williams Syndrome?", University of Massachusetts, Amherst, August 2001 and at the 2nd National Conference on Children's Language Disorders (ISES2), Potsdam, April 2002.

## Note

1. The effect is stronger in southern German speakers. This has probably to do with differences between the grammars of the German dialects concerned (see Bayer 1990).

## References

Barisnikov, K., Van Der Linden, M., & Poncelet, M. (1996). "Acquisition of new words and phonological working memory in Williams syndrome: A case study". *Neurocase, 2*, 395–404.

Bayer, J. (1990). "Notes on ECP in English and German". *Groninger Arbeiten zur Germanistischen Linguistik (GAGL), 30*, 1–55.

Cattell, R. B., Weiß, R. H., & Osterland, J. (1997). *CFT 1 – Grundintelligenztest Skala 1.* Goettingen: Hogrefe.

Clahsen, H. & Almazan, M. (1998). "Syntax and morphology in Williams syndrome". *Cognition, 68*, 167–198.

Clahsen, H. & Almazan, M. (2001). "Compounding and inflection in language impairment: Evidence from Williams syndrome (and SLI)". *Lingua, 110*(10), 729–757.

De Bleser, R., Cholewa, J., Stadie, N., & Tabatabaie, S. (t.a.). *LeMo – Lexikon.* München: Urban & Fischer.

De Villiers, J., Roeper, T., & Vainikka, A. (1990). "The acquisition of long-distance rules". In L. Frazier & J. de Villiers (Eds.), *Language Processing and Language Acquisition* (pp. 257–297). Dordrecht: Kluwer Academic.

De Villiers, J. & Roeper, T. (1996). "Questions after stories: On supplying context and eliminating it as a variable". In D. Mcdaniel, C. Mckee, & H. Smith Cairns (Eds.), *Methods for Assessing Children's Syntax* (pp. 163–187). Cambridge, MA: The MIT Press.

Frostig, M. (1968). *Frostigs Entwicklungstest der visuellen Wahrnehmung.* Göttingen: Beltz Test GmbH.

Glück, C. W. (1998). TASB – Test zur automatischen Schnellbenennung. München, non-puiblished diagnostic material.

Haegeman, L. (1994). *Introduction to Government and Binding Theory* (2nd edition). Oxford: Blackwell.

Karmiloff-Smith, A., Klima, E., Bellugi, U., Grant, J., & Baron-Cohen, S. (1997). "Language and Williams syndrome: how intact is intact?" *Child Development, 68*, 246–262.

Karmiloff-Smith, A., Brown, J. H., Grice, S., & Paterson, S. (submitted). "Dethroning the myth: cognitive dissociations and innate modularity in Williams syndrome". *Developmental Neuropsychology*.

Kauschke, C. & Siegmüller, J. (2002). *Patholinguistische Diagnostik bei Sprachentwicklungsstörungen*. München: Urban & Fischer.

Kiese, C. & Kozielski, P.-M. (1979). *AWST 3-6 – Aktiver Wortschatztest für drei bis sechsjährige Kinder*. Weinheim: Beltz Test GmbH.

Krause, M. & Penke, M. (2001). "Inflectional morphology in German Williams syndrome". *Brain and Cognition, 48*, 410–413.

McDaniel, D., Chiu, B., & Maxfield, T. L. (1995). "Parameters for WH-movement types: Evidence from child English". *Natural Language and Linguistic Theory, 13*, 709–753.

Mervis, C., Morris, C. A., Bertrand, J., & Robinson, B. F. (1999). Williams syndrome: Findings from an integrated program of research". In H. Tager-Flusberg (Ed.), *Neurodevelopmental Disorders: Contributions to a new framework from cognitive neuroscience* (pp. 65–110). Cambridge, MA: The MIT Press.

Penner, Z. & Kölliker Funk, M. (1998). *Therapie und Diagnose von Grammatikstörungen: Ein Arbeitsbuch*. Luzern: Edition SZH/SPC.

Penner, Z. (1999). *Screeningverfahren zur Feststellung von Störungen in der Grammatik*. Luzern: Edition SZH/SPC.

Ross, J. (1967). Constraints on Variables in Syntax. Ph.D. dissertation. Cambridge, MA: MIT.

Rubba, J. & Klima, E. (1991). "Preposition use in a speaker with Williams syndrome. Some cognitive grammar proposals". *Report, 5*(3), 1–12. Department of Linguistics, UCSD, San Diego.

Thomas, M. S. C., Grant, J., Barham, Z., Gsödl, M., Laing, E., Lakusta, L., Tyler, L. K. T., Grice, S., Paterson, S., & Karmiloff-Smith, A. (2001). "Past tense formation in Williams syndrome". *Language and Cognitive Processes, 16*, 143–176.

van der Lely, H. (in press). "Evidence for and implications of a domain-specific grammatical deficit." In L. Jenkins (Ed.), *Autonomy, Interaction or Cause: Evidence from regular and irregular morphology*. Oxford: Elsevier.

van der Lely, H. & Battel, J. (2003). Wh-movement in children with with grammatical- SLI: Atest of the RDDR hypothesis. *Language, 79*(1), 153–181.

Vicari, S., Brizzolara, D., Carlesimo, G.A., Pezzini, G., & Volterra, V. (1996a). "Memory abilities in children with Williams syndrome". *Cortex, 32*, 503–514.

Vicari, S., Carlesimo, G. A., Pezzini, G., & Volterra, V. (1996b). "Short-term memory in children with Williams syndrome: A reduced contribution of lexical-semantic knowledge to word span". *Neuropsychologia, 34*, 919–925.

Volterra, V., Capirci, O., Pezzini, G., Sabbadini, L., & Vicari, S. (1996). "Linguistic abilities in Italian children with Williams syndrome". *Cortex, 32*, 663–677.

Weiß, R. H. (1998). *Grundintelligenzskala 2, CFT 20*. Göttingen: Hogrefe.

Weissenborn, J., Roeper, T., & de Villiers, J. (1990). "The acquisition of WH-movement in German and French". In T. L. Maxfield & B. Plunkett (Eds.), *Papers in the acquisition of WH. Proceedings of the University of Massachusetts Roundtable* (pp. 43–73). Amherst: UMOP Special Edition.

Weissenborn, J., Roeper, T., & de Villiers, J. (1995). "Wh-acquisition in French and German: Connections between case, WH-features, and unique triggers". *Recherches Linguistique, 24*, 125–155.

Weissenborn, J. (2000). "Der Erwerb von Morphologie und Syntax". In H. Grimm (Ed.), *Sprachentwicklung. Enzyklopädie der Psychologie* (pp. 139–167). Göttingen: Hogrefe.

Zukowski, A. (2001). Uncovering Grammatical Competence in Children with Williams Syndrome. Boston University, Doctoral dissertation.

## Appendix

### List of trials: Complex wh-questions

1. (SCO-ARG)

| | |
|---|---|
| Lisa will im Kindergarten das Puppenhaus aufräumen. Es ist sehr unordentlich und Lisa will es nicht allein machen. Die Erzieherin fragt Jan, ob er Lisa dabei helfen kann. Jan sagt der Erzieherin: "Wenn ich die Autorennbahn fertig aufgebaut habe, werde ich Lisa helfen." | Lisa wants to tidy up the doll house. It is very untidy and Lisa does not intend to do it all by herself. The kindergarden teacher asks Jan, whether he could help Lisa. Jan says to the kindergarden teacher: "After I finished my car racing trail, I will help Lisa." |
| Was sagt Jan, wem er helfen will? | What does Jan say, whom he will help? |

2. (COPY-ARG)

| | |
|---|---|
| Peter will seine Oma besuchen. Bevor er losgeht, sagt die Mutter: "Bitte vergiss nicht, der Oma zu sagen, dass sie am Wochenende zum Kaffe zu uns kommen soll." Peter verspricht der Mutter: "Ich werde der Oma Bescheid sagen." | Peter wants to visit his grandmother. Before he leaves home, his mother says to him: "Please do not forget to remind Grandma that she is invited for tea at the weekend." Peter promises his mother: "I will remind Grandma." |
| Wem verspricht Peter, wem er Bescheid sagen will? | Whom does Peter promise, whom he will remind? |

3. (ARG-INV)

| | |
|---|---|
| Jans Kater ist durch die offene Balkontür gelaufen. Jan möchte mit ihm spielen, kann ihn in der Wohnung aber nicht finden. Er sagt zu seinem Papa: "Mein Kater muss in den Garten gelaufen sein. Ich werde ihm nachlaufen." | Jan's cat has run out of the balcony door. Jan wants to play with him, however cannot find him in the apartment. He tells his father: "My cat must have run in the garden. I will follow him." |
| Wem sagt Jan möchte er nachlaufen? | Whom does Jan tell he wants to run after? |

4. (ARG-ARG)
Der Hampelmann im Kindergarten ist kaputt. Ein Arm ist abgerissen. Lisa ist sehr traurig. Da zeigt ihr die Erzieherin, dass man den Hampelmann mit Klebstoff reparieren kann.
Wem zeigt die Erzeherin, was man reparieren kann?

The jumping jack in the kindergarden is broken. One arm is missing. Lisa finds this very sad. However, the kindergarden teacher shows her, how the jumping jack can be repaired with glue.
Whom does the kindergarden teacher show, what to repair?

5. (ADJ-ARG)
Jan besucht Lisa. Lisa möchte nicht, dass Jan mit ihrer neuen Puppe spielt und versteckt sie. Abends fragt die Mama, wo die Puppe ist. Lisa sagt: "Ich habe sie vorhin hinter meinem Schrank versteckt."
Wann sagt Lisa, wo sie die Puppe versteckt hat?

Jan visits Lisa. Lisa does not want Jan to play with her new doll. Therefore she hides the doll. In the evening, her mother asks, where she put her new doll. Lisa answers: "I have hidden my new doll behind my wardrobe."
When does Lisa say, where she had hidden her doll?

6. (ARG-ADJ)
Die Kinder sollen in der Schule ein Bild von ihrem besten Freund malen. Peter fragt die Lehrerin: "Wie soll ich das Bild denn malen?" Die Lehrerin sagt, er soll das Bild mit Buntstiften malen.
Wen fragt Peter, wie er malen soll?

In school, the children are drawing a picture from their best friends. Peter asks the teacher: "How am I supposed to draw the picture?" The teacher tells him to draw the picture with coloured pencils.
Who does Peter ask how to draw?

7. (SCO-ADJ)
Hier spielen Jan und Peter Fußball. Plötzlich schießt Peter den Ball in eine Fensterscheibe. Da sagt Jan wütend: "Du hast den Ball zu stark getreten."
Was sagt Jan, wie Peter den Ball getreten hat?

Here are Peter and Jan, playing soccer. Suddenly, Peter kicks the ball into a window. Jan says angry: "You have kicked the ball too hard."
What does Jan say, how Peter has kicked the ball?

8. (COPY-ADJ)
Peter klettert gern im Wald auf Bäume. Eines Nachmittags verliert er das Gleichgewicht und fällt vom Baum herunter. Am selben Abend nimmt er ein Bad und entdeckt einen blauen Fleck auf seinem Knie. Er sagt zu seinem Vater: "Ich glaube, ich habe mir heute Nachmittag wehgetan, als ich vom Baum gefallen bin."
Wann sagt Peter, wann er sich wehgetan hat?

Peter likes to climb on trees. One afternoon, he looses his balance and falls down from a big tree. At the evening of the same day he takes a bath and recognizes a wound on his knee. He says to his father: "I think, I have hurt myself this afternoon, when a fell from the tree."
When does Peter say, when he has hurt himself?

9. (ADJ-INV)

| | |
|---|---|
| Peter und Jan spielen auf dem Spielplatz. Im Sandkasten sagt Peter: "Ich werde nachher im Laden eine große Tüte Bonbons kaufen." | Peter and Jan are playing on a playground. In the sand pit Peter says: "Later on I will buy myself a big bag of sweets in the shop." |
| Wo sagt Peter kauft er die Bonbons? | Where does Peter say he buys the sweets? |

10. (ADJ-ARG)

| | |
|---|---|
| Peter will mit seiner Oma zum Einkaufen gehen. Die Oma sagt, er soll heute auch noch jemand anderem helfen. Peter fragt sie später im Supermarkt: "Wem soll ich denn heute noch helfen?" Die Oma sagt, er soll heute noch ihrer Nachbarin helfen. | Peter wants to go shopping with his Grandma. The Grandma says, that he is supposed to help someone else also. Peter asks her later in the supermarket: "Whom am I supposed to help?" Grandma answers, he shall help her neighbour. |
| Wo fragt Peter, wem er helfen soll? | Where does Peter ask whom he shall help? |

11. (SCO-ADJ)

| | |
|---|---|
| Jan lernt gerade Schlittschuhlaufen. Das will er seinem Freund Peter zeigen. Jan sagt zu ihm: "Ich kann schon richtig gut Schlittschuhlaufen!" Plumps! Da fällt er hin. | Jan learns to skate in the moment. He wants to show this to Peter. Jan says: "I am a good skater already!" Boom! There he falls on his back! |
| Was sagt Jan, wie er Schlittschuhlaufen kann? | What does Jan say, how he can skate? |

12. (COF-ARG)

| | |
|---|---|
| Peter und seine Mutter gehen durch die Stadt. Vor einem Kaufhaus stehen Musikanten, die Gitarre spielen und dazu singen. Peter gefällt die Musik. Er bleibt stehen und sagt zu seiner Mutter: "Ich möchte den Musikanten zuhören." | Peter and his mother walk through town. They notice a group of musicians, who sing and play the guitar in front of a shop. Peter likes the music. He stops and says to his mother: "I would like to listen to the musicians." |
| Wem sagt Peter, wem er zuhören möchte? | To whom does Peter say, whom he wants to listen? |

13. (ARG-INV)

| | |
|---|---|
| Peter hat zum Geburtstag ein Kaninchen geschenkt bekommen. Sein Vater ist im Garten, um einen Stall für das Kaninchen zu bauen. Peter sagt zu seiner Mutter: "Ich werde auch in den Garten gehen und Papa beim Bauen zuschauen." | Peter got a rabbit for his birthday. His father is building a stable for the rabbit in the garden. Peter says to his mother: "I will go in the garden and watch Dad." |
| Wem sagt Peter möchte er zuschauen? | To whom does Peter say he wants to watch? |

14. (ARG-ARG)

| | |
|---|---|
| Lisa hat den ganzen Tag im Kindergarten gebastelt. Dann kommt ihre Mutter und | Lisa has been painting and drawing the whole day in the kindergarden. Later on |

holt sie ab. Auf dem Nachhauseweg erzählt Lisa: "Ich habe für die Oma einen ganz großen Elefanten gebastelt."
Wem erzählt Lisa, was sie gebastelt hat?

her mother comes and picks her up. On the way home, Lisa tells her mother: "I have drawn a big elefant for Grandma."
Whom tells Lisa, what she has painted?

15. (ADJ-ARG)
Jan und Peter treffen sich auf der Straße. Sie wollen in die Stadt fahren. Im Bus sagt Jan: "Ich möchte nachher noch meine Oma besuchen."
Wo sagt Jan, wen er besuchen will?

Jan and Peter meet on the street. They want to got to town by bus. In the bus, Jan says: "Later this afternoon, I want to visit my Grandma."
Where does Jan say, whom he wants to visit?

16. (ARG-ADJ)
Lisa möchte für ihre Freunde im Kindergarten Kekse backen. Sie sagt zu ihrer Mutter. "Ich will die Kekse mit ganz viel Schokolade backen."
Wem sagt Lisa, wie sie die Kekse backen will?

Lisa wants to bake cookies for her friends in the kindergarden. She tells her mother: "I will bake the cookies with a lot of chocolate."
Whom does Lisa tell, how she will bake the cookies?

18. (COP-ADJ)
Peter ist mit seiner Mutter im Freibad. Er hat gerade schwimmen gelernt. Heute will er seiner Mutter zeigen, wie gut er das schon kann. Peter springt ins Wasser und schwimmt los. Die Mutter schaut vom Beckenrand aus zu und ruft sehr laut: "Du kannst aber schon toll schwimmen!"
Wie ruft die Mutter, wie Peter schwimmen kann?

Peter is in the swimming pool with his mother. Has has just learned to swim. Today, he want to show his mother, how good he is already able to swim. Peter jumps into the pool and starts swimming. His mother is watching him from the edge of the pool and shouts out very loud: "You swim very well!"
How does the mother shout how Peter is able to swim?

19. (ARG-INV)
Jan und Lisa besuchen ihre Oma. Beide haben großen Hunger und möchten etwas essen. Die Oma fragt Lisa, was sie denn heute kochen soll. Lisa sagt: "Ich möchte gern Nudeln mit Tomatensoße essen."
Was sagt Lisa soll die Oma kochen?

Jan and Lisa are visiting their grandmother. Both are very hungry. They want to eat something. Grandma asks Lisa what she shall cook today. Lisa says: "I would like to eat spaghetti bolognese."
What does Lisa say Grandma shall cook?

20. (ARG-ARG)
Peter kommt morgens in die Schule. Er ist ganz aufgeregt. Er läuft zu Jan und erzählt ihm: "Ich habe gerade im Park gesehen, wie ein Eichhörnchen eine Eichel gefressen hat."
Wem sagt Peter, was er gesehen hat?

Peter comes to school in the morning. He is very excited. He runs to Jan and tells him: "In the park I have just seen a squirrel eating an oak!"
To whom does Peter say, what he has seen?

| | |
|---|---|
| 21. (ADJ-ARG) | |
| Lisa hat eine neue Mütze. Auf der Straße bückt sie sich und die Mütze fällt herunter. Lisa geht aber weiter. Als sie abends nach Hause kommt, zieht sie ihre Jacke aus und merkt, dass die Mütze weg ist. Sie sagt zu ihrer Mutter: "Ich muss meine Mütze vorhin verloren haben." | Lisa has a new cap. On the street, she bends down and the cap falls off. However, Lisa keeps on walking. When she comes home in the evening, she takes off her coat and notices that her cap is lost. She tells her mother: "I must have lost my cap a little while ago." |
| Wann merkt Lisa, was sie verloren hat? | When does Lisa notice, what she has lost? |
| 22. (SCO-ARG) | |
| Lisas Mutter hat heute Geburtstag. Als Lisa mit Jan vom Kindergarten nach Hause geht, kauft sie einen großen Blumenstrauß. Sie sagt zu Jan: "Die Blumen will ich meiner Mutter zum Geburtstag schenken." | It's the birthday of Lisas mother today. When Lisa comes home from kindergarden together with Jan, she buys a big bunch of flowers. She says to Jan: "I will give the flowers to my mother for her birthday." |
| Was sagt Lisa, wem sie die Blumen schenken will? | What does Lisa say, to whom she will give the flowers? |
| 23. (COP-ADJ) | |
| Jan möchte Lisa zum Spielen abholen. Die Mutter möchte wissen, wann Lisa wieder zurückkommt. Beim Losgehen sagt Lisa: "Ich komme nach Hause, wenn es dunkel wird." | Jan wants to pick up Lisa for playing outside. Her mother wants to know, when Lisa will be home again. While walking off, Lisa says: "I will be home, when it gets dark." |
| Wann sagt Lisa, wann sie nach Hause kommt? | When does Lisa say, when she will return home? |
| 24. (ADJ-INV) | |
| Als Peter nach Hause kommt, legt er viele bunte Murmeln auf den Küchentisch. Die Mutter ruft: "Oh, wo hast du denn die tollen Murmeln her?" Peter sagt: "Ich habe sie heute Nachmittag im Sandkasten gefunden." | When Peter comes home, he puts some coloured marbles on the kitchen table. The mother calls: "Oo, where did you find these nice marbles?" Peter says: "I have found them this afternoon in the sand pit." |
| Wo sagt Peter hat er die Murmeln gefunden? | Where does Peter say, he has found the marbles? |
| 25. (ADl-ADJ) | |
| Peter hat in der Schule ein Lied gelernt. Als er am nächsten Tag Jan trifft, erzählt er: "Ich habe das neue Lied heute morgen unter der Dusche gesungen." | Peter has learned a song in school. When he meets Jan on the next day, he tells him: "I have sung the new song in the shower." |
| Wann sagt Peter, wo er das Lied gesungen hat? | When does Peter say, where he has sung the new song? |

27. (SCO-ADJ)

Lisa und Peter haben eine kleine Katze, um die sie sich gemeinsam kümmern. Als Peter mittags aus der Schule kommt, fragt er Lisa, wann sie die Katze gefüttert hat. Lisa sagt: "Ich habe ihr heute morgen etwas zu fressen gegeben."
Was sagt Lisa, wann sie die Katze gefüttert hat?

Lisa and Peter have a little cat, for which they have to look after. When Peter returns from school at lunchtime, he asks Lisa, when she has fed the cat. Lisa says: "I have given her something to eat in the morning."
What does Lisa say, when she has fed the cat?

28. (ADJ-INV)

Lisa und Peter spielen "Mensch ärger dich nicht". Lisa meint, dass es zu zweit nicht so viel Spaß macht und bestimmt bald langweilig wird. Als sie anfangen zu spielen, sagt Peter: "Wenn es langweilig wird, rufe ich Jan an und frage ihn, ob er mitspielen will."
Wann sagt Peter, will er Jan anrufen?

Lisa and Peter play a game. Lisa thinks that it might become boring playing only with Peter. When they start playing, Peter says: "When it gets boring, I call Jan and ask him, whether he would like to play with us."
When does Peter say he will call Jan?

29. (ADJ-ADJ)

Die Mädchen im Kindergarten spielen zusammen in der Puppenecke. Jan will aber nicht mitspielen. Deshalb sagt er wütend zu der Erzieherin: "Ich möchte viel lieber allein in der Puppenecke spielen!"
Wie sagt Jan, wo er spielen möchte?

The girls in the kindergarden play together with dolls in the doll house. Jan does not want to play with them. Angry he says to the kindergarden teacher: "I would like to play for myself in the doll house!"
How does Jan say, where he wants to play?

30. (ARG-ARG)

Im Kindergarten gibt es ein großes neues Puzzle. Lisa versucht, die passenden Teile zu finden. Das Puzzle ist aber sehr schwierig. Jan puzzelt auch sehr gern und sagt zu der Erzieherin: "Ich kann Lisa beim Puzzeln helfen."
Wem sagt Jan, wem er helfen kann?

In the kindergarden there is a huge puzzle. Lisa tries to put the right pieces together. However, the puzzle is very difficult. Jan likes to puzzle, too. He says to the kindergarden teacher: "I can help Lisa."
To whom does Jan say, whom he can help?

# Passives in German children with Williams syndrome*

Susanne Bartke
Justus-Liebig University Giessen

This paper investigates passive acquisition in exceptional developmental circumstances, the so-called Williams syndrome (WS). The purpose of this study is twofold. First, results add to the discussion whether individuals with WS will be able to analyse and use linguistic rules as claimed by Clahsen and colleagues (1998, 2001). Second, data provide insight into a special area of syntactic development. Participants consisted of ten individuals with WS (age range: 6–22 years; mental age range: 3;4–7;6). The control group included 103 normally developing children (3–8 years). The results of this picture-pointing task reveal that young WS children lag behind their control mates, but they catch up by a mental age of 5 years. Thus, WS children are able to analyse syntactic regularities. Further, language development in WS maybe interpreted in terms of a delay rather than a deviant path of development.

## 1. The two components of the language faculty: Rules and lexical storage

One main topic regarding the linguistic development and competence in Williams syndrome (WS) is the issue of whether individuals with WS are able to generalize grammatical phenomena or whether they are, in fact, very good rote learners. One test case has been the area of morphology as regular morphological forms are a field of generalizations as opposed to irregular morphological forms which are subject to rote learning and memory (lexical storage).

Although ample evidence has been reported, the majority of research results have argued for a strong ability of grammatical rule building in WS. Clahsen and Almazan (2001) reported for a group of four English children with WS (mental age: 5 and 7 years) a 100% performance on regular plural forms, but a failure of 55% on generating irregular plural forms (results are averaged over mental age groups; cf. details in Clahsen & Almazan 2001:739). The errors made by the two children with a mental age of 5 years consisted of 40% in the use of the regular plural case (i.e., *-s* marked forms represented by a (default) rule. For the 7-year-old children with WS, the overregularization rate was 20%. This was much higher than the rate observed in the control group matched for mental age. These results were interpreted as a very good ability in detecting and applying grammatical rules in WS. The low performance on irregular plural forms, in contrast, suggested that a lack within the lexical storage component exists.

The results obtained by Zukowski (2001) support the interpretation advocated by Clahsen and Almazan (2001). Her study included twelve individuals with WS, aged from 8 to 16 years (mental age range: 4–9 years). She observed a correctness score for irregular plurals of about 95%, while the correctness rate for irregular plurals reached only about 30%. Instead, about 25% of the irregular forms received the regular plural ending, namely the *-s* affix. Moreover, about 87% of the nonce words were pluralized with the *-s* affix; the remaining forms had been left unmarked. These results displayed a strong asymmetry of regular and irregular morphology with the rule system for regular morphology remaining intact (cf. Zukowski 2001:35, Table 7).

First results from a language with a somewhat richer inflectional system such as German confirmed these results (Krause & Penke 2001; Niedeggen-Bartke 2001). Krause and Penke (2001) observed 83% correct regular plural forms opposed to 67% correct irregular plural forms in two individuals with WS. Niedeggen-Bartke (2001), investigating data from 4 children with WS, noted a correctness rate of 94% for regular forms, but only 75% correct irregular forms. The incorrectly inflected irregular forms displayed a strong preference for the overregularization of the German default affix (*-s* allomorph).

In sum, considered from a cross-linguistic perspective, the analyses on morphological abilities in WS strongly suggest an intact rule system, while the lexical storage system is limited and disturbed. However, aside from morphological processes, rule-governed processes can also be found within the syntactic system. Analyses on these can add to the discussion on a preserved rule component in WS. One example might be movement operations for interpreting resp. generating passive sentences. In the first part of this article I will outline the grammatical characteristics of passives and present some acquisitional facts. In the second part I will present data of a picture pointing task carried out with ten children and adolescents each with WS, and mental ages ranging from about three up to about seven years. Note that this study is the first presenting elicited data on passives in a larger group of individuals with WS ranging from very young children to adults. The observation will be that the young children with WS up to a mental age of four years in comparison to children of typical development, show more difficulties with passives, whereas WS children with mental ages of 5 years and higher, perform comparable to their peers within the control group. The concluding section will relate the findings to the discussion of whether individuals with WS benefit from rules for compensating a lexical deficit.

## 2. Passive – its structure and acquisition

The model proposed by Chomsky (1995) is subdivided into two parts, one of them hosting the mental lexicon, the other one containing the computational system that generates complex words, phrases, and sentences.

Generating a passive sentence means to apply specific morphological changes and a movement rule. In German, for example, the verb changes its appearance: a simple verb is turned into a participle form and additionally receives an auxiliary. This auxiliary can be provided either by the verb *werden* ('to be', verbal passive reading) or by the verb *sein* ('to be', adjectival, static reading); compare the following examples:

(1) *Der Fußboden wird gewischt.* ('The floor is being wiped.')

(2) *Der Fußboden ist gewischt.* ('The floor is wiped.')

Note that the sentence in (2) has an ambiguous reading, because it can be read either from a static perspective or as a short cut for the verbal passive *Der Fußboden ist gewischt* <u>*worden*</u> ('The floor has been wiped'). The most important thing is a change at the syntactic level, namely a movement of the NP from the former object position into the subject position. The movement results in a chain and leaves a trace:

(3) a. *Moni wischt den Fußboden.* ('Moni wipes the floor$_{acc}$.')
b. [*Der Fußboden*]$_i$ *wird gewischt* $e_i$. ('The floor$_{nom}$ is being wiped.')

As can be seen from the examples given in (3), a further change is linked to the movement of the NP: the NP moving from the object position to the subject position is required to change case. The former object with accusative case marking undergoes case absorption, i.e. it is now being represented in the nominative case. The former subject, if inserted at all, can be inserted only by a prepositional phrase receiving the case from the preposition (either dative or accusative). The drop of the subject of the active sentence results in a short verbal passive (cf. example given in (1)), while insertion of the former subject via a prepositional phrase (*durch* resp. *von*, 'by') results in a long verbal passive as presented by the example in (4).

(4) *Der Fußboden wird von/durch Moni gewischt.* ('The floor is being wiped by Moni.')

Superficially, the sentences in (1) and (2) resemble copula structures as in (5) and (6):

(5) *Der Fußboden wird grün.* ('The floor is getting green.')

(6) *Der Fußboden ist grün.* ('The floor is green.')

The main criterion for distinguishing the sentence in (1) from the sentence in (5) is the identification of the verb, its grammatical features and the movement operation leading to a passive structure. Therefore, the most important prerequisite for interpreting passives is the ability to detect (rule-governed) traces indicating movement.

This competence is not easy to acquire. It is, in fact, accompanied by many errors which follow a certain system as described below. In addition to errors concerning an incorrect morphological form of the participle, children have made attempts to passivize verbs that usually cannot be passivized such as *He get died* (cf. Pinker et al. 1987: 204, Table 2) or *Hier ist Gold angestreift* ('Here the gold is being striped onto' meaning 'This is gold-striped/has gold stripes on it'; cf. Clark 1982:407). These examples display errors that are observed characteristically in production. Errors in comprehension are of a slightly different nature. As noted by Bever (1970), children tend to assign thematic roles to a passive sentence by a syntactically guided strategy (known by him as *Strategy D*, cf. Bever 1970: 298): "Any Noun-Verb-Noun (NVN) sequence within a potential internal unit in the surface structure corresponds to 'actor-action-object'."

The children's answer behavior results in a very predictable error pattern when presented with passive sentences: the situation acted out, the action performed or the picture selected by the child mirrors an answer with reversed roles in comparison to the sentence actually given. In a classic study carried out by de Villiers and de Villiers (1973), 33 children aged from 19 months to 36 months were tested on active sentences and long verbal passives, i.e. passive sentences with a *by* phrase. The children were asked to act out such sentences as, for example, *Make the dog be bitten by the cat* (de Villiers & de Villiers 1973: 334). As noted by de Villiers and de Villiers, the youngest children of this group even failed to perform above chance level on the active sentences. Considering the overall syntactic development of this stage, this observation was not very surprising. Children of the late MLU-stage I have mostly mastered the actives while they still struggle with passives. For actives an increasing performance rate could be observed: in the early stage I, 31% of the sentences were answered correctly, while at the age of 26–36 months, i.e. at the early stage V, children responded correctly in 83% of the cases. The correctness scores for passive sentences increased less dramatically. Instead, an interesting change in error pattern could be observed over time. When focusing on the incorrect answers for passives only, the results obtained by de Villiers and de Villiers (1973: 335) reveal the following pattern (cf. Table 1).

**Table 1.** Incorrect responses observed by de Villiers and de Villiers (1973: 335)

| | n | Passives reversed | child as actor | refusals |
|---|---|---|---|---|
| Early stage I (MLU 1.00–1.50) | 7 | 37% | 43% | 20% |
| Late stage I (MLU 1.50–2.00) | 3 | 42% | 42% | 16% |
| Stage II (MLU 2.00–2.50) | 7 | 69% | 27% | 4% |
| Stage III (MLU 2.50–3.00) | 7 | 74% | 22% | 4% |
| Early stage IV (MLU 3.00–3.50) | 4 | 100% | – | – |
| Late st. IV & early st. V (MLU 3.50–4.25) | 5 | 83% | 5% | 11% |

Beginning with the MLU-stage II, for interpreting passives, children increasingly apply the word order strategy as described by Bever (1970). At the age of 26–36 months resp. at the transition to MLU-stage V, children still acted out over 83% of the sentences incorrectly by applying the word order strategy.

To sum up the observations so far, if children have not detected syntactic chains indicating movement that in turn indicates a syntactic structure different from an active sentence, they make use of a rule that maps syntactic units onto thematic roles in a canonical fashion. For the purpose of this paper, I will call the interpretation of passives by the usage of a syntactic rule as the *deep structure strategy* (leading to correct responses), while I will call the compensation strategy (being semantically guided and leading to reversed and therefore incorrect responses) the *actor-action-object strategy*.

Bever (1970) acknowledged the fact that some passive sentences are more vulnerable than others to misinterpretation because of their semantic context. Due to probabilistic constraints, a sentence like (7) is more likely to evoke a reversed response than a sentence like (8) (examples adapted from Bever 1970).

(7) *The cow is kissed by the horse.*

(8) *The mother is patted by the dog.*

Investigating the data of children aged from 2 to 5 years of age, he observed a steady increase in performance when the children were presented with reversible sentences until roughly 4 years of age. Then suddenly, a drop in performance could be observed, followed by an increase in performance again. Bever interprets the temporary decrease as '… the phase in which he [the child, SB] depends relatively heavily on something like Strategy D for the comprehension of sentences that do not have semantic constraints' (Bever 1970: 306f.).

Investigating the development of passives in German children, Schaner-Wolles and her collaborators (1986, 1989) took a closer look at this phenomenon of reversible and non-reversible sentences. They presented 27 children aged from 3;2 to 5;9 years of age with three types of verbs or, rather, sentences: (i) reversible sentences, (ii) potentially reversible sentences, i.e. those with a low pragmatic likelihood which should influence the children's decision, and (iii) irreversible sentences, i.e. agent and patient are determined by the verb in a way that they cannot get exchanged (for details cf. Schaner-Wolles 1989: 143). The set of passive sentences consisted of six short verbal passives and six full verbal passives. The sentences were read aloud to the children. The children's task consisted of selecting the best fitting picture from an array of three pictures. Overall, the number of correct responses was higher than expected from the results of former studies. Furthermore, errors based on the so-called strategy D (Bever 1970) occurred rather rarely. Therefore, Schaner-Wolles states '[...] it is safe to hypothesize that an agent-first strategy plays no or only an inferior role in the interpretation skills of our German speaking subjects' (Schaner-Wolles 1989: 149).

To conclude, the results of the German study allow assuming that German children as young as 3 years of age are capable of decoding the syntax behind a passive sentence. The semantic context has a rather low disturbing influence.

## 3. Passive in English-speaking individuals with Williams syndrome

Most studies investigating language development in Williams syndrome were dealing with the English language. Among the first was the study by Bellugi et al. (1990). In this investigation, six children with Williams syndrome (mental age: 6–7 years) took part. The test included semantically reversible passive sentences of which between 80% and 100% were answered correctly. This remarkable result was confirmed by further studies, although unfortunately no further details were provided (cf. Wang & Bellugi 1993; Bellugi et al. 2000).

First quantitative results were provided by Clahsen and Almazan (1998) and Karmiloff-Smith et al. (1998). Karmiloff-Smith et al. tested eight individuals with Williams syndrome (mental age: 14;9 to 34;8 years) and 18 normal adults (age range: 19–29 years) on the Birkbeck Reversible Sentences Test (Black et al. 1991). The test included seven different sentence types: (i) an active sentence with an agentive verb; (ii) an active sentence with a non-agentive verb; (iii) a passive sentence with an agentive verb; (iv) a passive sentence with a non-agentive verb; (v) a sentence containing an adjective; (vi) a sentence containing a deverbal adjective;

(vii) a sentence containing a locative. While the results of the controls are reported as 'virtually error-free on this task' (cf. Karmiloff-Smith et al. 1998: 347), the individuals with Williams syndrome performed less well. They reached correctness scores ranging between 63 and 86%, mean error was given as 24%.[1] Unfortunately, no information is given on the kind of these errors (either selecting the picture showing the action with reverse roles or the picture with a distractor, i.e. showing an action different from the presented sentence). Therefore, it remains unclear if a system other than a syntactic one led to incorrect answers. In sum, the observations made by Karmiloff-Smith et al. suggested that individuals with Williams syndrome have difficulties acquiring the syntax of passives.

A detailed quantitative analysis is presented by Clahsen and Almazan (1998). They presented the children (mental age: 5 and 7 years) with four different types of sentences: (i) an active sentence; (ii) a short progressive passive sentence; (iii) a long verbal passive sentence; (iv) a sentence with ambiguous reading, with either a verbal or an adjectival interpretation. In a picturepointing task the children had to identify from an array of pictures the picture best matching the sentence that was read aloud to them. The results obtained in the group with Williams syndrome showed a performance better than the results obtained in the control groups, namely children of the same mental age: the answers of the children with Williams syndrome were correct in 96–100%. In other words, the children with Williams syndrome reached adult performance (for details cf. Clahsen & Almazan 1998: 180, Table 4). In comparison, specifically of language impaired children (SLI) at the mental age of 5 to 7 years (cf. details in van der Lely 1996: 253f.) did show significant difficulties on decoding full and short verbal passives. Similar results were obtained in a study carried out by Bishop et al. (2000). As emphasized by Clahsen and Almazan, the SLI children displayed an error pattern not observed in the children with Williams syndrome, i.e. selecting a reversal answer.

Although Karmiloff-Smith et al. and Clahsen and Almazan used a similar method (sentence-picture matching task), they obtained diverging results. The reasons are not clear and open to speculation. Perhaps these differing results were based on the differences in linguistic material. It is possible that the verbs used may differ in familiarity, so that less familiarity might lead to more errors in the study by Karmiloff-Smith et al. (1998). Perhaps, some of the verbs used by Clahsen and Almazan (1998) are semantically less ambiguous, leading to a performance at ceiling. In contrast, Karmiloff-Smith et al. have used without exception reversible sentences. In sum, this would suggest that the study carried out by Clahsen and Almazan tested predominantly grammatical knowledge concerning the underlying syntactic structure of passives, while the task carried out by Karmiloff-Smith et al. tested predominantly the influence of semantics. This, in turn, would imply that grammatical knowledge on passives is present and available, but that grammatical processing can be influenced easily by the semantics of the verb. If supposed that features of the verb, such as number and kind of theta roles, is part of the verb's lexical entry, this might hint at lexical problems. This would be in line with further observations of an aberrant lexical organization in Williams syndrome as indicated by difficulties with vocabulary acquisition (cf. Böhning & Weissenborn 2003) and difficulties with respect to irregular morphological processes (cf. Clahsen & Almazan 2001; Levy & Hermon 2000; Niedeggen-Bartke 2001; Penke & Krause this volume; Zukowski 2001).

In sum, the studies presented to date suggest strongly that older children and adults with Williams syndrome have acquired the rules of the syntax of passives. Consequently, the guiding questions will be:

1. Will German children with WS provide incorrect answers that might reflect difficulties in decoding passives? Former studies have revealed a high performance on passives, but the participants have been more advanced than the four youngest participants of the present study.
2. What kind of errors can be observed? While some studies on English speaking children report a predominance of interpreting passives with reversed roles, Schaner-Wolles could not confirm this observation for her group of German children with typical development.
3. An additional question would be whether reversible sentences are more affected than irreversible sentences.

## 4. Passive in German children with Williams syndrome

The study presented here investigates the knowledge of passives in Williams syndrome by administering a sentence-picture matching task. Following the procedure of van der Lely and Stollwerck (1996) and Clahsen and Almazan (1998), four different types of sentences are chosen to present 20 different verbs, half of the verbs resp. sentences are reversible from a semantic point of view. From a syntactic point of view, only transitive verbs are selected, i.e. technically each verb allows a passive sentence structure (cf. list of verbs in Appendix 1).

Results from two groups of children and adolescents with Williams syndrome are to be presented. These are compared to results obtained from a large group of typically developing children.

### 4.1 Participants

The group of individuals with Williams syndrome consisted of ten participants. Four of them had been tested on the Hamburg-Wechsler-Intelligence Scale III (Tewes & Wechsler 2001) which allowed a closer analysis of verbal and non-verbal

**Table 2.** Children with Williams syndrome tested on HAWIK-III

| | Julia | Maria | Laura | Robert |
|---|---|---|---|---|
| chronological age | 6;11 | 8;11 | 8;9 | 9;0 |
| IQ | 69 | 66 | 61 | 69 |
| performance IQ | 48 | 46 | 48 | 61 |
| verbal IQ | 86 | 74 | 76 | 79 |
| verbal age-equivalent | 4;1 | 4;0 | 4;5 | 4;9 |
| mental age-equivalent | 3;4 | 3;4 | 3;7 | 4;7 |

**Table 3.** Children and adolescents with Williams syndrome; IQ scores based on CFT

| | Frauke | Karla | Martin | Ansgar | Johanna | Lena |
|---|---|---|---|---|---|---|
| chronological age | 9;2 | 13;2 | 12;0 | 18;2 | 22;0 | 9;8 |
| mental age-equivalent | 5;8 | 6;0 | 6;6 | 7;6 | 7;6 | 7;6 |

abilities. The mental age-equivalents for verbal and performance IQ's demonstrate clearly the uneven, but characteristic cognitive profile (cf. Table 2). The second group consisted of adolescents of higher age with respect to the chronological age as well as with respect to mental age-equivalents. These adolescents had been tested on the Grundintelligenztest Skala (CFT 1, Weiß 1997 resp. CFT 20 Weiß 1998; cf. Table 3).[2]

In sum, data of individuals with Williams syndrome covering the mental age range from 3 years of age to 7 years of age were considered for analyses.

All children had been diagnosed genetically or clinically as carrying the Williams syndrome.

The control group consisted of 103 typically developing children, eleven 3 year olds, 18 4 year olds, 26 5 year olds, 13 7 year olds, and nine 8 year olds. They were selected in order to match the group with Williams syndrome with respect to mental age-equivalents. For the children of the control group no history of any language impairment was reported. All children were monolingual German, acquiring Standard German.

### 4.2 Materials and procedure

Four different sentence types were selected: (i) an active sentence; (ii) a long verbal passive sentence; (iii) a short verbal passive sentence; (iv) a short sentence with an ambiguous reading (either a static reading or an abbreviated verbal reading). Twenty verbs were selected belonging to one of the following two types of verbs: (i) a reversible reading is possible; (ii) a reversible reading is not possible. In each group, half of the verbs were of low frequency, the other half of high frequency

(1 Million lemma corpus according to the CELEX database (Baayen et al. 1993)). The full list of verbs can be found in Appendix 1. Each verb is presented with each sentence type, resulting in a final set of 80 test sentences. Examples are given in (9) to (12); an example of a picture set can be found in Appendix 2.

(9) Type 1: active sentences
   a. Michael grillt das Würstchen. ('Michael barbecues the sausage.')
   b. Der Helfer pudert die Schauspielerin. ('The assistant powders the actress.')

(10) Type 2: short verbal passives
   a. *Das Würstchen wird gegrillt.* (The sausage is being barbecued)
   b. *Die Schauspielerin wird gepudert.* ('The actress is being powdered.')

(11) Type 3: long verbal passives
   a. *Das Würstchen wird von Michael gegrillt.* ('The sausage is barbecued by Michael.')
   b. *Die Schauspielerin wird von dem Helfer gepudert.* ('The actress is powdered by the assistant.')

(12) Type 4: ambiguous reading
   a. *Das Würstchen ist gegrillt.* ('The sausage is barbecued.')
   b. *Die Schauspielerin ist gepudert.* ('The actress is powdered.')

For each single sentence, a set of four pictures have been conducted. One of the pictures displays the action as given by the sentence types 1 to 3, e.g. a man introduced as Michael is barbecuing a sausage. But this picture also matches the situation introduced by sentence type 4, because the ambiguous reading allows this sentence to be interpreted as a short-cut of a verbal reading (cf. discussion above). A second picture displays this action with reversed roles, e.g. a sausage is barbecuing a man-like puppet named Michael. A third picture, matching one of the possible situations of sentences type 4, displays a static result, e.g. a barbecued sausage is being served. A fourth picture mirrors a semantic distractor, e.g. a man named Michael is playing a flute. Because each verb is presented four times, though in a different sentential context, each set of pictures is presented equally often. To prevent children from developing a strategy of selection, no picture appears more than once at the same spot of the set.

To motivate the children for 80 test sentences, a little story was set up: A picture book writer has written an awful lot of little stories which he has enriched with little pictures. Unfortunately, a wind gust has made a mess. Everything is confused now and the child has been asked to help out by sorting the correct picture to the little story (the sentence) read aloud to her.

The children were tested individually. There was no time limit; in case a child had not understood a sentence, the sentence was repeated. The answers were noted on an individual record sheet. Children received tea lights for their participation.

## 4.3 Results

As mentioned above, guiding questions concern quantity as well as quality of incorrect answers according to mental age of the participants with WS. I will begin with presenting a quantitative analysis, i.e. a general survey of correct and incorrect answers. Subsequently, I will present the results in detail by reporting breakdowns of answers to each of the four sentence types. The answers to irreversible and reversible sentences will be presented in the same figure. The respective answers of the individuals with WS will always be compared instantly to the answers given by the children of the control group.

Because the mental age groups of children with Williams syndrome are very small (n range: 1 to 3), I will refrain from statistical analyses; instead, percentages of correctness will be presented and compared.

### 4.3.1 *Overall correctness scores*

A first survey as illustrated in Figure 1a reveals that even the typically developing children produce erroneous answers, although these erroneous answers occur significantly less than correct answers.[3] Probably extending the set of pictures from three (as preferred by Schaner-Wolles 1986, 1989) to four pictures per array might increase the non-linguistic demands of the task and therefore lead to an overall lower performance. As can be seen further in Figure 1a, there is an advantage for irreversible sentences over reversible ones.[4] This is in line with previous observations, namely that even young children acknowledge the fact that verbs can place certain demands regarding their semantic roles.

The break down for sentence types (cf. Figure 1b) demonstrates that the sentences are not equally affected, but that the correctness scores for active sentences increases from 72% (3 year olds) up to 96% (8 year olds). This development is closely followed by the correct answers to ambiguous sentences, where transitive as well as static choices are counted as correct answers.

Most interesting to note is the increase in performance on passives. Both long and short verbal passives are equally well, or less well mastered, respectively. The youngest children respond roughly half of the time correctly (50% for long verbal passives, 46% for short verbal passives), while the oldest children respond correctly near ceiling (93% for long verbal passives; 94% for short verbal passives).[5]

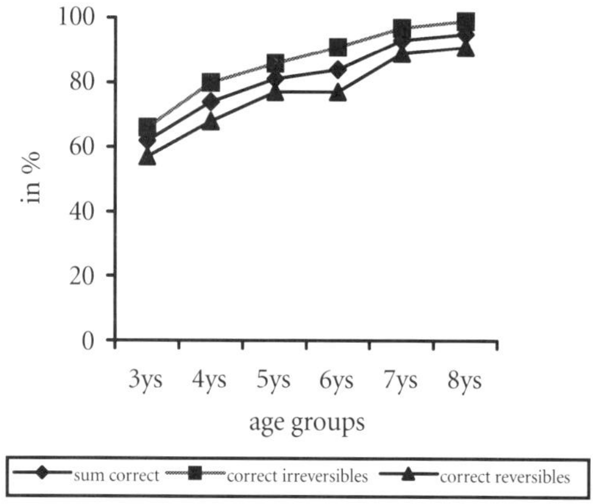


**Figure 1a.** Overall correctness scores: control group

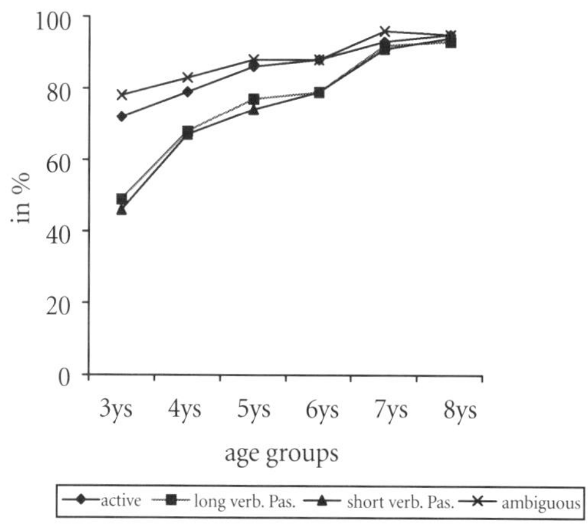


**Figure 1b.** Overall correctness scores: break down for sentence types (control group)

The data observed for the group of subjects with Williams syndrome (cf. Figures 2a and 2b) look less linear than the results obtained by the control group. Note that the general tendency of development is the same. The youngest group of children with Williams syndrome reaches correctness scores of 52% which is 10% below the performance of the 3 year olds of the control group. However, the children with a mental age equivalent of 7 years catch up with the control group: their performance of 90% nearly reaches the 94% of the 7 year olds of the control group.

Furthermore, it is interesting to note that the relation between irreversible and reversible sentences is the same for the Williams group: reversible sentences are more vulnerable to misinterpretation than irreversible sentences. This might imply

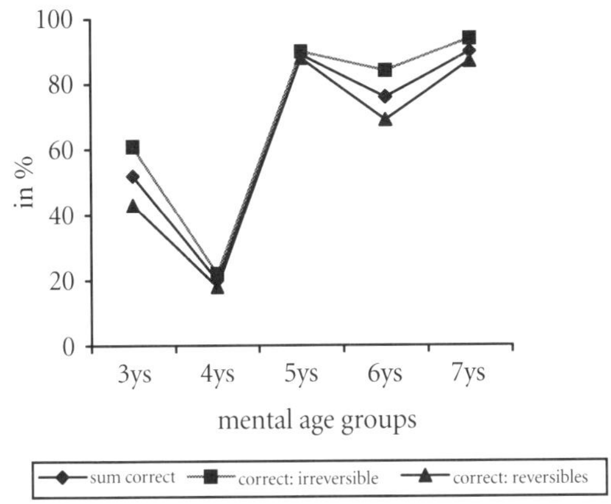


**Figure 2a.** Overall correctness scores: participants with WS

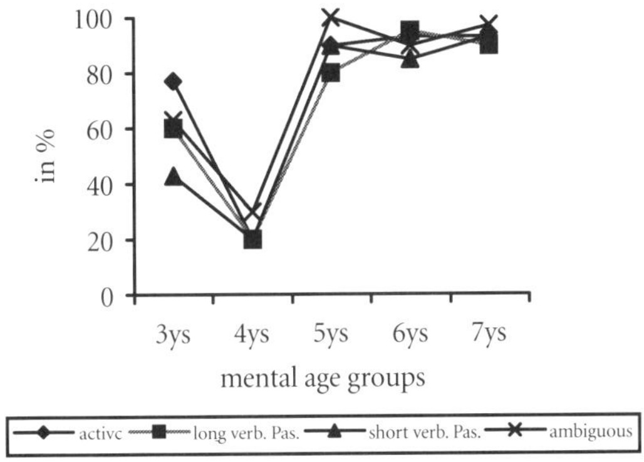


**Figure 2b.** Overall correctness scores: break down for sentence types (participants with WS)

that the participants with Williams syndrome also have acquired some knowledge about the verb's demands on semantic roles.

The performance rates regarding the four different sentence types, too, resemble the data observed in the control group, with regard to the older age equivalent groups (5 to 7 years) (Figure 2b). An increase of performance for all sentence types over age can be seen. As in the control group, active sentences and ambiguous sentences are mastered better than any passive structure.

This break down already suggests that children with WS do not equal their mental age mates all the time; but rather the 3 and 4 year olds of the WS group performed notably below their typically developing age mates, the data obtained by the Williams child at the mental age of 4 years especially illustrate the difference very clearly. The severity of decrease in performance at the mental age group of 4 years may well be an artifact, since just a single child could be sorted into this group. Nevertheless, a clear break in performance could be observed between the WS children of mental age groups of 3 and 4 years of age on the one side and the WS children at the mental age group of 5 years of age and older. Thus, beginning at the age equivalent of 5 years the children with WS start to perform better than their peers of the control group: 90% correct for long verbal passives and 85% correct for short verbal passives at the mental age group of 5 years in the group of WS children to 86% for long verbal passives and 77% for short verbal passives obtained by the 5 year olds of the control group.

To sum up and to answer the first of the guiding questions mentioned above, WS children as well as children with typical development do produce erroneous responses. WS children older than the age equivalent of 5 years outperform their mental age matched controls while younger WS children perform clearly below their age-matched controls. Nevertheless it is important to note that the same relations exist for the typically developing children and the individuals with WS. In particular, reversible sentences are more difficult than irreversible ones for each participating group regardless of (mental) age. Further, passive sentences led more often to erroneous answers than active sentences.

To answer the second guiding question concerning the type of errors, a detailed analysis of the error pattern will be provided in the subsequent sections. I will present the results for (i) active and ambiguous sentences, (ii) long verbal passives, and (iii) short verbal passives successively. Each result section will be completed using bar graphs that are organized as follows: There are separate bar graphs for the control group and the WS group. The bar graphs will consider the two sentence conditions, irreversible and reversible sentences. Therefore, answers to irreversible sentences are noted in the left half of each bar graph, related to (mental) age groups; in the right half of each bar graph answers to reversible sentences related to (mental) age groups are noted.

#### 4.3.2 *Active and ambiguous sentences*

The performance regarding active and ambiguous sentences has been quite good (except for the WS child at the mental age of 4 years). The few errors on active sentences have mainly consisted of static responses, in which only very few reversed pictures or distractors have been chosen.

For the ambiguous sentences the transitive as well as the static response have been counted as correct answers because the sentence structure allows for both interpretations. As can be seen from Figure 3a, the children of the control group have responded similarly to irreversible and reversible sentences, whereas there are significantly more correct responses to irreversible sentences than to reversible ones.[6]

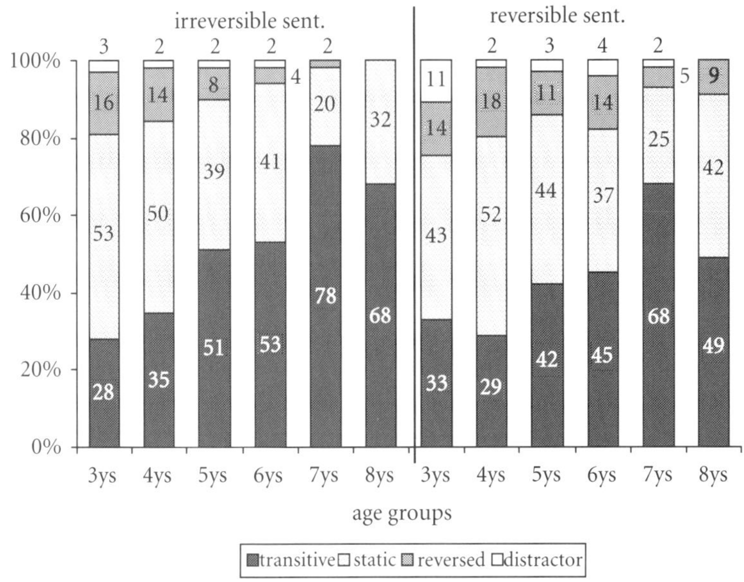


Figure 3a. Responses to ambiguous sentences, control group

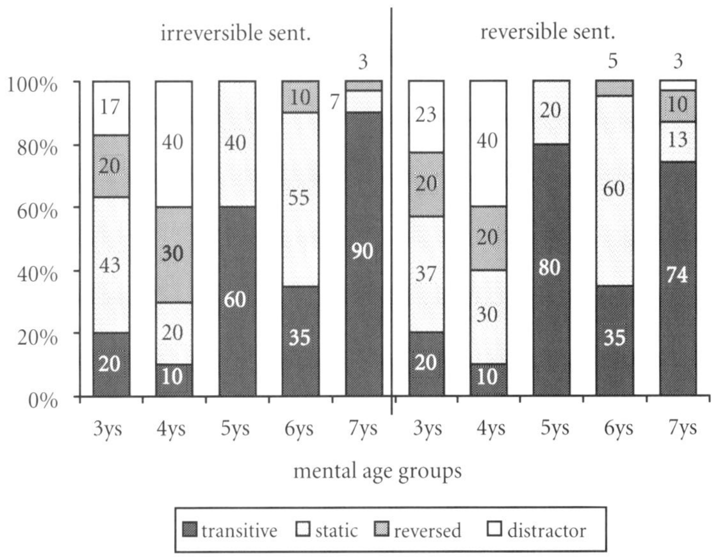


Figure 3b. Responses to ambiguous sentences, participants with WS

Despite the high rate of performance, a shift of answer pattern depending on a change of age can be noted (cf. Figure 3a); for irreversible sentences as well as for reversible ones the transitive answers have increased depending on change of age.[7] However, surprisingly, even the 8 year olds opted very often for the static response, while reversible sentences are more often answered with a static response than irreversible sentences. Maybe, reversible sentences are more easily read as a short cut to a passive construction than it might be the case for irreversible sentences. A similar observation, although less linear, can be made for the group of children with WS as illustrated in Figure 3b.

Aside from the drop of performance by the child at the mental age of 4 years, the response pattern of the WS group resembles that of the control group. However, the shift from a preference for a static response in the mental age group of 6 year olds to a preference for a transitive response in the mental age group of 7 year olds cannot yet be explained, and has to be subject for further research.

#### 4.3.3 *Long verbal passives*

The response pattern to long verbal passives is characterized by an increase in performance according to age, while the overall level of performance for irreversible sentences is higher (cf. left part of Figure 4a) than for reversible ones (cf. right part of Figure 4a). The youngest typically developing children respond correctly to irreversible sentences in 54% (45% for reversible sentences), while the oldest children of the control group answer correctly in 99% resp. 88% (cf. Figure 4a).

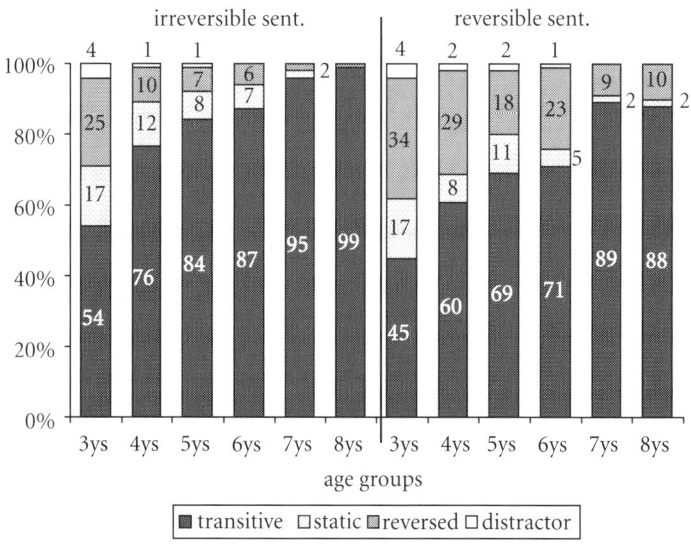


**Figure 4a.** Responses to long verbal passives, control group

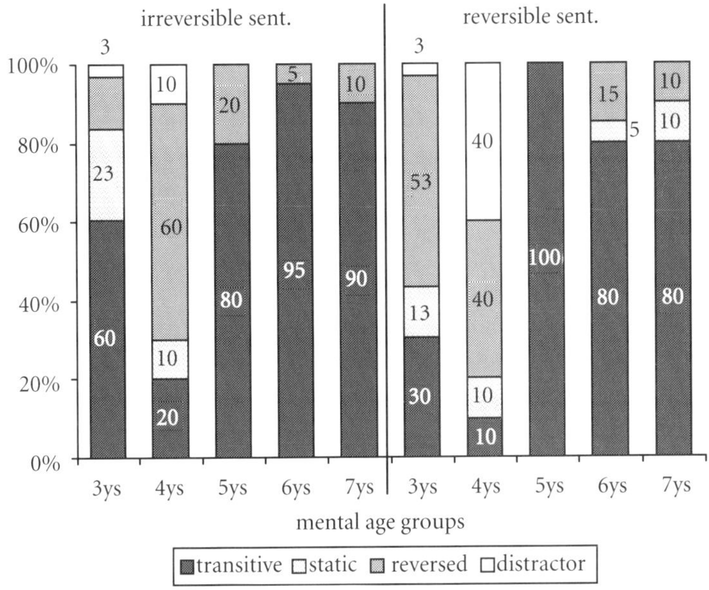


**Figure 4b.** Reponses to long passives, participants with WS

The higher correctness scores for the irreversible sentences clearly show that the children make a distinction between irreversible and reversible sentences, which in turn leads to the assumption that the children acquire knowledge on semantic roles.[8] Next to error quantity, error quality is also dependent on the type of sentences. In the cases in which the children select an incorrect response, they tend to choose a reversed response over any other incorrect answer possibility (depending on age).[9]

As displayed in Figure 4b, for the irreversible sentences the performance of the children with WS equals the performance of control children except for the WS child at the mental age of 4 years. But the results for irreversible sentences suggest a subdivision into two groups: the children of the mental age groups of 3 and 4 years perform worse than their mental age peers, while the WS children of higher mental ages resemble the control children. This might be interpreted in a way that the WS children up to a mental age of 4 years remain behind their mental age peers. Since this lack of competence was obviously overcome by the children of the higher mental age groups, the difficulties of WS children could be best captured by the notion of a delay in language development.

When analyzing the error pattern, though not in all mental age groups, it is striking that the children with WS tend to use the reversed response more often than the control children. This holds for both conditions, the irreversible as well as the reversible sentences. A first guess might suggest that because of the general high level of performance the WS children have mastered the syntax of passives, but that WS children are more vulnerable to semantic influences by the verb which is reflected by the high rate of reversed responses. If this conclusion is right, a similar result should be observed in the responses to short verbal passives, because semantic influences should be independent of the overt appearance of syntactic components.

### 4.3.4 *Short verbal passives*

The children of the control group respond to short verbal passives in a nearly identical way as to when responding to long verbal passives. This holds for irreversible sentences (cf. left part of Figure 5a) in the same way as for reversible sentences (cf. right part of Figure 5a), although, again, the reversible sentences are more vulnerable to incorrect responses than irreversible sentences.[10] Thus, a semantic influence can be observed in the control group, too.

Not only is the performance rate very similar, but error quality, too. Depending on age, performance level increases, while for incorrect responses a preference for reversed responses can be observed.[11]

The children of the WS group, in general, also respond similarly to short verbal passives as they do when being presented with long verbal passives (cf. Figure 5b).

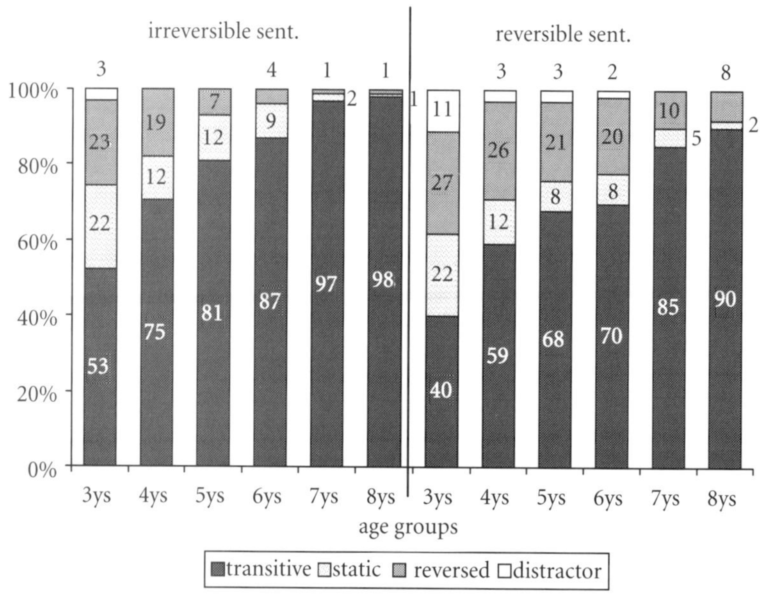


**Figure 5a.** Responses to short verbal passives, control group

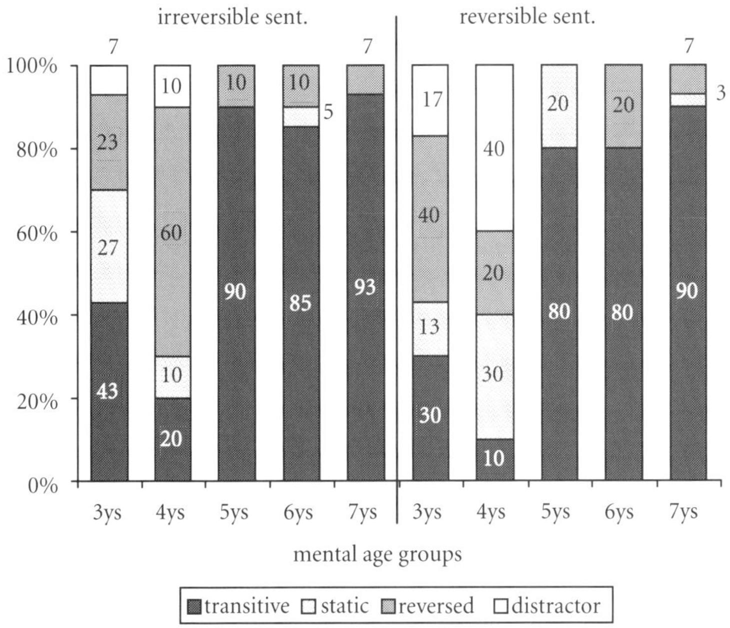


**Figure 5b.** Responses to short verbal passives, participants with WS

Interestingly, the difference between younger and older children with WS now becomes apparent in the 'irreversible' condition, too: the children of the mental age groups of 3 and 4 years lag behind their mental age peers in general. As illustrated by Figure 5b, WS children can overcome the severe difficulties in early stages of language acquisition in a remarkable fashion which further strengthens the interpretation of a delay rather than a deviance.

The error pattern in short verbal passives is less even than in long verbal passives. Although children of some mental age groups respond to short verbal passives preferably with the static picture, for most mental age groups the reversed picture can be determined as the most frequent error.

This result suggests that WS children are influenced partly by the syntactic shape, namely the short sentence leading to a static response. But they are also influenced by the semantic roles of the verb, because reversed answers are observed more often than other incorrect responses.

## 5. Discussion and summary: Deep structure strategy or actor-action-object strategy?

The results to be discussed with respect to the initial guiding questions can be summarized as follows.

1. The typically developing children show a continuous increase in rate of performance for all four sentence types as well as for both conditions, irreversible and reversible sentences, depending on a change of age. Irreversible sentences are more often connected correctly to a picture.
2. In the control group, when responding to passive sentences erroneously, the main error consists of selecting a picture showing the reversed action. No difference between long and short verbal passives could be observed.
3. The children of the WS group show a less continuous increase in overall performance. Instead, a sharp distinction can be drawn between young children with WS (mental age equivalent of 3 and 4 years) and older children resp. adolescents (of higher age than mental age equivalent of 5 years). The performance on irreversible sentences is better than on reversible ones.
4. In the WS group, too, the main error when being presented with passive sentences consists of selecting a picture displaying the reversed action. Only a minor difference between long and short verbal passives can be observed: the number of static responses increases slightly.

These results show that German children with typical development as young as 3 years do not perform the tests using mere chance when presented with verbal passives, but they also show a level of performance far from perfect mastery. This level of performance is lower than in the study carried out by Schaner-Wolles (1989). The reason might be that the array of pictures consisted of three pictures in the previous study, but of four pictures in the present study.

More interesting in this case is the type of errors. The majority of errors with a verbal passive consisted of selecting the picture with the reversed action. In other words, the children opted for the *actor-action-object strategy* when interpreting verbal passives. This response behavior was observed more often in reversible sentences than in irreversible ones. This can be interpreted as evidence for the acquisition of the syntactic rules underlying passive sentences. The higher error rate on reversibles can be explained as follows: When not interpreting eventual case markers, the reversible sentences represent a case of ambiguous sentences which initiate a default reading as formulated by Bever (1970), i.e. the first NP is interpreted as the agent controlling the action. This agent then is assigned to the syntactically characterized subject position. Thus, a second NP is assigned to the object position serving as patients, experiencer, or some thing accordingly.

It remains to draw attention to another result, namely that the children from early on analyze the passives as well as the ambiguous sentences as verbal sentences and less often as adjectival sentences. This can be seen as further evidence for the point of view advocated by Eisenbeiss (1994) who argues against the maturational approach proposed by Borer and Wexler (1987a, b).

The results of the children and adolescents with WS have to be discussed in two steps. While the participants of the WS group from the mental age of 5 years and older perform at least in the same way as the control children who are matched for their mental ages, the youngest children with WS perform noticeably worse than their mental age peers. Note that except for the child with a mental age equivalent of 4 years the main error consists of selecting the reversed response picture. The children with WS, too, opt for the *actor-action-object strategy* like their mental age peers did. In sum, the difference between the very young children with WS and mental age matched controls consists of a quantitative difference rather than a qualitative difference. Since this difference disappears at the mental age of 5 years, the learning of syntactical rules in WS is to be thought of in terms of a delay.

However, the view of a relatively intact language capacity as put forward from early on by Bellugi and her collaborators (e.g. Bellugi et. al. 1993; Bellugi et al. 2000) has to be rejected, since studies illustrating difficulties concerning lexical retrieval (Clahsen & Almazan 1998; Krause & Penke 2001; Monnery et al. 2002; Niedeggen-Bartke 2000; Zukowski 2001) clearly document the selective deficit of the language competence in Williams syndrome.

## Notes

* For comments on an earlier version of this paper I thank Julia Siegmüller, Chris Schaner-Wolles, David Ingram, Richard Wiese, and Franz Josef Stachowiak as well as the audience of the ISES2 held in Potsdam 2002. For very helpful assistance with the statistics I thank Marita Böhning cordially. Special thanks go to all the children and their families who supported this research by their patient and lively participation.

1. A second control group consisted of elderly participants at the ages of 60 and 75 years with low educational level. They, too, made many errors: mean 17%, range 4–30%. This result is below that of the younger controls, but still above the performance of the Williams group. Since no further details are provided concerning this control group, it is difficult to evaluate these results. This second control group was selected on the criterion of educational level. Perhaps, age-dependent attention difficulties and other things have influenced negatively the results.

2. Thanks for carrying out some of the data on passives of the group of children and adolescents with a mental age of 5 years and higher go to Julia Siegmüller. Some of the participants introduced here also participated in the study carried out by J. Siegmüller and

J. Weissenborn (this volume) and carry the following abbreviations. Frauke: JF; Martin: PM; Ansgar: MA; Lena: PL, Johanna: SJ; Karla: GC.

3. Correct answers are given significantly more often than incorrect ones ($t$ (102) = 22,722, $p < 0.001$).

4. Irreversible sentences are significantly more often answered correctly than reversible ones ($t$ (102) = 9,108 $p < 0.001$).

5. For each sentence type a significant increase of correct answers depending on age can be observed: 1) correct answers to actives F (5,97) = 8,494, $p < 0{,}001$; 2) short verbal passives F (5,97) = 15,261, $p < 0{,}001$; 3) long verbal passives F (5,97) = 14,029, $p < 0{,}001$; 4) ambiguous sentences F (5,97) = 6,981, $p < 0{,}001$ (one-way ANOVA).

6. No main effect for age; main effect for type of error F (7,679) = 97,920, $p < 0{,}001$; interaction for age and type of error F (7,679) = 4,232, $p < 0{,}001$ (one-way ANOVA). Post hoc t-tests comparing correct responses to irreversible versus reversible sentences reveal a significant difference for the 4 year olds, $t(35) = -2{,}528$, $p = 0{,}016$, for the 5 year olds, $t(51) = 2{,}7691$, $p = 0{,}007$, and for the 6 year olds, $t(51) = -2{,}232$, $p = 0{,}030$.

7. Irreversible sentences: No main effect for age; main effect for type of answer: F (3,291) = 119, 189, $p < 0, 001$; interaction for age and type of answer F (3,291) = 5, 205, $p < 0{,}001$ (one-way ANOVA). Post hoc t-tests reveal a significant difference for transitive choices on irreversible sentences: 5year olds vs. 6year olds, $t(24) = 2{,}085$, $p = 0{,}048$; for the 7year olds vs. 8year olds: $t(7) = 2{,}679$, $p = 0{,}032$. Post hoc t-tests reveal a significant difference for static choices on irreversible sentences: 5year olds vs. 6year olds, $t(24) = 2{,}790$, $p = 0{,}010$; for the 7year olds vs. 8year olds, $t(7) = 4{,}240$, $p = 0{,}004$. Reversible sentences: No main effect for age; main effect for type of answer: F (3,291) = 84,651, $p < 0{,}001$; interaction for age and type of answer F (3,291) = 3,389, $p < 0{,}001$ (one-way ANOVA). Post hoc t-tests reveal a significant difference for transitive choices on reversible sentences: 6year olds vs. 8year olds, $t(7) = 3{,}120$, $p = 0{,}017$. Post hoc t-tests reveal a significant difference for static choices on reversible sentences: 5year olds vs. 6year olds, $t(24) = 2{,}473$, $p = 0{,}021$. Post hoc t-tests reveal a significant difference for reversed choices on reversible sentences: 3year olds vs. 4year olds, $t(9) = -3{,}320$, $p = 0{,}009$; for the 4year olds vs. 8year olds, $t(7) = 2{,}376$, $p = 0{,}049$; for the 6year olds vs. 7year olds, $t(11) = 3{,}261$, $p = 0{,}008$. Post hoc t-tests reveal a significant difference for distractor choices on reversible sentences for 4year olds vs. 5year olds, $t(16) = 2{,}138$, $p = 0{,}048$.

8. No main effect for age; main effect for type of answer: F (7,679) = 516, 268, $p < 0{,}001$; interaction for age and type of answer F (7,679) = 7,342, $p < 0{,}001$ (one-way ANOVA). Post hoc t-tests comparing correct responses to irreversible versus reversible sentences reveal a significant difference for the 4 year olds, $t(17) = 2{,}927$, $p = 0{,}009$, for the 5 year olds, $t(25) = 3{,}994$, $p = 0{,}001$, for the 6 year olds, $t(25) = 4{,}386$, $p < 0{,}001$, and for the 8 year olds, $t(8) = 2{,}857$, $p = 0{,}021$.

9. Irreversible sentences: No main effect for age; main effect for type of answer: F (3,291) = 778,805, $p < 0{,}001$; interaction for age and type of answer F (3,291) = 8,793, $p < 0{,}001$ (one-way ANOVA). Post hoc t-tests reveal a significant difference for static choices on irreversible sentences: 3year olds vs. 4year olds, $t(9) = 4{,}523$, $p = 0{,}001$; Post hoc t-tests reveal a significan difference for reversed choices on irreversible sentences for the 3year olds vs. 6year olds,

$t(9) = 2{,}629$, $p = 0{,}027$; 5year olds vs. 7year olds $t(11) = 2{,}281$, $p = 0{,}043$. Reversible sentences: No main effect for age; main effect for type of answer: F (3,291) = 341, 150, $p < 0{,}001$; interaction for age and type of answer F (3,291) = 6,375, $p < 0{,}001$ (one-way ANOVA). Post hoc t-tests reveal a significant difference for transitive choices on reversible sentences: 6year olds vs. 8year olds, $t(7) = 4{,}982$, $p = 0{,}002$. Post hoc t-tests reveal a significant difference for static choices on reversible sentences: 3year olds vs. 8year olds, $t(7) = 2{,}742$, $p = 0{,}029$; for 5year olds vs. 7year olds, $t(11) = -2{,}674$, $p = 0{,}022$; 6year olds vs. 7year olds, $t(11) = 3{,}233$, $p = 0{,}008$. Post hoc t-tests reveal a significant difference for reversed choices on reversible sentences: 3year olds vs. 8year olds, $t(7) = 4{,}378$, $p = 0{,}003$.

10. No main effect for age; main effect for type of answer: F (7,679) = 519, 118, $p < 0{,}001$; interaction for age and type of answer F (7,679) = 8,359, $p < 0{,}001$ (one-way ANOVA). Post hoc t-tests comparing correct responses to irreversible versus reversible sentences reveal a significant difference Post hoc t-tests reveal a significant difference for the 4 year olds: $t(17) = 3{,}154$, $p = 0{,}006$, for the 5 year olds: $t(25) = 3{,}304$, $p = 0{,}003$, for the 6 year olds: $t(25) = 4{,}014$, $p < 0{,}001$, and for the 7 year olds: $t(12) = 2{,}645$, $p = 0{,}021$.

11. Irreversible sentences: No main effect for age; main effect for type of answer: F (3,291) = 833,629, $p < 0{,}001$; interaction for age and type of answer F (3,291) = 10,408, $p < 0{,}001$ (one-way ANOVA). Post hoc t-tests reveal a significant difference for static choices on irreversible sentences: 4year olds vs. 6year olds,: $t(16) = 2{,}566$, $p = 0{,}020$. Reversible sentences: No main effect for age; main effect for type of answer: F (3,291) = 321,974, $p < 0{,}001$; interaction for age and type of answer F (3,291) = 7,075, $p < 0{,}001$ (one-way ANOVA). Post hoc t-tests reveal a significant difference for transitive choices on reversible sentences: 3year olds vs. 6year olds, $t(9) = 2{,}548$, $p = 0{,}031$; for the 3year olds vs. 8year olds, $t(7) = 2{,}729$, $p = 0{,}029$; for the 6year olds vs. 7year olds, $t(11) = 4{,}106$, $p = 0{,}002$; for the 6year olds vs. 8year olds, $t(7) = 2{,}787$, $p = 0{,}027$. Post hoc t-tests reveal a significant difference for reversed choices on reversible sentences: 3year olds vs. 7year olds, $t(9) = 2{,}566$, $p = 0{,}030$. Post hoc t-tests recveal signifcant differences for distractor choices on reversible sentences for the 3year olds vs. 4year olds, $t(9) = 4{,}358$, $p = 0{,}002$; for the 3year olds vs. 6year olds, $t(9) = 2585$, $p = 0{,}029$.

## References


Baayen, H., Piepenbrock, R., & van Rijn, H. (1993). *The CELEX Lexical Database.* Philadelphia, PA: Linguistic Data Consortium, University of Pennsylvania.

Bellugi, U., Bihrle, A., Jernigan, T., Trauner, D., & Doherty, S. (1990). "Neuropsychological, neurological and neuroanatomical profile of Williams syndrome". *American Journal of Medical Genetics Supplement,* 6, 764–768.

Bellugi, U., Marks, S., Bihrle, A., & Sabo, H. (1993). "Dissociation between language and cognitive functions in Williams syndrome". In D. Bishop & K. Mogford (Eds.), *Language Development in Exceptional Circumstances* (pp. 177–189). Hillsdale, NJ: LEA.

Bellugi, U., Lichtenberger, L., Jones, W. Lai, Z., & St. George, M. (2000). "The neurocognitive profile of Williams syndrome: A complex pattern of strengths and weaknesses". *Journal of Cognitive Neuroscience, 12* (Supplement 1), 7–29.

Bever, Th. G. (1970). "The cognitive basis for linguistic structures". In J. R. Hayes (Ed.), *Cognition and the Development of Language* (pp. 279–362). New York, NY: Wiley.

Bishop, D. V. M., Bright, P., James, C., Bishop, S. J., & van der Lely, H. K. J. (2000). "Grammatical SLI: A distinct subtype of developmental language impairment?" *Applied Psycholinguistics, 21*, 159–181.

Böhning, M., Starke, F., & Weissenborn, J. (this volume). "Fast mapping in Williams syndrome: A single case study". In S. Bartke & J. Siegmüller (Eds.), *Williams Syndrome across Languages*. Amsterdam: John Benjamins.

Borer, H. & Wexler, K. (1987a). "A principle-based theory of the structure and growth of passive". Ms.

Borer, H. & Wexler, K. (1987b). "The maturation of syntax". In T. Roeper & E. Williams (Eds.), *Parameter Setting and Language Acquisition* (pp. 123–172). Dordrecht: Reidel.

Chomsky, N. (1995). *The Minimalist Programme*. Cambridge, MA: The MIT Press.

Clahsen, H. & Almazan, M. (1998). "Syntax and morphology in Williams syndrome". *Cognition, 68*, 167–198.

Clahsen, H. & Almazan, M. (2001). "Compounding and inflection in language impairment: Evidence from Williams syndrome (and SLI)". *Lingua, 111*, 729–757.

Clark, E. (1982). "The young word maker: A case study of innovation in the child's lexicon". In E. Wanner & L. R. Gleitman (Eds.), *Language Acquisition. The state of the art* (pp. 390–425). Cambridge: CUP.

de Villiers, J. G. & de Villiers, P. A. (1973). "Development of the use of word order in comprehension". *Journal of Psycholinguistic Research, 2*(4), 331–341.

Eisenbeiß, S. (1994). "Auxiliaries and the acquisition of the passive". In E. Clark (Ed.), *The Proceedings of the 25th Annual Child Language Research Forum. CSLI* (pp. 235–242). Stanford, CA: CSLI.

Karmiloff-Smith, A., Tyler, L. K., Voice, K., Sims, K., Udwin, O., Howlin, P., & Davies, M. (1998). "Linguistic dissociations in Williams syndrome: Evaluating receptive syntax in on-line and off-line tasks". *Neuropsychologia, 36*(4), 343–351.

Krause, M. & Penke, M. (2002). "Inflectional morphology in German Williams syndrome". *Brain and Cognition, 48*(2–3), 410–413.

Levy, Y. & Hermon, S. (2000). "Morphology in children with Williams syndrome. Evidence from Hebrew". In S. A. Fish & T. Keith-Lucas (Eds.), *Proceedings of the 24th Annual Boston University Conference on Language Development*, Vol. 2 (pp. 498–509). Somerville, MA: Cascadilla Press.

Monnery, S., Seigneuric, A., Zagar, D., & Robichon, F. (2002). "A linguistic dissociation in Williams syndrome: Good at gender agreement but poor at lexical retrieval". *Reading and Writing: An Interdisciplinary Journal, 15*, 589–612.

Niedeggen-Bartke, S. (2001). "The default-rule, subregularities, and irregulars in the morphology of German Williams syndrome". Paper presented at the 26th Annual Boston University Conference on Language Development 2001.

Pinker, S., Lebeaux, D. S., & Frost, L. A. (1987). "Productivity and constraints in the acquisition of the passive". *Cognition, 26*, 195–267.

Penke, M. & Krause, M. (this volume). "Regular and irregular inflectional morphology in Williams syndrome". In S. Bartke & J. Siegmüller (Eds.), *Williams Syndrome across Languages*. Amsterdam: John Benjamins.

Schaner-Wolles, C., Binder, H., & Tamchina. D. (1986)."Frühes Leid mit der Leideform. Zum Passiverwerb des Deutschen". *Wiener Linguistische Gazette, 37*, 5–38.

Schaner-Wolles, C. (1989). "Strategies in acquiring grammatical relations in German: Word order or case marking?" *Folia Linguistica, 13*(1–2), 131–156.

Tewes, U. & Wechsler, D. (2001). *HAWIK-III: Hamburg-Wechsler-Intelligenztest für Kinder*. Bern: Huber.

van der Lely, H. (1996). "Specifically language impaired and typically developing children: Verbal passive vs. adjectival passive sentence interpretation". *Lingua, 98*, 243–272.

Van der Lely, H. & Stollwerck, L. (1996). "Binding theory and grammatical specific language impairment in children". *Cognition, 62*, 245–290.

Wang, P. P. & Bellugi, U. (1993). "Williams syndrome, Down syndrome, and cognitive neuroscience". *American Journal of Disabled Children, 147*, 1246–1251.

Weiß, R. & Osterland, J. (1997). *CFT 1 – Grundintelligenztest Skala 1*. Göttingen: Hogrefe.

Weiß, R. (1998). *Grundintelligenztest Skala 2 CFT 20*. Göttingen: Hogrefe.

Zukowski, Andrea (2001). Uncovering Grammatical Competence in Children with Williams Syndrome. Unpublished doctoral dissertation, Boston University.

## Appendix 1

List of verbs

| non-reversible | | | | reversible | | | |
|---|---|---|---|---|---|---|---|
| low-frequent | | high-frequent | | low-frequent | | high-frequent | |
| baggern | *to dredge* | rühren | *to stirr* | bürsten | *to brush* | wecken | *to wake* |
| bügeln | *to ironing* | sieben | *to sift* | fönen | *to blow-dry* | jagen | *to chase* |
| grillen | *to barbecue* | wischen | *to wipe* | lausen | *to louse* | küssen | *to kiss* |
| pflücken | *to pick* | leeren | *to empty* | pudern | *to powder* | retten | *to rescue* |
| wickeln* | *to swaddle* | löschen | *to extinguish* | zwacken | *to pinch* | zerren | *to jerk* |

*This verb could be analysed as potentially reversible, but this is from a semantic perspective totally impossible.

## Appendix 2

Picture sample for the verb *grillen* 'to barbeque'

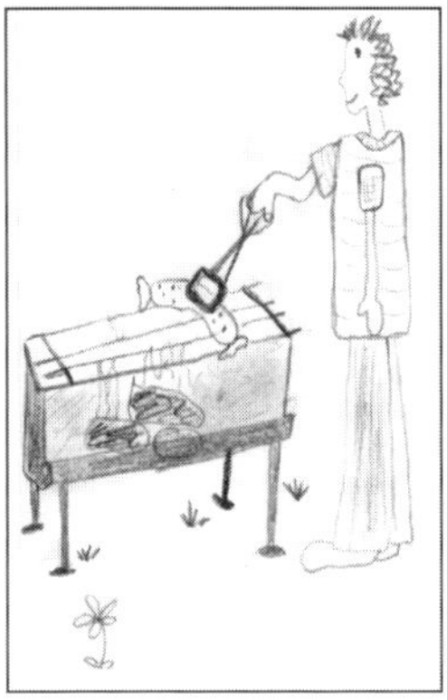

A picture with a transitive reading.

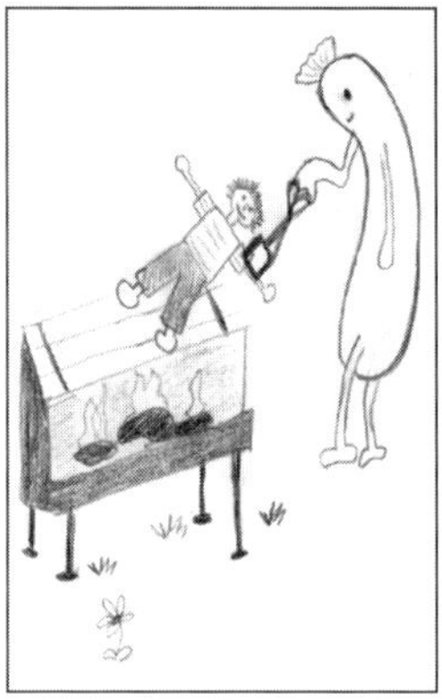

A picture displaying the reversed action.

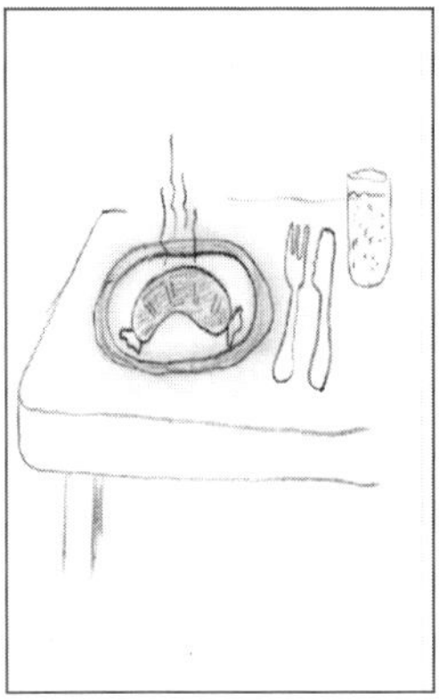

A picture showing the static perspective.

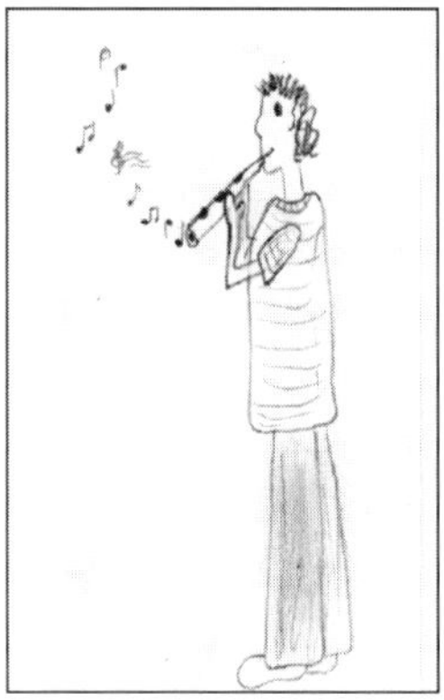

The picture with the distractor.

# Index of tests

# Index of subjects

In the series *Language Acquisition and Language Disorders* the following titles have been published thus far or are scheduled for publication:

1 **WHITE, Lydia:** Universal Grammar and Second Language Acquisition. 1989. xii, 198 pp.

2 **HUEBNER, Thom and Charles A. FERGUSON (eds.):** Cross Currents in Second Language Acquisition and Linguistic Theory. 1991. viii, 435 pp.

3 **EUBANK, Lynn (ed.):** Point Counterpoint. Universal Grammar in the second language. 1991. x, 439 pp.

4 **ECKMAN, Fred R. (ed.):** Confluence. Linguistics, L2 acquisition and speech pathology. 1993. xvi, 260 pp.

5 **GASS, Susan M. and Larry SELINKER (eds.):** Language Transfer in Language Learning. Revised edition. 1992. x, 236 pp.

6 **THOMAS, Margaret:** Knowledge of Reflexives in a Second Language. 1993. x, 234 pp.

7 **MEISEL, Jürgen M. (ed.):** Bilingual First Language Acquisition. French and German grammatical development. 1994. vi, 282 pp.

8 **HOEKSTRA, Teun and Bonnie D. SCHWARTZ (eds.):** Language Acquisition Studies in Generative Grammar. 1994. xii, 401 pp.

9 **ADONE, Dany:** The Acquisition of Mauritian Creole. 1994. xii, 167 pp.

10 **LAKSHMANAN, Usha:** Universal Grammar in Child Second Language Acquisition. Null subjects and morphological uniformity. 1994. x, 162 pp.

11 **YIP, Virginia:** Interlanguage and Learnability. From Chinese to English. 1995. xvi, 247 pp.

12 **JUFFS, Alan:** Learnability and the Lexicon. Theories and second language acquisition research. 1996. xi, 277 pp.

13 **ALLEN, Shanley E.M.:** Aspects of Argument Structure Acquisition in Inuktitut. 1996. xvi, 244 pp.

14 **CLAHSEN, Harald (ed.):** Generative Perspectives on Language Acquisition. Empirical findings, theoretical considerations and crosslinguistic comparisons. 1996. xxviii, 499 pp.

15 **BRINKMANN, Ursula:** The Locative Alternation in German. Its structure and acquisition. 1997. x, 289 pp.

16 **HANNAHS, S.J. and Martha YOUNG-SCHOLTEN (eds.):** Focus on Phonological Acquisition. 1997. v, 289 pp.

17 **ARCHIBALD, John:** Second Language Phonology. 1998. xii, 313 pp.

18 **KLEIN, Elaine C. and Gita MARTOHARDJONO (eds.):** The Development of Second Language Grammars. A generative approach. 1999. vi, 412 pp.

19 **BECK, Maria-Luise (ed.):** Morphology and its Interfaces in Second Language Knowledge. 1998. x, 387 pp.

20 **KANNO, Kazue (ed.):** The Acquisition of Japanese as a Second Language. 1999. xii, 180 pp.

21 **HERSCHENSOHN, Julia:** The Second Time Around – Minimalism and L2 Acquisition. 2000. xiv, 287 pp.

22 **SCHAEFFER, Jeanette C.:** The Acquisition of Direct Object Scrambling and Clitic Placement. Syntax and pragmatics. 2000. xii, 187 pp.

23 **WEISSENBORN, Jürgen and Barbara HÖHLE (eds.):** Approaches to Bootstrapping. Phonological, lexical, syntactic and neurophysiological aspects of early language acquisition. Volume 1. 2001. xviii, 299 pp.

24 **WEISSENBORN, Jürgen and Barbara HÖHLE (eds.):** Approaches to Bootstrapping. Phonological, lexical, syntactic and neurophysiological aspects of early language acquisition. Volume 2. 2001. viii, 337 pp.

25 **CARROLL, Susanne E.:** Input and Evidence. The raw material of second language acquisition. 2001. xviii, 461 pp.

26 **SLABAKOVA, Roumyana:** Telicity in the Second Language. 2001. xii, 236 pp.

27 **SALABERRY, M. Rafael and Yasuhiro SHIRAI (eds.):** The L2 Acquisition of Tense–Aspect Morphology. 2002. x, 489 pp.

28 **SHIMRON, Joseph (ed.):** Language Processing and Acquisition in Languages of Semitic, Root-Based, Morphology. 2003. vi, 394 pp.

29 **FERNÁNDEZ, Eva M.:** Bilingual Sentence Processing. Relative clause attachment in English and Spanish. 2003. xx, 294 pp.

30 **HOUT, Roeland van, Aafke HULK, Folkert KUIKEN and Richard J. TOWELL (eds.):** The Lexicon–Syntax Interface in Second Language Acquisition. 2003. viii, 234 pp.

31 **MARINIS, Theodoros:** The Acquisition of the DP in Modern Greek. 2003. xiv, 261 pp.

32 **PRÉVOST, Philippe and Johanne PARADIS (eds.):** The Acquisition of French in Different Contexts. Focus on functional categories. 2004. viii, 384 pp.

33 **JOSEFSSON, Gunlög, Christer PLATZACK and Gisela HÅKANSSON (eds.):** The Acquisition of Swedish Grammar. 2004. vi, 298 pp. + index.

34 **OTA, Mitsuhiko:** The Development of Prosodic Structure in Early Words. Continuity, divergence and change. 2003. xii, 224 pp.

35 **SÁNCHEZ, Liliana:** Quechua-Spanish Bilingualism. Interference and convergence in functional categories. 2003. x, 189 pp.

36 **BARTKE, Susanne and Julia SIEGMÜLLER (eds.):** Williams Syndrome across Languages. 2004. xii, 370 pp. + index.